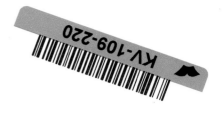
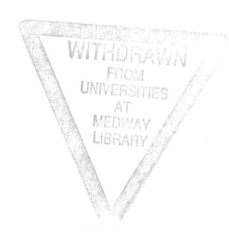

Nutrition and Physical Activity

Nicole Wolfram • Michael Rigby
Michael Sjöström • Rosa Giuseppa Frazzica
Wilhelm Kirch

Editors

Nutrition and Physical Activity

Health Information Sources in EU Member States,
and Activities in the Commission, WHO,
and European Networks

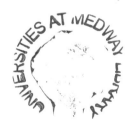

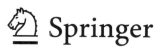

Springer

Editors

Nicole Wolfram
TU Dresden, Medizinische Fakultät
Forschungsverbund Public Health Saxony
  and Saxony Anhalt
Fiedlerstr. 33
01307 Dresden
Germany

Michael Rigby
Centre for Health Planning
  and Management
Darwin Building
Keele University
Keele, Staffordshire, ST5 5BG
United Kingdom

Michael Sjöström
Unit of Preventive Nutrition
Department of Biosciences and Nutrition
  at Novum Karolinska Institutet
Hälsovägen 7
SE-141 57 Huddinge
Sweden

Rosa Giuseppa Frazzica
CEFPAS
Centre for Training and Research
  in Public Health
via G. Mulè, 1
I - 93100 - Caltanissetta
Italy

Wilhelm Kirch
TU Dresden, Medizinische Fakultät
Forschungsverbund Public Health Saxony
  and Saxony Anhalt
Fiedlerstr. 33
01307 Dresden
Germany

The close of entries and text was in 2006.
The Scientific Platform of the Working Party on Information on Lifestyle and Specific Subpopulations, Grant agreement 2005111, and the current publication received funding from the European Union/DG Health and Consumer Protection/Health Programme. The sole responsibility for the content of this book lies with the authors and not the European Commission. The European Commission is not responsible for any use that may be made of the information contained in the book.

ISBN: 978-0-387-74840-5   e-ISBN: 978-0-387-74841-2
DOI: 10.1007/978-0-387-74841-2

Library of Congress Control Number: 2007940372

Preface

Many Health Information Activities related to nutrition and physical activity have been initiated during the past years by several institutions at national and international level as well as by several European networks. A multitude of projects with different scopes and methodologies has arisen. This variety makes it necessary to bring the results of these activities into a coordinated framework.

The report aims to give a structured overview on the availability of routinely repeated or repeatable data on the health determinants nutrition and physical activity in European countries. An Inventory of Health Information Activities on nutrition and physical activity was built up, which summarizes activities carried out by the European Commission, WHO, various European networks, as well as national examples.

The Health Information Activities collected as national examples assess data for all countries belonging to the European Union up to 2006, the European Economic Area (EEA), and all candidate countries. The Inventory considers activities that started in 1990 or later, which were still running or were approved but have not yet started. Food safety and food labeling are not constituent subjects of the report.

The report analyses institutional initiatives of the European Commission, WHO, selected European networks as well as examples of health information activities at national level. A network of European public health professionals identified available national health information activities and survey data, which were summarised in a structured online database.

The results section presents the analysis of the database, which summarises health information activities in European countries. The database is freely accessible at the Web site of the Working Party on Information on Lifestyle and Specific Subpopulations. Additionally, the printed report provides a summary of all project database entries in the form of *Project Identity Cards*. For each country, Health Information Activities have been summarised in *Country Profile* Sheets.

The report provides a general overview on Health Information Activities related to nutrition and physical activity as well as a state-of-the-art investigation about available data in European countries. The concluding section of the report aims to recommend future Health Information actions that outline open issues.

The Scientific Platform of the Working Party on Information on Lifestyle and Specific Subpopulations has compiled this project report on Health Information Activities on nutrition and physical activity on request of DG SANCO of the European Commission.

Dresden   Grit Neumann, M.A.
July 2008   Prof. Dr. Dr. Wilhelm Kirch

Contents

List of Figures and Tables

Contributors

Javier Aranceta
Community Nutrition Unit Bilbao, Department of Public Health, Luis Brinas 18,
Bilbao, Spain, jaranceta@unav.es

Wojciech Drygas
Department of Social and Preventive Medicine, Medical University,
ul. Zeligowskiego 7/9, 90–643 Łódź, Poland, office@cindi.org.pl,
wdrygas@ikard.waw.pl

Rosa Giuseppa Frazzica
CEFPAS, Centre for Training and Research in Public Health, via G. Mulè 1
93100, Caltanissetta, Italy, frazzica@cefpas.it

Serge Hercberg
National Institute for Public Health Surveillance (InVS), 74 rue Marcel Cachin,
93317 Bobigny, Cedex, France, hercberg@cnam.fr

Jautrite Karashkevica
Health Statistics and Medical Technologies, State Agency, Duntes Street 12/22,
Riga, LV 1005, Latvia, jautrite.karaskevica@vsmtva.gov.lv

Wilhelm Kirch
Faculty of Medicine, Carl Gustav Carus Research Association Public Health
Saxony and Saxony-Anhalt, Technische Universität, Fiedlerstraße 33,
01307 Dresden, Germany, Public.Health@mailbox.tu-dresden.de

Lijana Kragelj-Zaletel
Medical Faculty, Department of Public Health, University of Ljubljana,
Zaloška 4, SI-1000 Ljubljana, Slovenia, lijana.kragelj@mf.uni-lj.si

Marie Kunesova
Obesity Management Centre, Institute of Endocrinology, Czech Society
for the Study of Obesity, Narodni 8, 116 94 Prague 2, Czech Republic,
mkunesova@endo.cz

Athena Linos
Environmental and Occupational Health, Institute of Preventive Medicine,
Prolepsis, 2A Athinas str., 14671 Kastri, Athens, Greece, info@prolepsis.gr

Sven Majerus
Direction de la Santè, Villa Louvigny, Allèe Macroni, LU- 2120 Luxembourg,
Luxembourg, Sven.Majerus@ms.etat.lu

Eliza Markidou
Department of Medical and Public Health Services, Ministry of Health
of the Republic of Cyprus, 10 Markou Drakou str., Pallouiotisse, Cyprus,
eliza@spidernet.com.cy

Neda Milevska
Center for Regional Policy Research and Cooperation "Studiorum",
Department of Public Health, Pirinska BB, POB 484, 1000 Skopje,
Macedonia, milevska@studiorum.org.mk

Irena Misevičiene
Institute for Biomedical Research, Kaunas University of Medicine,
Eineniu Str. 4, 50009 Kaunas 7, Lithuania, irenmisev@kmu.lt

Cemil Özcan
Faculty of Medicine, Department of Public Health, Celal Bayar University,
45020 Manisa, Turkey, halksagligi@bayar.edu.tr

Stoyanka Popova
Dean of FPH, Faculty of Public Health, Medical University of Varna, 55 Marin
Drinov Str., 9002 Varna, Bulgaria, phealth@vizicomp.com

Michael Rigby
The Centre for Health Planning and Management, Keele University, Newcastle-
under-Lyme, Staffordshire, ST5 5BG, Great Britain, m.j.rigby@hpm.keele.ac.uk

Michael Sjöström
Unit for Preventive Nutrition; Institute of Biosciences and Nutrition,
Karolinska Institute Sweden, Novum Research Park, 141 57 Huddinge, Sweden,
michael.sjostrom@prevnut.ki.se

Florian Valentin Sologiuc
National School of Public Health and Health Services Management- NSPHHSM,
Department of Health System Research, Vaselor Street 31, Sector 2, 021253
Bucharest, Romania, contact@incds.ro

István György Tóth
TÁRKI Social Research Institute Inc., Budaörsi út 45, 1112 Budapest,
Hungary, toth@tarki.hu

Herman Van Oyen
Scientific Institute of Public Health, Unit of Epidemiology, J. Wytsmanstraat 14, 1050 Brussels, hvanoyen@iph.fgov.be

Cindy Veenhof
Department of Allied Health Care, Netherlands Institute for Health Services Research NIVEL, Postbus 15683500 BN, The Netherlands, c.veenhof@nivel.nl

Toomas Veidebaum
National Institute for Health Development, Hiiu 42, 11619 Tallinn, Estonia, Toomas.veidebaum@tai.ee

Acknowledgement

Acknowledgement is given to all partners, whose knowledge contributed to this publication:

Technische Universität Dresden, Germany
Nicole Wolfram, Grit Neumann, Christiane Hillger
Doreen Klein

CEFPAS - Centre for Training and Research in Public Health, Caltanissetta, Italy
Pasquale Di Mattia, Roberta Arnone, Marilena Pinco, Danilo Greco

Unit for Preventive Nutrition; Institute of Biosciences and Nutrition, Karolinska Institute, Sweden
Sanna Sorasto

Medical University of Varna, Faculty of Public Health, Bulgaria
Iskra Mircheva

Ministry of Health of the Republic of Cyprus; Department of Medical and Public Health Services, Cyprus
Eliza Markidou

National Institute for Health Development, Estonia
Leila Oja

National Institute for Public Health Surveillance (InVS), France
Michel Vernay

Institute of Preventive Medicine, Environmental and Occupational Health, Prolepsis, Greece
Panajiota Karnaki

TÁRKI Social Research Institute Inc., Hungary
József Vitrai;
Csilla Kaposvari

Landspitali University Hospital, Unit for Nutrition Research, Iceland
Inga Thorsdottier; Ingibjorg Gunnarsdottir;
Alfons Ramel

Health Statistics and Medical Technologies, State Agency; Latvia
Iveta Pudule

Institute for Biomedical Research, Kaunas University of Medicine, Lithuania
Jurate Klumbiene

Direction de la Santè, Luxembourg
Sven Majerus

Center for Regional Policy Research and Cooperation "Studiorum"
Department Public Health, Macedonia
Vera Dimitrievska

National School of Public Health and Health Services Management- NSPHHSM,
Department of Health System Research, Romania
Silvia Florescu; Mihaela Stoican

Department of Health Promotion
National Public Health Authority, Slovak Republic
Tomás Kúdela

Community Nutrition Unit Bilbao
Department of Public Health; Spain
Carmen Pérez Rodrigo

Celal Bayar University; Faculty of Medicine, Department of Public Health,
Turkey
Gonul Dinc

1
Background and Purpose

Analysing people's health and reporting on health have become increasingly important for a large number of EU Member States. Health reporting is defined as "a system of different products and measures aiming at creating knowledge and awareness of important Public Health problems and their determinants (in different population groups) among policy makers and others involved in organisations that can influence the health of a population." [6] Health reporting systems are intended to monitor the status of health, health behaviour, and risk factors as well as the health care system at national level. Politicians, scientists, and stakeholders are thus offered an information background. Accordingly, effective health monitoring is an important instrument for health policy decisions and support for national health policy. Furthermore, it can lead to the identification of health data needs and health research priorities.

In the past, the European Commission has supported several activities to measure health in Europe and to implement a unique and comparable health monitoring system at the level of the European Union that allows for the measurement of health status, trends, and determinants throughout the community. First steps have been taken, but to ensure that health monitoring fulfils these functions at a national as well as at international level, future efforts are necessary.

On 23 September 2002, the European Parliament and the Council adopted a new Community Action Programme for Public Health. The programme started on 1 January 2003 and was originally intended to run for a 6-year period until 31 December 2008. This programme was designed to complement national policies; its overall aim was to protect human health and improve public health. There were three general objectives:

- To improve information and knowledge for the development of public health (health information)
- To enhance the capability of responding rapidly and in a coordinated fashion to threats to health (health threats)
- To promote health and prevent disease through addressing health determinants across all policies and activities (health determinants) [7, 8]

Under the thematic priority *health information* within the Community Public Health Programme 2003–2008, the European Commission is launching public

N. Wolfram et al. (eds.) *Nutrition and Physical Activity*,
© Springer Science + Business Media, LLC 2008

health monitoring projects. This thematic strand sets the objective of establishing and operating a sustainable health monitoring system. The system aims at producing comparable information on health and health-related behavior of the European population, on diseases and health systems.

This will be based on European-wide common agreed indicators with regard to their definition, data collection, and use [9]. The system is to be established on the basis of the previous work in former Community Health Programmes and will now be continued intensively under the new Public Health Programme, which starts in 2007 and runs till 2013. The new Public Health Programme will substitute the old programme (2003–2008).

One of the key priorities in the EU Public Health Action Programme is the life-style-related health determinants of nutrition and physical activity, not least because of the linkage to the growing problem of overweight and obesity. During the past years, many Health Information Activities related to nutrition and physical activity have been initiated by several institutions on the national and international level as well as by European networks.

The majority of research activities in this field have been initiated because nutrition and inappropriate physical activity are significant risk factors for many common noncommunicable diseases. The top noncommunicable health problems (cardiovascular disease, obesity, diabetes, osteoporosis, and cancer) are life-style-related diseases and share common risk factors. These are unhealthy nutrition, lack of physical activity, smoking, and heavy drinking. For the majority of adults in Europe who neither smoke nor drink excessively, what they eat, and how physically active they are, are the most significant controllable risk factors affecting their long-term health. During the past decades, physical inactivity and high dietary fat intakes have becoming increasingly prevalent in people's daily living in industrialised countries [20, 23].

The awareness of the importance of nutrition and physical activity on health status has given rise to a multitude of projects with different scopes and methodologies. Until now the European Commission's aim to produce comparable information on health and health-related behavior of the population has not been fulfilled. The measurement of comparable health status, trends, and determinants throughout the Community is not yet possible.

One important reason that hampers the production of comparable data in the field of the lifestyle indicators nutrition and physical activity is the absence of agreed measures and related data definitions within Europe. As mentioned earlier, a considerable number of projects have been initiated. They used different definitions, indicators, and methods, which made the production of comparable data difficult.

First steps in the field to harmonise and compare health information activities have already been taken. A first set of European Community Health Indicators was produced by the European Community Health Indicators (ECHI) project in its first and second phases (ECHI 1 and ECHI 2), which included indicators on nutrition and physical activity. The objective of this project was to continue the work on specific indicators to complete the European Community Health Indicators list that will serve as a basis for the European health information system including their operational definitions.

The project "Monitoring Public Health Nutrition in Europe" also contributed to comparable health indicator definitions across member states. This project aimed to clearly define the indicators for nutrition and physical activity that should be monitored for nutrition-related health outcomes [24].

To tie up to these efforts of harmonisation and standardisation, it is necessary to bring together into a coordinating framework the results of past activities related to nutrition and physical activity, with their different scopes and methodologies. In this context, a report on the availability of national data sources since 1990 concerning the health determinants, nutrition and physical activity has been initiated; at the same time, it should be noted that food safety and food labeling are not covered in this report.

The report also presents an Inventory of Health Information Activities on Nutrition and Physical Activity, which summarizes National Examples and activities carried out by the European Commission, the WHO, and selected European Networks. Therefore, the report provides a general overview on Health Information Activities, which are related to nutrition and physical activity, and thus provides a state-of-the-art investigation. The report aims to analyse which existing resources can be linked into one coordinated database. The concluding section of the report aims to recommend future Health Information Actions, which would address issues that have not yet been covered.

2
Objective

Many Health Information Activities, which provide data on people's nutrition and physical activity, have been initiated during the past years by several institutions at national and international level as well as by various European networks. This results in a multitude of projects with different scopes and methodologies. This circumstance of variety makes it necessary to bring activities into a coordinated framework.

The main objective of this report is to provide an overview about the availability of routinely repeated or repeatable Health Information Activities in the form of *National Examples*.

The Health Information Activities collected within this report assess data for:

- All countries belonging to the European Union up to 2006
- The European Economic Area (EEA) countries
- All candidate countries

This report is intended to give a general overview about available Health Information Activities, which are topically related to *nutrition* and to *physical activity*. This overview includes projects and activities that have been carried out by:

- The European Commission
- The World Health Organisation
- Various European Networks

The national examples include research projects and surveys that started in 1990 or later, which were still running or were approved but have not yet started.

The report's aim is to identify available health-related activities and survey data in Europe containing data on nutrition and physical activity. For that purpose, a network of public health professionals for data collection was established.

Identified Health Information Activities were entered into a structured database by scientists. While including projects into the database, all scientific coworkers who contributed to the report concentrated on Health Information Activities in general. Health Information Activities in this report cover a broad scope and are defined in "Defining Concepts."

The inventory contains information about the projects' contents, methods used, and towards which indicators the activities provide data. It is especially interesting

N. Wolfram et al. (eds.) *Nutrition and Physical Activity*,
© Springer Science + Business Media, LLC 2008

how far this multitude of projects that have been initiated in the timeframe since 1990 produced comparable data in the field of nutrition and physical activity. The results of data collection within this report are the basis for further discussion and steps that have to be considered. Thus, the report aims to recommend future Health Information Actions that outline open issues.

The report is limited to data availability in the countries covered. Health reporting activities at national level are summarised in *Country Profile Sheets* (pp. 52–86). Individual activities are additionally listed in *Project Identity Cards* in the appendix (pp. 141–477). All activities are available in the online database, which is freely accessible at the web page of the Working Party (http://www.public-health. tu-dresden.de/Query001/). Thus, the inventory provides a structured framework for Health Information Activities on nutrition and physical activity. Assessments of data quality and data usability are not within the scope of this report. Also, this is a *snap shot* study given the one-off resourcing – though the database will continue to be available for consultation, it will not be updated.

3
Background Information

3.1. Defining Concepts

Nutrition

Within Europe there are no established definitions of nutrition or of physical activity. The project, therefore, devised the following definitions, which were used throughout the project

Nutrition can be defined as the interactions that occur between living organisms and food. It studies the psychological, social, cultural, economic, and technological factors that influence which food we choose to eat. The science of nutrition also studies the biological process by which we consume food and utilize the nutrients it contains [25].

Public Health Nutrition focuses on the promotion of good health through healthy food habits and a physically active lifestyle and the prevention of illness in the population [23].

Physical Activity

Physical activity can be defined as "any bodily movement produced by skeletal muscle that results in energy expenditure" [2]. Physical activity is closely related to, but distinct from, exercise and physical fitness. It can be categorized as occupational, leisure, sports, household, or other forms of activity.

Exercise is a subset of physical activity that is "planned, structured and repetitive bodily movement, done to improve or maintain one or more components of physical fitness" [2].

Fitness is "a set of attributes that people have or achieve that relates to the ability to perform physical activity" [2].

Health-related fitness broadens the traditional concept of fitness to include the functional capacity needed for everyday life and health. It includes the characteristics of functional capacity that are affected positively by physical activity or negatively by the lack of physical activity and are, at the same time, associated with health status. Good

N. Wolfram et al. (eds.) *Nutrition and Physical Activity*,
© Springer Science + Business Media, LLC 2008

health-related fitness is composed of endurance, bodily control, muscular strength, joint mobility, and suitable weight. A person who is sufficiently healthy can cope with everyday activities without overtiring [20].

Health Information Activities

Health Information Activities within this report cover a broad scope. They are defined as published activities, such as projects or surveys, related to nutrition and physical activity on a population level. There was no limitation as regards age of project target groups. Activities focusing on all age groups were included.

Information on European and national projects and activities as well as projects with a regional scope were collected. Although regional projects were included, data from national and international projects were the prime focus. There were no limitations to projects with a specific study design. Though the prime intention was to identify ongoing data sources, in the report studies that were only conducted once were also included, because in many countries, there were data sources with no repetition so far, but they do currently provide useful data for the national health monitoring system.

Activities that do not produce data, or merely promote and implement projects, were not considered eligible Health Information Activities. The same is true for prevention programmes, intervention studies, Health Information Activities on food safety and projects published as textbooks. The purpose of this study was focussed solely on building up a picture of data availability from routinely repeated or repeatable sources, which could inform national policy makers; and secondly to highlight areas where further national or European action on data gathering and information presentation is needed.

At a meeting, subcontracted partners were trained and informed about the definition of Health Information Activities. They were furthermore invited to contact the main partner in case of questions. Those partners who could not attend the meeting were given detailed instructions and were encouraged to closely cooperate with the main partner.

Indicator

It was intended to find a generally binding definition for "indicator," but the references proved to be very inconsistent. For this reason, we provide in this report definitions from various partners.

An indicator is an informative presentation of the status of an empirically-based and scientifically-framed measure of a detailed subject of interest [22].

In general, indicators are identified as variables that help to measure changes. Furthermore, indicators facilitate the current status and the future actions illustrated from the underlying goal. Finally, they are a simplified representation of measurements used for example to answer scientific questions in the process of monitoring as well as evaluating health promoting activities.

Color Plate

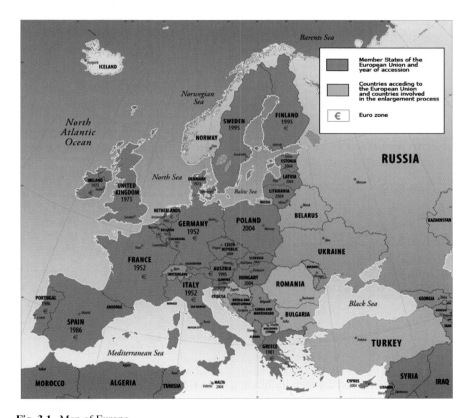

Fig. 3.1 Map of Europe
Reference: http://euramis.org/abc/maps/index_en.htm

In the main, WHO defined indicators as: "… variables which help to measure changes. Indicators are an indication of a given situation, or a reflection of that situation. Often they are used particularly when these changes cannot be measured directly … They are indirect or partial measures of a complex situation, but if measured sequentially over time they can indicate direction and speed of change and serve to compare different areas or groups of people at the same moment in time" [37].

Indicators represent the relationship between rather abstract or theoretical terms, such as health, and measurements, which are linked directly to the concept of "health". For this reason, indicators should at best conform to the quality measures of scientific testing instruments: "… the ideal indicators should be valid – that is, they should actually measure what they are supposed to measure; they should be objective – the answer should be the same if measured by different people in similar circumstances; they should be sensitive – that is, they should, be sensitive to the changes in the situation; and they should be specific – that is, they should reflect changes only in the situation concerned. In real life there are very few indicators that comply with all these criteria" [37].

Regarding the selection of recommended indicators for a comparable measurement of health, this project included relevant work from the project "Monitoring Public Health Nutrition in Europe" [24]. This project was part of the EU Programme on Health Monitoring, which aimed to establish a Community Health Monitoring System for the measurement of health status, trends and determinants throughout the community. The project "Monitoring Public Health Nutrition in Europe" defined indicators for nutrition and physical activity that should be monitored across all member states to achieve maximum comparison. The project recommended ideally those indicators that are already being collected in the majority of member states or those that can be added easily to current data collection systems in the member states [24]. According to the proposed context, three different groups of indicators were defined:

(A) Nutrition related indicators
(B) Indicators related to physical activity
(C) Miscellaneous indicators

To establish the inventory on available health information on nutrition and physical activity in Europe, this report uses the recommended indicators of the project "Monitoring Public Health Nutrition in Europe" and analyzes how far the available health data sources provide information on the recommended indicators and ensure comparability.

Methods of Data Collection

Information on the method of data collection applied in the health information projects was gathered. For this purpose, methods used to collect data on nutrition and/ or physical activity were grouped into the following categories and included in the project database:

(A) Methods measuring food consumption/availability
(B) Methods measuring physical activity
(C) Other methods

Age Groups

There are a multitude of definitions on age groups in scientific literature across Europe. They vary to a considerable extent with respect to individual age groups and whether age groups in themselves are further divided into subgroups or classi-fied as age-gender-groups. The decision as to where to draw the line between one age group and another is determined by the actual content of a study as well as social and biological factors.

3.2.   Geographical Coverage

Figure 3.1 below shows the Member States and Candidate Countries of the European Union. In Table 3.1, the countries that have been considered in this report are listed. This report provides national data for all the 25 Member States of the European Union as of 2006. Furthermore, all candidate countries have been included in the report. These were – with reference to the year 2006 – Bulgaria, Croatia, Macedonia, Romania, and Turkey. Since 1 January 2007, Romania and Bulgaria have become new Member States of the European Union. Health Information

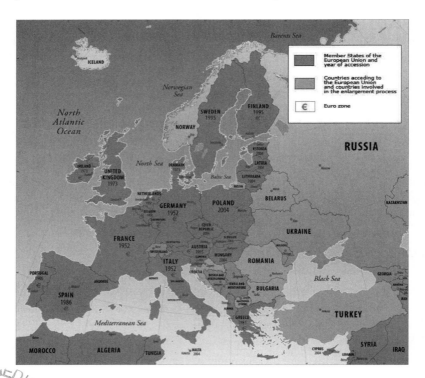

Fig. 3.1 Map Europe (*see Color Plate*)
Reference: http://euramis.org/abc/maps/index_en.htm

Activities collected within this report assess also data for countries of the European Economic Area, namely Iceland, Liechtenstein, and Norway.

Furthermore, Table 3.1 provides information on the project partners' responsibilities regarding geographical coverage. Experts in the field of Health Information Activity were contacted to do research on available health data sources in either one or several countries.

Table 3.1 Partners' responsibility regarding geographical coverage

Geographical Coverage	Responsible Instiution	Represented by	Country
Austria	Technische Universität Dresden; Faculty of Medicine Carl Gustav Carus; Research Association Public Health Saxony and Saxony-Anhalt	Prof. Wilhelm Kirch	Germany
Belgium	Netherlands Institute for Health Services Research NIVEL, Dept. Allied Health Care	Dr. Cindy Veenhof	The Netherlands
	Scientific Institute of Public Health, Unit of Epidemiology	Prof. Herman Van Oyen	Belgium
Bulgaria	Medical University of Varna, Faculty of Public Health	Prof. Stoyanka Cvetkova Popova	Bulgaria
Croatia	Dept. of Public Health, Medical Faculty of University of Ljubljana, Slovenia	Dr. Lijana Kragelj-Zaletel	Slovenia
Cyprus	Ministry of Health of the Republic of Cyprus, Dept. of Medical and Public Health Services	Dr. Androulle Agnoti; Eliza Markidou	Cyprus
Czech Republic	Czech Society for the Study of Obesity, Obesity Management Centre, Institute of Endocrinology	Prof. Marie Kunesova	Czech Republic
Denmark	Unit for Preventive Nutrition, Institute of Biosciences and Nutrition, Karolinska Institute Sweden	Prof. Michael Sjöström	Sweden
Estonia	National Institute for Health Development	Prof. Toomas Veidebaum	Estonia
Finland	Unit for Preventive Nutrition, Institute of Biosciences and Nutrition, Karolinska Institute Sweden	Prof. Michael Sjöström	Sweden
France	National Institute for Public Health Surveillance (InVS)	Prof. Serge Hercberg	France
Germany	Technische Universität Dresden; Faculty of Medicine Carl Gustav Carus; Research Association Public Health Saxony and Saxony-Anhalt	Prof. Wilhelm Kirch	Germany

(continued)

Table 3.1 (continued)

Geographical Coverage	Responsible Instiution	Represented by	Country
Great Britain	The Centre for Health Planning and Management; KEELE University	Prof. Michael Rigby	Great Britain
Greece	Institute of Preventive Medicine, Environmental and Occupational Health, Prolepsis	Prof. Athena Linos	Greece
Hungary	TÁRKI Social Research Institute Inc.	Prof. István György Tóth	Hungary
Iceland	Landspitali University Hospital, Unit for Nutrition Research	Dr. Torfi Magnússon	Iceland
Ireland	The Centre for Health Planning and Management; KEELE University	Prof. Michael Rigby	Great Britain
Italy	CEFPAS; Centre for Training and Research in Public Health	Dr. Rosa Giuseppa Frazzica	Italy
Latvia	Health Statistics and Medical Technologies, State Agency	Dr. Jautrite Karashkevica	Latvia
Liechtenstein	Technische Universität Dresden; Faculty of Medicine Carl Gustav Carus; Research Association Public Health Saxony and Saxony-Anhalt	Prof. Wilhelm Kirch	Germany
Lithuania	Institute for Biomedical Research, Kaunas University of Medicine	Prof. Irena Misevičiene	Lithuania
Luxembourg	Technische Universität Dresden, Faculty of Medicine Carl Gustav Carus, Research Association Public Health Saxony and Saxony-Anhalt,	Prof. Wilhelm Kirch	Germany
	Direction de la Santè	Sven Majerus	Luxembourg
Macedonia	Center for Regional Policy Research and Cooperation "Studiorum,"Dept. Public Health	Neda Milevska, MSc, MCPPM	Macedonia
Malta	The Centre for Health Planning and Management; KEELE University	Prof. Michael Rigby	Great Britain
Norway	Unit for Preventive Nutrition, Institute of Biosciences and Nutrition, Karolinska Institute Sweden	Prof. Michael Sjöström	Sweden
Poland	Department of Social and Preventive Medicine, Medical University	Prof. Wojciech Drygas	Poland
Portugal	Community Nutrition Unit Bilbao, Dept. of Public Health	Dr. Javier Aranceta	Spain
Romania	National School of Public Health and Health Services Management- NSPHHSM,Dept. of Health System Research	Dr. Florian Valentin Sologiuc	Romania
Slovakia	Dept. of Health Promotion, National Public Health Authority of the Slovak Republic	Dr. Tomás Kúdela	Slovakia

(continued)

Table 3.1 (continued)

Geographical Coverage	Responsible Instiution	Represented by	Country
Slovenia	Dept. of Public Health, Medical Faculty of University of Ljubljana, Slovenia	Dr. Lijana Kragelj-Zaletel	Slovenia
Spain	Community Nutrition Unit Bilbao, Dept. of Public Health	Dr. Javier Aranceta	Spain
Sweden	Unit for Preventive Nutrition, Institute of Biosciences and Nutrition, Karolinska Institute Sweden	Prof. Michael Sjöström	Sweden
The Netherlands	Netherlands Institute for Health Services Research NIVEL, Dept. Allied Health Care	Dr. Cindy Veenhof	The Netherlands
Turkey	Celal Bayar University, Faculty of Medicine, Dept. of Public Health	Prof. Cemil Ozcan	Turkey

4
Methods

Investigation for Health Information Activities in the four categorised levels was implemented as follows:

4.1. National Data

For the collection of national data sources containing data on nutrition and physical activity, a competent institution was identified for each country. Table 4.1 in Sect. 4.2 provided an overview about the subcontracted partners that contributed to data collection. One national expert or organisation per country was commissioned to gather information on the project specification. This did not apply for those countries where a project partner was asked to undertake the data collection role.

Working together with local scientists and experts in the field of nutrition and physical activity implied a more effective handling of language barriers and ensured obtaining local data. Additionally, the contributions from national experts helped to understand the way national Health Information Activities are organized, as well as helped to understand cultural and political developments in national settings.

After first explanations through telephone between the subcontracted partners and the main partners, a comprehensive information meeting took place with the intention of introducing the project and its objectives. Furthermore, methods (regarding the database) and their use were presented. Subcontracted partners were introduced to their research tasks and were trained. Questions were answered. The principal aim for all partners was to identify national Health Information Activities with population scope. All partners were invited to contact the main partner to clarify open issues that might occur during the research process.

For national data collection, a database was created with Microsoft Access. In a fixed time period, starting from June 2006 and ending in November 2006, all partners were invited to enter their research findings into the database via a Web interface. By using the database, available national data sources related to nutrition and physical activity could be collected in a standardized manner to ensure comparability.

N. Wolfram et al. (eds.) *Nutrition and Physical Activity*,
© Springer Science + Business Media, LLC 2008

The database entries concentrated on the following aspects:

- General project Information (e.g., executive institution, project leader, funding agency)
- Employed methods and published literature referring to the Health Information Activity
- Description of employed methodology
- Geographical coverage of the data generated by the Health Information Activity
- Collected indicators on nutrition and physical activity
- Age groups covered

The database for collecting national Health Information Activities in European countries is shown in Appendix A.

Regarding the collection of national data sources and their entries into the database, the aim was to find as many Health Information Activities as possible. However, it could not guarantee the compilation of a fully comprehensive picture of implemented Health Information Activities in each European country. As the purpose of the report indicates, the report sets out to give an overview about national *examples*.

First, to arrange collected data more clearly and in a structured way, the database entries were additionally summarised in *Project Identity Cards*. Project Identity Cards comprise main background information for each project that was entered into the database (e.g., project leader and executing institution, short project description, keywords, and age groups). The summary is presented in Appendix C for European Projects and in Appendix D for national projects.

Second, subcontracted partners were asked to give an overview about the way national health reporting is organized in general and with special focus on the health determinants nutrition and physical activity. Furthermore, fundamental changes in the health monitoring system that took place during the reporting period (1990–2006) were asked about as well as a listing of national institutions that are involved in health reporting activities. The overview of health reporting in each country is summarized in *Country Profile Sheets*.

Keywords

A maximum of six published keywords per health information project was included in the project database and project identity cards. Project partners collected keywords from publications on the individual Health Information Activities. In cases where no keywords were published, this part was left blank in the project database and project identity cards.

The keywords provide a thematic structure for the Health Information Activities included in this report. Thus, they help the reader to research the project database.

Age Groups

To ensure usability of the inventory across definitions, ages of study subjects were entered into the database. Where several groups of different ages were included in a study, age was entered separately for any of the groups. The age of the youngest and the oldest participants was stated for every participant group. With the help of a description field, further information about subgroups or age-gender-classifications could be entered as text. The database thus provides the opportunity to identify exactly the age groups used in different health information activities. These details can then be matched with the definitions on age groups.

4.2. DG's at the European Commission (by M. Sjöström)

For the section of the different DG's at the European Commission, several representatives were contacted. Furthermore all available documents of the DG's were used to get all necessary information relating to this report.

4.3. WHO Section (by M. Rigby)

The section on WHO activities related to information on nutrition and physical activity at the population level was compiled by mixed methods on the basis of primarily an amalgam of personal knowledge not least through previous collaboration with WHO, direct contact, personal visit, and WHO projects as profiled on the WHO Internet pages.

Material was assembled and refined through the following steps:

- Personal knowledge of principal relevant activities
- Search of WHO Web pages (both European and headquarters) for relevant projects
- Email explaining the nature of the project sent to senior WHO contacts in both Copenhagen and Rome offices; included in this approach were contacts in nutrition, physical activity, noncommunicable disease policy, information and databases, and health reporting
- The author offered to visit both the Copenhagen and Rome offices for direct discussion with relevant officers to pick up information beyond that formally published
- A visit was made to Copenhagen in December 2006, coordinated by a senior officer to which several others contributed material; it was felt that aspects from the Rome office were clear from published material
- The draft completed chapter was circulated to all contacts, and improvements were consequently made.

This section seeks to indicate WHO activities within Europe providing, or contributing to national activities supplying, information on nutrition and physical activity in Europe, and also to capture professional views on key issues.

4.4. European Networks (by P. Di Mattia)

Different electronic scientific databases were used entering "European networks" as keywords. This strategy achieved no meaningful results.

Further searching was done with the following strategies:

- Different generic electronic databases were used (Google, arianna, etc.) entering "nutrition" and "physical activity" as keywords. Thousands of results were obtained, both relevant and not. A manual purposeful screening was done for European Networks Web sites
- From the literature review, a search was manually done looking for articles mentioning European Networks
- All official EU and USA Web sites on "Nutrition and Physical Activity" were consulted for "Useful links"

Following the above methodology, a number of European Networks involved in "Nutrition and Physical Activity" were identified.

5
Results

5.1. National Examples

5.1.1. Introduction

Data on national Health Information Activities have been collected in two ways. The country profile sheets provide a summary on health reporting for each country within the geographical coverage of this report. Project data on individual Health Information Activities have been entered into a project database and serve as national examples in this report.

In the country profile sheets, partners were asked to provide a general overview on Health Information Activities carried out on a national and regional level. Furthermore, they were requested to include institutions involved in health reporting and to outline any fundamental changes that took place in health reporting during the reporting period 1990–2006. Some examples of Health Information Activities were also included. All partners were encouraged to contact the main partner in case clarification on any open issue was required.

The country profile sheets reflect the multitude of activities and differences among EU member states, the European Economic Area and candidate countries. Factors, such as country size, constitutional and institutional structure influence health reporting activities. In some countries, Health Information Activities are exclusively carried out on a regional basis, whereas in other countries there are national activities. The size of the regions varies to a considerable extent among countries and in some cases even includes municipal level. In Turkey, for example, municipally administered health authorities report data to the Turkish Ministry of Health. However, the data are not reported back to municipal level.

Health reporting activities differ furthermore with respect to the frequency of data collection and how scientific findings are further communicated and published.

N. Wolfram et al. (eds.) *Nutrition and Physical Activity*,
© Springer Science+Business Media, LLC 2008

5.1.2. Country Profile Sheets

Austria

General Overview of Health Reporting Activities

Austrian health reporting activities document and analyse the population health status in regionally defined areas, e.g., municipalities, regions, federal states, and national state, with respect to the kind and size of stationary and ambulant facilities. Furthermore, health reports consider health determining factors, such as the environment and behavior. Health reporting aims at identifying deficits, preparing measures to improve the situation, and to observe effectiveness and efficiency of these measures. Health reporting is thus a permanent process that should be carried out at national, federal state, and national level.

The Austrian Federal Institute for Health Care is responsible for collection, analyses, and evaluation of data, which are of importance to the health status of the population. The Health Department of the Austrian Federal Institute for Health Care commissioned the establishment of the Austrian Health Information System, which was established for data collection and administration of data on the health status of the population and health framework. Health prevention measures, on the basis of the analysis of health-related data and information, contribute to the prevention and the establishment of best possible health in the whole population. Evaluations of the population health status, facilities of the health care system, and many health promotion and prevention measures can be obtained from the Health Information System any time.

Health Reporting Activities on Nutrition and Physical Activity at National Level

The Austrian Institute of Health Care is in charge.

Health Reporting Activities on Nutrition and Physical Activity at Regional Level

There are regional activities.

Institutions Involved in Health Reporting Activities

The Austrian Federal Institute for Health Care.

Examples of Health Reporting Activities

REGIS. REGIS is a free service of the Austrian Federal Institute for Health Care, which provides regionally comparable evaluation on health-related issues. REGIS targets all professionals and institutions in the health sector or interested in this sector.

Changes in the Health Reporting System Between 1990 and 2006

Federal state harmonization of health reporting, via a modular approach, in alignment with the WHO and EU guidelines.

Belgium

General Overview of Health Reporting Activities

The Scientific Institute of Public Health, Unit of Epidemiology, is responsible for reporting on national and international level. It works together with European institutions dealing with health reporting, like the World Health Organisation (WHO), Organisation for Economic Co-operation and Development (OECD), and the European Commission. The Scientific Institute of Public Health has several tasks, varying from the National Health Interview Surveys, and the National Food Consumption Survey, to evaluating and recommending methods for health interviews for the European Community Member States.

Health Reporting Activities on Nutrition and Physical Activity at National Level

The Scientific Institute of Public Health is responsible for the National Health Interview Survey (1997, 2001, 2004, 2008; see http://www.iph.fgov.be/epidemio/epien/index4.htm) and the Food Consumption Survey (2004; see http://www.iph.fgov.be/epidemio/epien/index5.htm). The HIS has a food frequency, the WHO question on PA and the IPAC. BMI is obtained through self reporting as is information on weight control. The FCS has a food frequency and two repeated 24-h-dietary recall. Waist circumference is measured, and BMI is obtained through self reporting as is information on weight control. The Scientific Institute of Public Health (different departments together) publish on nutrition-linked infections and zoonosis. Another institution is the Federal Administration of Health, which produced a health and nutrition plan in 2006. The High Council on Health publish the nutrition and physical activity-related recommendations.

Health Reporting Activities on Nutrition and Physical Activity at Regional Level

Flemish Community level

Besides the Scientific Institute of Public Health, numerous further institutions provide information about health on the Flemish Community level, for example:

- The Policy Research Centre "Sport, Beweging en Gezondheid"
- RIZIV (Rijksdienst voor ziekte en invaliditeitsverzekering) reports regularly on health-related costs and investigating policy measures
- The Flemish institute for health promotion (Vlaams Instituut voor gezondheids-promotie)
- Regional committees to follow up and built an inventory on all health promotion activities (http://www.wvc.vlaanderen.be/gezondheidsbevordering)

In addition, universities also contribute data to health reporting in numerous research projects on a national and international level. The Katholieke Universiteit

Leuven (K.U. Leuven), the Vrije Universiteit Brussel (VUB), and Ghent University are joined in a consortium: the Policy Research Centre "Sport, Beweging en Gezondheid." Health reporting is also performed by the University of Antwerp and University of Hasselt.

French Community level

The province of Henaut publish yearly health reports, including information collected by different sources such as the National HIS and presents provincial data on nutrition and health habits.

As in the Flemish community, many universities are involved in nutrition research. Focusing on public health and nutrition is the School of Public Health of the ULB.

Institutions Involved in Health Reporting Activities

The Scientific Institute of Public Health
The Federal Administration of Health

Examples of Health Reporting Activities

National Health Interview Survey
National Food Consumption Survey
Health and nutrition plan in 2006

Changes in the Health Reporting System Between 1990 and 2006

None reported

Bulgaria

General Overview of Health Reporting Activities

Health reporting in Bulgaria occurs comprehensively on a state authority basis through 28 regional health centers and 28 regional inspectorates for public health protection and control.

Health reporting in Bulgaria is subdivided in state health reporting and regional health reporting. The central health reporting institution in Bulgaria is the National Center of Health Informatics along with the National Center of Public Health Protection.

Health Reporting Activities on Nutrition and Physical Activity at National Level

The National Center of Public Health Protection is in charge.

Health Reporting Activities on Nutrition and Physical Activity at Regional Level

Regional health centers feed their information into the National Center for Informatics. The National Center of Health Informatics is a specialized authority of the Ministry of Health responsible for the provision of information on healthcare. Some of its major tasks are as follows:

- The creation and support of information bases on health-demographic status of the population, resources, and activities of the healthcare system
- Investigations on the needs of information in the medical practice and its documentation support
- Preparation of medico-statistical information and specialized analyses on the problems of healthcare system, etc.

It works together with the National Center of Public Health Protection, the National Statistical Institute, the National Social Security Institute and 28 regional health centers and 28 regional inspectorates for public health protection and control.

Institutions Involved in Health Reporting Activities

The national center of Public Health Protection
Five medical universities
The Bulgarian Academy of sciences

Examples of Health Reporting Activities

Reports on national health surveys

Research projects

Changes in the Health Reporting System Between 1990 and 2006

Working together with the WHO and the European Commission

Croatia

Health Reporting Activities with Respect to Nutrition and Physical Activity
at National Level (Including Examples)

The Croatian Adult Health Survey (CAHS) was conducted in 2003 as a part of an
overall strategy for health system reforms in Croatia. This survey was carried out
on the national level. Through the cooperation of the Croatian Central Bureau of
Statistics, the CAHS sample of dwellings was selected from the 2001 Census of
Households under a multistage stratified cluster design. At the final stage 11, 250
dwellings were selected. The households in the selected dwellings formed the sample of households. One person aged 18 or over per household was randomly
selected using a simple random sampling approach. Response was obtained for
9,070 individuals (response rate of 84.3%). Survey was done by the CAHS Team
(A. Stampar School of Public Health staff) in collaboration with the National
Institute of Public Health and under the management of the Canadian Society of
International Health. Data were collected by well-trained public health nurses.
They conducted interviews by formatted paper questionnaire and collected anthropometric measures such as height, weight, and blood pressure at the end of the
interview for all respondents. The questionnaire included topics like health status,
determinants of health (smoking, physical activity, nutrition, alcohol use) and use
of health care services. The questions on nutrition and physical activity were based
on existing studies (CINDI/WHO) and SF-36.

WHO Countrywide Integrated Noncommunicable Diseases Intervention (CINDI)
Health Monitor Surveys was conducted from 2002 to 2005 in four areas (communities and counties/districts) both rural and urban (Pozega, Gospic, Vinkovci, Daruvar).
These surveys are conceptually a part of a wider international project in the frame of
the WHO CINDI programme and run by the Andrija Stampar School of Public
Health. A random sample was drawn from the local population registries. In the district of Pozega, all adults (over 18 years) were included. The total number of adults
was 5,600 and the response rates varied from 54 to 68%. The questionnaire was used,
on the basis of the CINDI Health Monitor Core Questionnaire. The questions on
behavioral risk factors included several questions on nutrition and physical activity.
The interviews at home were conducted by trained medical students.

Changes in the Health Reporting System Between 1990 and 2006

There is no regular reporting on nutrition or physical activities (except for children
and youth – related to the regular measurement at schools). Data obtained from the
Croatian Adult Health Survey (CAHS) are available and published.

Further Scientific Institutions Involved in Health Reporting Activities

- Andrija Stampar School of Public Health, Medical School Zagreb (development, implementation, monitoring, evaluation and reporting both surveys)
- National Institute of Public Health (collaborator in CAHS involved in data collection), at present regular source of data obtained
- Ministry of Health and Social Welfare (formal supporter)
- Croatian Central Bureau of Statistics and local government (population register)
- International Health Canada and Statistics Canada (advisor for CAHS,)
- Community Health Centres in demonstration areas (supporter in CINDI program)
- CINDI Croatia (formal supporter in CINDI Health Monitor Surveys)

Cyprus

General Overview of Health Reporting Activities

The Health Services in Cyprus are divided into two sectors, i.e., the public health sector and the private sector. The Ministry of Health is responsible for both the public and the private sector. The public sector is considered more important as the main source of information and implementing policies.

Health Reporting Activities on Nutrition and Physical Activity at National Level

The Department of Medical and Public Health Services is mainly responsible for providing information about the health determinants, nutrition, and physical activity at national level. The Ministry of Health is responsible for reporting this information on a national and international level. The Ministry works mainly with the World Health Organization (WHO) and the European Commission. Both organizations mainly collaborate in research as well as in applying policies and political decisions that deal with health in our country.

Concerning nutrition and physical activity, there are two types of data collection projects, i.e., projects that focus on research on nutrition and lifestyle and those on surveillance systems that have anthropometric results and questions on nutrition.

Health Reporting Activities on Nutrition and Physical Activity at Regional Level

Not applicable

Institutions Involved in Health Reporting Activities

The Department of Medical and Public Health Services
The Ministry of Health

Examples of Health Reporting Activities

The Ministry of Health publishes an annual report on various aspects of public health in Cyprus, i.e., activities and information concerning all departments.

Changes in the Health Reporting System Between 1990 and 2006

Most of the research done in the area of nutrition, diet, and physical activity took place after 1995. During the reporting period, a great interest in nutrition and physical activity has been established, and the health reporting system during this period has improved dramatically as the national interest in nutrition and physical activity has increased considerably.

Czech Republic

General Overview of Health Reporting Activities

Health reporting in the Czech Republic is provided on the national level, the regional level and as a part of research projects of universities and research institutes.

Health Reporting Activities on Nutrition and Physical Activity at National Level

Systematic monitoring of diseases related to nutrition and physical activity is provided by the Institute of Health Information and Statistics (Ustav zdravotnickych informaci a statistiky, UZIS), a government organisation established by the Ministry of Health. In children and adolescents, obesity (E66) is one of the diagnoses followed together with other types of overnutrition (hypervitaminosis A and D) and also with consequences of overnutrition (E68).

The National Institute of Health (Statni zdravotni ustav, SZU) is also responsible for health reporting. The SZU performs systematic monitoring of the environmental impact on population health in the Czech Republic, preparation of legislation in the field of health protection, including harmonization of Czech legislation with the norms of the European Commission. The Institute operates the Environmental Health Monitoring System.

Health Reporting Activities on Nutrition and Physical Activity at Regional Level

The Public Health Institutes conduct regional data sampling on Nutrition and Physical activity.

Institutions Involved in Health Reporting Activities

The Institute of Health Information and Statistics (Ustav zdravotnickych informaci a statistiky, UZIS)
The National Institute of Health (Statni zdravotni ustav, SZU)

Examples of Health Reporting Activities

Both Institutes are responsible for reporting on national and international level and collaborate on common programmes and projects with World Health Organization and European Commission. National Board of Obesity (advisory board of Ministry of Health) participates in creating of the surveillance system of consequences of over nutrition and poor physical activity. Universities and Health Institutes contribute to reporting by their research programmes.

Changes in the Health Reporting System Between 1990 and 2006

Since 1994 an independent Total Diet Study (TDS) has been organized by the National Institute of Public Health, and it has been an important data source for risk management. The longitudinal national anthropological survey is conducted by the Institute in collaboration and alignment with the WHO and EU guidelines.

Denmark

General Overview of Health Reporting Activities

The National Institute of Public Health (NIPH) is the main institute providing information about the health-determinants nutrition and physical activity on international, national, and regional level in Denmark. The NIPH is an independent sectorial research institute under the Danish Ministry of the Interior and Health. Nutrition and physical activity are two focus areas of research and publications of the institute. The NIPH cooperates with other European institutions such as the European Commission and the World Health Organization (WHO). Research is organized in seven research programmes, which all provide health information and involve determinants nutrition and physical activity in a variety of ways. The National Board of Health is also responsible for health reporting in Denmark.

Health Reporting Activities on Nutrition and Physical Activity at National Level

The National Health Interview Surveys (SUSY) is one of the most common national surveys carried out by the NIPH. The overall aim of this programme is the establishment of a set of indicators that describe the health status of the Danish population as a whole and of various population groups. Some of the performed studies focus on nutrition and physical activity as main determinants whereas other studies concentrate on a larger perspective and consider nutrition and physical activity among other determinants.

Health Reporting Activities on Nutrition and Physical Activity at Regional Level

None reported

Institutions Involved in Health Reporting Activities

The National Institute for Public Health (NIPH)
The National Board of Health

Examples of Health Reporting Activities

Examples of the NIPH's research projects are as follows:

- The National Health Interview Surveys (SUSY)
- Arctic public health research
- The Danish Nurse Cohort Study 1993
- Children, food, and exercise
- Frame and presumption for diet and physical activity in 3- to 10-year-old children

Changes in the Health Reporting System Between 1990 and 2006

The National Board of Health cooperates with a number of health professional forums mainly within the framework of the European Union, the World Health Organization, the Nordic Council of Ministers, and the Council of Europe.

Estonia

Health Reporting Activities on Nutrition and Physical Activity at National Level

The Estonian Social Survey (ESS), the Estonian Family and Fertility Survey (ESTONIAN FFS), the national-based health status information has been collected using several interview surveys, such as the Estonian Health Interview Survey 1996 and the Estonian Health Behavior Survey of Adult Population (HBAP) using the postal survey. All mentioned surveys include either some questions or question-naire parts about nutrition or physical activity.

Health Reporting Activities on Nutrition and Physical Activity at Regional Level

None Reported

Institutions Involved in Health Reporting Activities

1. Estonian Statistical Office: Estonian Social Survey (ESS)
2. Estonian Demographic Association, Estonian Demographic Institute: Estonian Family and Fertility Survey (ESTONIAN FFS)
3. Institute for Epidemiological and Clinical Research, reorganized for now – National Institute for Health Development:

    (a) Estonian Health Interview Survey 1996
    (b) Estonian Health Behaviour Survey of Adult Population (HBAP)

Examples of Health Reporting Activities

The Estonian Social Survey (ESS)
The Estonian Family and Fertility Survey (ESTONIAN FFS)
The Estonian Health Interview Survey 1996
The Estonian Health Behaviour Survey of Adult Population (HBAP), using the postal survey

Changes in the Health Reporting System Between 1990 and 2006

The Estonian health system has undergone significant changes since the country's independence in 1991. Reforms took place in two waves: a first wave of "big bang" reforms introduced major changes during the early 1990s, while a second wave introduced more incremental developments during the late 1990s. More information about health care systems in transition can be found at http://www.euro.who.int/Document/E85516.pdf

Reforms in all Estonian health systems influenced also the health reporting system. Until 1996, the National Health Information independently collected health information following the procedure of the Statistical Office of Estonia. Since 1997 the health information have been collected and coordinated by Ministry of Social Affairs.

Finland

General Overview of Health Reporting Activities

National health reporting in Finland is mainly provided by the National Public Health Institute (KTL). It provides information about the health-determinants nutrition and physical activity at international, national, and regional level in Finland. Working under the jurisdiction of the Ministry of Social Affairs and Health, KTL provides public decision makers, other stakeholders, and the general public with reliable information on public health. KTL is responsible for the control of infectious and for the prevention of chronic diseases in collaboration with the health care system. KTL cooperates with a number of health professional forums such as the European Commission and the World Health Organization. The institute has an important role in shaping Finnish public health work and health policies.

Health Reporting Activities on Nutrition and Physical Activity at National Level

Every year, several reports are published by KTL on various aspects of public health in Finland. There are reports that concentrate specifically on physical activity and/or nutrition in the Finnish population. Some of the reports focus on a broader topic, like health in general in Finland, but include physical activity and/or nutrition as one of the determinants.

Health Reporting Activities on Nutrition and Physical Activity at Regional Level

None reported

Institutions Involved in Health Reporting Activities

National Public Health Institute (KTL)
    National Research and Development Centre for Welfare and Health (STAKES)
    STAKES is an expert agency in the field of social welfare and health care in Finland. STAKES is a sector research institute under the Ministry of Social Affairs and Health. Its core functions are research, development, information production and producing information and expertise for policymakers and other stakeholders. It promotes the welfare and health of the population and develops social and health services. STAKES maintains statistics and registers within its sphere of activities. STAKES annually runs a wide range of projects in cooperation with different actors in the public sector in Finland. Nutrition and physical activity are one part of different national registers and annual publications.

Examples of Health Reporting Activities

Health Behavior and Health among the Finnish Adult Population
    The National FINRISK Study
    The National Findiet Study
    Nutrition report
    School Health Promotion (SHP) Study
    FINBALT Health Monitor

Changes in the Health Reporting System Between 1990 and 2006

None reported

France

General Overview of Health Reporting Activities

The French nutritional status monitoring system was created in 2001 upon implementation of the National Nutrition and Health Programme (Programme National
Nutrition Santé, PNNS) by the Ministry of Health. This public health program is
based on nine principal health objectives which focus on:

- Food consumption (increase in consumption of fruits and vegetables, calcium
  and reduce in alcohol and fat intakes).
- Nutritional status (reduce in average adult cholesterol levels by 5%, reduce in
  average adult systolic blood pressure by 10 mmHg, reduce in the prevalence of
  overweight and obesity (BMI > 25 kg/m^2) by 20% among adults and preventing
  the increase in prevalence of childhood obesity).
- Physical activity (increase in daily physical activity).

Health Reporting Activities on Nutrition and Physical Activity at National Level

Current data on obesity, food consumption, physical activity, or nutritional status of
the population at the national level primarily come from four large studies. These
studies are shown below as examples of health reporting activities. In addition, the
National Nutrition and Health Survey (ENNS) which is currently in progress with
the first results available in 2007. The objectives of the ENNS include describing
food consumption, nutritional status and physical activity of a representative sample of 2,000 children aged 3–17 years and 4,000 adults aged 17–74 years.

Other studies are also regularly conducted at schools in collaboration with the
Ministry of Education in order to collect data on childhood obesity.

Health Reporting Activities on Nutrition and Physical Activity at Regional Level

None reported

Institutions Involved in Health Reporting Activities

National Institute for Health Surveillance (Institut de Veille Sanitaire, InVS)
French Agency for Food Security (Agence Française de Sécurité Sanitaire des
    Aliments, AFSSA)
National Institute for Health Prevention and Education (Institut National de
    Prévention et d'Education pour la Santé, INPES)

Examples of Health Reporting Activities

- The National Individual Food Consumption Survey (Enquête Individuelle
  Nationale sur les Consommations Alimentaires, INCA-1) conducted for the first
  time in 1998–1999 – a second survey is currently in progress – by the French
  Agency for Food Security

- The Health Nutrition Barometer carried out by the National Institute for Health Prevention and Education
- The ObEpi study conducted by the Roche Institute on obesity in collaboration with INSERM (Institut National de la Santé et de la Recherche Médicale)
- The SUVIMAX study

Changes in the Health Reporting System Between 1990 and 2006

The National Institute for Health Surveillance (InVS), in partnership with the Conservatoire National des Arts et Métiers (CNAM) and the University of Paris 13, created a Surveillance and Nutritional Epidemiology Unit (Unité de Surveillance et d'Epidémiologie Nutritionnelle, USEN) in 2001, which is intended to:

- Assure the monitoring of nutritional status of the population living in France
- Evaluate the effectiveness of adopted measures with regard to the PNNS objectives
- Support the standardization of data collection methods (physical activity, dietary intakes, etc.) with respect to European and international methods

Germany

General Overview of Health Reporting Activities

Health reporting in Germany is heterogeneous. It is influenced, predominantly by two factors namely: the reunification in 1990 and the federal structure of the German Republic, which has had fundamental influence on health reporting. Health reporting in Germany is conducted at a national, regional, and local level.

Health Reporting Activities on Nutrition and Physical Activity at National Level

The Federal Health Reporting Service (Gesundheitsberichterstattung des Bundes, GBE) is a joined task of the Robert Koch Institute and the Federal Statistical Office. The Robert Koch Institute is responsible for the scientific input and coordination of the Federal Health Reporting service. The Federal Statistical Office is in charge of gathering data and operating the information system. The political responsibility for the Federal Health Reporting service lies with the Federal Ministry of Health.

The three pillars of the Federal Health Reporting service are reports either published as booklets (Themenhefte, e.g., GBE-Booklet 26: Physical activity) or as Focus Reports. Additionally to this the Information System provides health-related information in all fields of health reporting in the form of an online database.

Existing data form the basis for the Federal Health Reporting service. It systematically collects scattered information from the multitude of institutions in the health sector. These data are harmonized to present a comprehensive overview on the health sector. Official statistics as well as data of cross sectional or longitudinal studies are used for this purpose. The German Health Survey 1998, which contains the Nutrition Survey carried out by the Robert Koch Institute, provides the most important and most extensive database considering the lifestyle indicators nutrition and physical activity.

The information offered by the Federal Health Reporting service focuses on the national level and provides reference for the health reporting activities of the German Federal States (Bundesländer).

Health Reporting Activities on Nutrition and Physical Activity at Regional Level

An important basis for national health reporting activities has been established with the common indicator set for health reporting activities of the German Federal States (Indikatorensatz für die Gesundheitsberichterstattung der Länder). This catalogue covers about 300 indicators for different health-related issues, which allows comparisons at national level. The thematic domain "health-relevant behavior" contains indicators to monitor smoking, drinking behavior, nutrition, body mass index (BMI), and physical activity.

Two laender, Bavaria and Saxony, conducted nutrition surveys on the federal state level. An increase of the sample size of the German Health Survey allowed for state specific analyses for Bavaria and North Rhine-Westphalia.

At municipal level, there are several health reports considering special local health issues. Usually, the health offices take a leading role in these reporting activities. The outcomes of municipal health reports can rarely be transferred to the national level. Lifestyle indicators are rarely recorded and are often not comparable.

Institutions Involved in Health Reporting Activities

The Federal Ministry of Health
The Robert Koch Institute
The Federal Statistics Office

Examples of Health Reporting Activities

The German Health Survey 1998
Nutrition Survey within the German Health Survey 1998

Changes in the Health Reporting System Between 1990 and 2006

Before the Federal Health Reporting Service in its present form was institutional-ized, in 1999, basic guidelines and concepts had been developed in a perennial research period. This research project was financed by the Federal Ministry of Education and Research (former Federal Ministry of Education, Science, Research and Technology) together with the Federal Ministry of Health. The general research objective was to improve the incomplete database concerning German health care as well as to produce a data infrastructure, which can be used as valid information background by politicians, scientists, researchers, and interested stakeholders.

Greece

General Overview of Health Reporting Activities

The collection of national health data in Greece is primarily conducted by the National Statistical Service. The state, and in particular the Ministry of Health and Welfare, is the main user of this data and the indices produced, which guide decision makers in the development of health-related policies and health-related interventions. Nevertheless, the Statistical Service does not conduct systematic surveys to obtain reliable and nationally representative data on nutrition and physical activity patterns.

Health Reporting Activities on Nutrition and Physical Activity at National Level

The only available data on a national scale concern data are on nutrition, which are extracted from the national Household Budget Surveys (HBS) periodically conducted in most Member States of the European Union including Greece. In Greece, HBS are conducted every 5 years among a country representative household sample. HBS among other items measure values and quantities of food purchased by households, which are then used by various public health institutions to depict dietary patterns of the Greek population. This information can be easily examined in relation to demographic and other socioeconomic data captured in the same survey and used to create the nutritional profile of the Greek consumer.

Health Reporting Activities on Nutrition and Physical Activity at Regional Level

Some health reporting activities with respect to nutrition and physical activity are conducted only at regional level in Greece. These data selected through these activities cover only specific regions of the country and cannot be applied to the Greek population.

Some of the institutions that carry out such activities are the following:

- Department of Nutrition and Dietetics, Harokopio University of Athens. The department collects information on nutritional patterns (mostly local) through various research projects namely CARDIO 2000, the ATTICA study, GREEKS, and others
- Public Health Nutritional and Epidemiology Unit, Department of Hygiene and Epidemiology, University of Athens, which is also the WHO Collaborating Center for Nutrition and coordinates EU funded projects such as DAFNE (which uses HBS data), EPIC, EPIC ELDERLY providing among other issues a wealth of information on socio-demographic and healthrelated factors, including diet habits
- Laboratory of Operations Research, Health Policy and Planning Unit, University of Patras, which has conducted studies on a local level on the dietary and physical exercise habits of the people of the city of Patras

- Department of Preventive Medicine and Nutritional clinic, Medical School, University of Crete, which is involved in various nutritional-related studies
- Department of Physical Education and Sports Science, Democritus University of Thrace, which has conducted research on physical activity patterns
- National School of Public Health
- The National Centre for Social Research

Institutions Involved in Health Reporting Activities

The Ministry of Health and Welfare
The National Statistical Service

Examples of Health Reporting Activities

Household budget survey carried out every 4 years

Hungary

Health Reporting Activities with Respect to Nutrition and Physical Activity on a National and Regional Level (Including Examples)

In Hungary, the National Public Health and Medical Officer Service (NPHMOS) is the state organ responsible for public health. The NPHMOS carries out its tasks at national and local level via its national centers, county, and town institutions. Among other various activities set out by law, the responsibilities of the NPHMOS are to collect, study, analyze, and disseminate data and information on the health status of the population and its determinants. Health reporting by the NPHMOS is operated at national and county levels. Data collections and reporting by national professional institutes within the NPHMOS most importantly involve the health status of the population, work health, nutrition, and environmental factors.

Other state institutions whose activities involve routine data collection on health determinants and health care also do regular and ad hoc health reporting. The most important institutes are the following:

- The Hungarian Central Statistical Office (official source of demographic and mortality data) routinely collects data such as demographic, health care, and population surveys routinely on determinants and occasionally on health
- The Health Insurance Fund collects routine health care data for financing purposes
- Other professional institutes under the Ministry of Health, e.g., Institute of Child Health (HBSC studies)

A project was launched in 1999 by the Ministry of Health to improve the Hungarian health monitoring system. In line with international recommendations, the project developed a standard methodology for population-based health surveys, standard health indicators, a national health database and health reporting at national, regional, and county levels. The project was coordinated by the National Center for Epidemiology within the NPHMOS.

Pillars of the health monitoring system established during the above project:

- The National Health Interview Surveys in 2000 and 2003 (latest available year) among others provide data on health status, functionality, smoking, drinking, consumption of fruit and vegetables (in 2003 a nutrition diary was also included), social and economic determinants, and use of health services.
- The National Health Database was assembled, regularly maintained, and made available online.
- A comprehensive public health report for experts was published in 2004 on the health status of the population and its determinants. Brief annual reports were published specifically targeting policy-makers.

In 2005 regional public health reports targeting county and regional policy makers and professionals were published. These reports analyzed and interpreted data

mainly from the National Health Interview Surveys, routine data from the mentioned sources and any other relevant and high quality data.

Further Scientific Institutions Involved in Health Reporting Activities

Universities and a few private research institutes also contribute important data and
health reports from research projects on national and subnational levels.
  Links to said institutions, health reports available in English:

- NPHMOS – http://www.antsz.hu
- National Center for Epidemiology – http://www.oek.hu
- National Health Interview Surveys Hungary 2000 and 2003 – https://www.iph.
  fgov.be/hishes/
- National Health Database – http://www.eski.hu
- National Health Reports – http://www.oek.hu/oek.web?to=8,722,979&nid=393
  &pid=1&lang=hun

Iceland

Health Reporting Activities with Respect to Nutrition and Physical Activity
at National Level

Several institutions provide information about the health-determinants nutrition and
physical activity at national level.

Statistics Iceland

Statistics Iceland is the National Statistical Institute of Iceland and was
founded in 1914. Statistics Iceland operates in accordance with the United
Nations Fundamental Principles of Official Statistics, the European Statistcs
Code of Practice as well as the Act on the Protection of Privacy regarding the
processing of personal data. The division of social statistics comprises four
departments, one of them, the department of labor market and social statistics,
deals with statistics on employment, living conditions and social matters,
health, gender, justice, and environment statistics. Statistical reports are published
on a regular base.

The Public Health Institute of Iceland

The Public Health Institute of Iceland was officially established on 1 July 2003 and
is answerable to the Ministry of Health and Social Security. The policy and function
of the Institute is in accordance with Icelandic National Health Plan to the year
2010 and the guide lines set down by the World Health Organization. Matters dealt
with by the Institute include alcohol and drug abuse prevention, nutrition, accident
prevention, mental health and physical activity, dental health, and tobacco use prevention. Before 1 July 2003, several smaller institutes dealt with public health
issues. In 2006, the new Icelandic nutrition recommendations were published by
The Public Health Institute of Iceland.

The Medical Director of Health

The Medical Director of Health serves as adviser to the Minister and to the government on everything concerning health. He supervises the activities and the working
facilities of health professionals, collects statistical reports, and is in charge of the
publication of the country's health statistics.

The Icelandic Heart Association

The Icelandic Heart Association (IHA) was founded 1964 around an initiative to battle increasing cardiovascular death in Iceland. One of its purpose is to promote and conduct studies and reasearch of heart diseases in Iceland, risk factors, and preventive methods. The IHA participated in the MONICA project.

The Icelandic Cancer Society

The Icelandic Cancer Society was established on 27 June 1951, now being an association of 24 local voluntary cancer divisions, chapters, in various parts of the country and five voluntary organizations of former cancer patients. The Icelandic Cancer Society is one of five members of the Nordic Cancer Union (NCU), since 1952 a member of the International Union Against Cancer (UICC) and also an active member of Association of European Cancer Leagues (ECL).

Further Scientific Institutions Involved in Health Reporting Activities

Universities also contribute data to health reporting in numerous research projects on a national and international level. Some large studies on health and health indicators (e.g., studies on child nutrition, maternal nutrition, and birth outcomes) have been performed in the area of Reykjavík by the local universities.

Ireland

Ireland is a unitary state occupying some 80% of the land mass of the island of Ireland, and a similar proportion of the population. The remaining six Northern Counties are part of the United Kingdom, constituting the UK "home country" of Northern Ireland.

The Republic of Ireland has a largely publicly funded national health service. Hospitals, community health services, ambulance services, and the public health functions are provided by public services and basically are free at the point of use, though there are some user charges. Primary medical care is provided by general practitioners operating in independent medical practices. These are private in the sense that patients pay per consultation, though there is a national medical card system whereby the state directly meets the charges for specific groups including the very elderly and those with low incomes. There are national schemes whereby the state picks up the cost of prescribed medicines for these groups, in another scheme whereby the state meets the balance above a monthly contribution for persons with chronic conditions or multiple medications; otherwise, patients pay the full cost of prescribed medicines. There is provision of private hospitals, some based in the grounds of public hospitals. There is also an active, but declining, not-for-profit sector, particularly in mental health and services for those with intellectual disability or chronic conditions – these independent providers may be contracted by the public sector to provide the local public service; they may also provide a traditional private service funded by full economic charges.

A recent development is the provision of cross-border services between Northern Ireland and the Republic of Ireland. This is part of a philosophy contained within the Peace Agreement, which sought to end the conflict in Northern Ireland, whereby a number of initiatives are provided on an Island of Ireland basis, or specifically to foster harmony and mutual understanding across the land border. Thus, for instance, some specialist medical services for residents of the North West of Ireland are provided from Northern Ireland. This may complicate the statistics for these specific services.

The Ministry responsible for health services in Ireland is the Department of Health and Children. Until 2004, the public health services were run by a series of Area Health Boards (and one Regional Health Authority in the East of the country). These covered specific geographical areas, which were reasonably aligned to social services districts. However, in 2004, a major reorganisation of the health services saw the creation of the autonomous Health Services Executive, with a Chief Executive and a team of Directors, who now manage all health services. Thus, there is a totally national health system, though with operational management delegated to a smaller number of local offices. The full impact of these reforms is still working through the system. Social care is the responsibility of the Department of Social and Family Affairs.

Introduction of Health Reporting Activities and Important Institutions

Statistical provision broadly divides between vital statistics and activity statistics. Vital statistics are the responsibility of government. The Department of Health and Children is the primary repository for health and health activity data. There is also a strong tradition of public health research, through university departments and through bodies such as the Health Research Board.

Italy

General Overview of Health Reporting Activities

In Italy, there are many important public and private institutions which realize, at different levels, research about food, nutrition, and the influence of physical activity on quality of life. Their studies, anyway, are not systematic even if they are very interesting and useful. Some of these institutions, for example, are:

– Universities that contribute data to health reporting in numerous research projects
– The Center for Social Studies and Policies (CENSIS), who realizes research commissioned primarily by ministries, regions, provinces, municipalities, chambers of commerce, business and professional associations, banks, private companies, network managers, and international organisations, as well as various European Union programmes

As far as the systematic research is concerned, in Italy there are two kinds of reporting activities, at national, regional, and local level.

Health Reporting Activities on Nutrition and Physical Activity at National Level

At national level, the Italian Institute of Statistical Research (ISTAT) is the main supplier for official statistical information in Italy. ISTAT, among other kinds of research, collects health data concerning nutrition and physical activity.

"The Istituto Superiore di Sanità" (ISS) is the leading technical and scientific public body of the Italian National Health Service. Its activities include research, control, training, and consultation in the interest of public health protection." (http://www.iss.it/).

The ISS is realizing the "PASSI Study" (the Study of Progresses of Local Health Organizations for the Italian Health) collaborating with "Tor Vergata" University, Rome, and the National Center for Epidemiology, Supervision, and Health promotion (CNESPS) of the ISS. The PASSI Study is a national study with the aim to supervise the Italian health status by monitoring habits, lifestyles, and programs that the country carried out to modify risk behaviors. The PASSI Study, among the other themes, focuses on the study of physical activity, smoking, nutrition, and alcohol consumption.

The Ministry of Health is responsible for reporting at a national level and it is in charge of approving the National Health Plan, which is redefined every 3 years and states the general Public Health objectives to be achieved. One of the main objectives of the National Health Plan 2005–2008 is the prevention of women and child obesity, through the promotion of sports and physical activity.

Health Reporting Activities with Respect to Nutrition and Physical Activity at Regional Level

Regional and Local level

The Regional Ministry for Health and Local Health Organizations collect, in each region, data concerning nutrition and physical activity the PASSI Study.

Furthermore, ISTAT has many offices in each region where health data are collected. These data are then analyzed at regional and national level.

More details on Italian research about nutrition and physical activity are included in the project database.

Latvia

Health Reporting Activities on Nutrition and Physical Activity at National Level

In Latvia health statistics data are collected either as routine statistics or from statistical surveys. Routine statistics provide information on demographics (e.g., births, deaths, and population), death causes, morbidity, healthcare resources, inpatient, and outpatient health care, maternal and infant health care, emergency care, disability, injuries, and accidents. Routine statistics are obtained on both national and regional level as well as by cities and districts.

However, some statistical data can be obtained from statistical surveys, only. The most important groups are smoking, nutrition, physical activity, alcohol consumption, body mass, spread of most chronic diseases, activity limitations, etc.

In Latvia statistical information on nutrition and physical activity can be obtained from such surveys:

- *Health Behavior among Latvian Adult Population:* a regular survey is performed by the National Public Health Institute of Finland and the Health Promotion Centre of Latvia every second year. The first survey was carried out in 1998, the next surveys – in 2000, 2002, 2004 and 2006.
- *Health Survey of Latvian Population 2003:* a single survey performed by Central Statistical Bureau of Latvia in 2003.

Most of these data are at national level as well as subdivided by urban and rural population. Only the Health Survey of the Latvian population presents data by five regions of Latvia.

Both of these surveys have data on different health-related topics including nutrition and physical activity.

In 1993 a statistical survey, *The Most Prevalent Chronic Diseases in Latvia,* was carried out in Latvia. This survey was based on the World Health Organisation's programmes *INTERHEALTH, CINDI* and *MONICA.* The structure of this survey was similar to the surveys mentioned earlier.

Liechtenstein

General Overview of Health Reporting Activities

The Princedom of Liechtenstein is a member of the UN and has been in close union with Switzerland as regards currency, economy, and social union since the 1920s.

The assumption is near that Liechtenstein participates in Swiss surveys but according to the "Fürstlichen Amtes für Volkswirtschaft Liechtenstein" (Liechtenstein Department of Economics) has neither taken part in the Swiss microcensus or health surveys of the Swiss Federal Statistical Office nor in Swiss panels or any other European Activities that Switzerland is involved in.

There is no representative data collection apart from continuous registration of birth and death rate by state authorities.

The renewed structure of the health insurance system has resulted in increased responsibilities of health insurances as regards data collection and data transfer to official statistics.

The government of Liechtenstein started the campaign "bewusst**er**leben" ("Live More Consciously") in 2006, which aimed at strengthening health awareness and individual responsibility.

Within the frame of this campaign, a survey on prevention and individual prevention was carried out in summer 2006. "Live More Consciously" will be continued for three years and more output is expected.

Lithuania

Health Reporting Activities with Respect to Nutrition And Physical Activity
at National Level (Including Examples)

- The Department of Statistics to the Government of the Republic of Lithuania
  and the Lithuanian Health Information Centre (WHO Collaborating Center) are
  the main health reporting institutions. These data are published in the Statistical
  Yearbooks annually.
- The Department of Statistics provides data on food availability obtained from
  food balance sheets and household budget surveys annually.
- The National Nutrition Center is responsible for national dietary surveys.
  Dietary surveys on national random samples of population aged 20–64 were
  conducted in 1997 and 2002 (to be on target in 2007). These data were presented
  in the reports.
- Kaunas University of Medicine is carrying out Lithuanian health behavior monitoring
  among adult population and health behavior surveys among Lithuanian school children.
  These data, including nutrition and physical activity, are presented in the reports.

Health Reporting Activities with Respect to Nutrition and Physical Activity
at Regional Level

None reported

Institutions involved in health reporting activities

Universities and research institutes conduct the research projects on nutrition and
physical activity. Examples of institutions and their research projects are:

The Report of the Nordic Council of Ministers, 2002: NORBAGREEN study:
The consumption of vegetables, potatoes, fruit, bread and fish was assessed in eight
Nordic and Baltic countries (national level).

Kaunas University of Medicine:

School Children Nutrition Survey (national level). Kaunas University of
Medicine conducted the survey among school lchildren of the 9th and 11th grade.

Dietary and physical activity surveys within the framework of the WHO Countrywide
Integrated Non-communicable Diseases Intervention (CINDI) Programme (regional
level). The surveys were carried out in 1987, 1993, 1999, and 2006/2007. Kaunas
University of Medicine is responsible for data collection and management.

Lithuanian Academy of Physical Education: Physical activity of Lithuanian
school children (regional level). Lithuanian Academy of Physical Education carried
out the study among school children of five largest cities of Lithuania.

Department of Physical Education and Sports: The Department analyses the attitudes of the Lithuanian population toward physical exercises and engagement into physical activity (national level). Department of Physical Education and Sports belongs to the Government of the Republic of Lithuania and carried out the study.

Department of Statistics: Health survey of Lithuanian adult population (national level). In 2005, Department of Statistics carried out a study using the guidelines of Eurostat for the European Health Interview Survey. Data on physical activity (IPAQ questionnaire), weight, and height were collected.

Luxembourg

General overview of health reporting activities

Following the first National Health Conference in November 2005, the initiative was taken by the Ministry of Health to elaborate a national programme for healthy nutrition and physical activity. Some of the most important goals were the constitution of an interdisciplinary expert group for the elaboration, the regular updates, and the surveillance of national recommendations in the given areas. Furthermore, the elaboration of strong networks for the implementation of actions, the coordination of existing scattered projects, the identification of population groups and areas with special needs were focused. Finally, the improvement of statistical information on determinants of nutrition and physical status of the population and the evaluation of actions were also in the center of attention.

By the means of the study "Motricity among 9, 14, and 18-Year-Old Children and Adolescents," published in spring 2006, the collaboration between the Ministries of Health, Education, Sports, and Family was intensified. A common policy and a coherent, complementary action plan in favor of healthy nutrition and physical activity have been worked out. At the beginning of July 2006, the four ministers presented a common declaration for their commitment to promote this initiative and for the implementation of concrete and complementary actions in their respective fields of responsibility. (Particular attention will be given to children and adolescents).

Health Reporting Activities with Respect to Nutrition and Physical Activity at National Level (Including Examples)

At national level, few data exist for the moment about the population status in the field of nutrition or physical activity. Representative data about adolescents are available, coming from the international studies "Health behavior in School-aged Children" (HBSC 2002, 2004) in which Luxembourg participates. A representative evaluation on the BMI of the adolescents of Luxembourg has been carried out in 2000. The motricity study also includes data on general health determinants and nutrition behaviors.

The improvement of data includes the improvement of the quality, the collection, and the evaluation of national data collected by school medical services in charge of the systematic surveillance of the school aged children.

Specific nutritional questions have been addressed in specific projects, e.g., Iodine supplementation, breastfeeding, and drinking habits.

Elaboration of a module on healthy lifestyles, including nutrition and physical activity behaviors to be added to the regular household surveys is in discussion.

Another option would be a consumption survey at a large scale (representative of the entire population like the Belgian Food Consumption Survey 2004). However, there is no adequate infrastructure and not enough qualified manpower to manage a survey of this dimension. Besides, the population is highly diversified regarding cultural background (so there are also a lot of different consumption habits) and that would make it very complicated for getting a representative sample of the whole population.

At European level the publications by "Eurostat – Key data on health 2002 – FAOSTAT Database – United Nations Food and Agricultural Organisation" which provide data about energy and macronutrient intake (Kcal, P, L) should be mentioned. There is also the Pan-EU Survey on Consumer Attitudes to Physical Activity, Body-weight, and Health from the European Commission 1999, which gives information about body mass index. Finally, there is also the Eurobarometer (collected in Luxembourg by tns-ilres) on Physical activity (2003), Health, Food and Alcohol and Safety (2003), Health and Food (November 2006).

Macedonia

General Overview of Health Reporting Activities

Health reporting in the Republic of Macedonia is regulated by the Law for Health Protection and its amendments (Official gazette of the Republic of Macedonia, No. 38/91-613, 84/05-44,111/05-2). According to the Article 110, the Republic Institute for Health protection is responsible for monitoring, reporting and analysing the health situation of the population, the causes and phenomena of spread of infectious diseases.

The main functions of the Institute for Health Protection are collection of data for Health for all indicators; monitoring the health status of the population, reports, and analyses of the health status; organization of the health care system, epidemiological surveillance, immunization, environmental monitoring, drug control; and advising the Ministry of Health on matters related to health policy.

Health Reporting Activities on Nutrition and Physical Activity at National Level

The Republic Institute of Health Protection is the national reference center for health statistics and the official partner of national and international organizations in this field. The Republic Institute and the ten regional Institutes of Health Protection partially possess the necessary hardware and software for this purpose, but there is no integrated system that connects the 11 institutes with each other and with other relevant organizations such as the Ministry of Health, the Health Insurance Fund (HIF), and health care facilities.

There are a number of centrally funded vertical programs also, which are for the most part, delivered by primary care staff. Ongoing programs include:

- General check-ups of school children and students
- Mother and child health care
- Blood donation
- Immunization (compulsory)

These programs are funded centrally by the Ministry of Health and international organizations.

Health Reporting Activities on Nutrition and Physical Activity at Regional Level

Universities of applied science also contribute data to heath reporting in numerous research projects on national and international level.

Institutions Involved in Health Reporting Activities

The Ministry of Health
The Republic Institute for Health Protection

Examples of Health Reporting Activities

The status and organization of the health care system
Epidemiological surveillance
Immunization

Changes in the Health Reporting System Between 1990 and 2006

The Government of the Republic of Macedonia intends to adopt a Strategy for the Development of an Integrated Health Information System (IHIS) in 2006. This strategy will recommend the necessary actions to rectify present deficiencies in health information systems and to put in place the framework to ensure the optimal development and utilisation of health information, leading to an IHIS.

Malta

General Overview of Health Reporting Activities

The Ministry of Health is responsible for the overall provision of health care in Malta. It is also responsible for running the public health care services – hospitals, health centres, and Directorates of Information and of Health Promotion.

Health Reporting Activities on Nutrition and Physical Activity at National Level

There is no health reporting in Malta as defined within the frame of this report.

Malta is the smallest Member State of the European Community, with a population of approaching 400,000. It comprises the main island and the smaller islands of Gozo and Comino. Because of the smallness of the islands, the population density of the country is one of the highest in the world. Because of its location, it is also one of the most physically distanced members of the Community. It has its own language, Maltese, though English is also widely used.

The island primarily has a publicly provided health care system, which for Maltese nationals is generally free at the point of consumption. Hospital facilities are provided on the main island, but also with a hospital on Gozo. There is a primary care system and also polyclinics. Alongside, there is a private sector of both private clinics and private hospitals.

Because of its physical isolation, Malta has to be largely autonomous for healthcare, though with external agreements for specified tertiary services. In particular, there is a reciprocal agreement with the United Kingdom to accept cases needing specialist tertiary care in return for free emergency care for United Kingdom tourists and other visitors (other nonresidents except refugees being charged for services).

There is a National Statistics Office. Malta also has a strong tradition of academic public health, through the University of Malta.

Health Reporting Activities on Nutrition and Physical Activity at Regional Level

None reported. Because of the small size of the Maltese population, it is dealt with as one department.

Institutions Involved in Health Reporting Activities

The Ministry of health
The national Statistics Office

Examples of Health Reporting Activities

None reported

Changes in the Health Reporting System Between 1990 and 2006

None reported

The Netherlands

General Overview of Health Reporting Activities

Health reporting in the Netherlands is divided into national health reporting and municipal health reporting. Several institutions provide information about the health-determinants nutrition and physical activity at national level.

Health Reporting Activities on Nutrition and Physical Activity at National Level

The National Institute for Public Health and the Environment (RIVM) is responsible for reporting at national and international level. The RIVM works together with European institutions dealing with health reporting, such as the World Health Organization (WHO) and the European Commission. Every four years, a report is published by the RIVM on various aspects of public health in the Netherlands. For this report, data are collected and integrated from several sources/organizations. Among others, the determinants nutrition and physical activity and their impact on health are included in this report. Various organizations deliver data for the report as they collect health data on a national or international level. Concerning nutrition and physical activity, data collection is subdivided in two types of projects. First, projects that focus specifically on physical activity and/or nutrition. Second, projects that focus on a broader topic (e.g., consumer data panel, health in general) but include some questions on physical activity and/or nutrition. Examples of institutions and their research projects are:

- TNO Quality of Life/Nutrition:
  - Monitor Physical Activity and Health
  - National Food Consumption Survey (in collaboration with RIVM)
- Statistics Netherlands (CBS):
  - Health and Labor of the Integrated System of Social Survey (POLS)
- The Netherlands Institute for Health Services Research (NIVEL):
  - The Second Dutch National Survey of General Practice (in collaboration with RIVM)
  - Consumer Data Panel
  - National Panel of Chronically Ill and Disabled (NPCG)
- Social and Cultural Planning Office of the Netherlands (SCP), which performs various surveys such as the Time Use Survey and the Amenities and Services Utilization Survey.

Health Reporting Activities on Nutrition and Physical Activity at Regional Level

None reported

Institutions Involved in Health Reporting Activities

The national Institute for Public Health and Environment RIVM and all other mentioned organizations. Also, universities are involved in health reporting activities.

Examples of Health Reporting Activities

RIVM Four yearly report on various aspects of public health in the Netherlands

Changes in the Health Reporting System Between 1990 and 2006

None reported

Norway

General Overview of Health Reporting Activities

There are two national institutes in Norway, which provide health reporting, the Norwegian Institute of Public Health (NIPH), and the Norwegian Board of Health.

Health Reporting Activities on Nutrition and Physical Activity at National Level

The Norwegian Institute of Public Health (NIPH) is responsible for six of the seven central health registers in Norway. The NIPH bears the responsibility for ensuring good utilisation, high quality, and simple access to the data in the registers, as well as assuring that health information is treated in accordance with the rules for basic protection of privacy. The NIPH cooperates closely with leading professional and technical environments in Norway that provide health information. In Europe, collaborating partners are the European Commission and the World Health Organization (WHO) among others. Health information is reported and published annually both on a national and a regional level by the NIPH. Most of the studies consider nutrition and physical activity as two of the main determinants among others. Data from different Norwegian health surveys constitutes the health register CONOR.

The Norwegian Board of Health is an important national institute providing health reporting in Norway. The institute is an independent supervision authority, with responsibility for general supervision of health and social services in the country. The Norwegian Board of Health directs the supervision authorities at the county level: county governors' offices supervise social services and the Norwegian Board of Health in the county, which supervises health services and health care personnel. The National Board of Health cooperates with a number of health professional forums in Europe as with the European Union, the World Health Organization, the Nordic Council of Ministers and the Council of Europe.

Health Reporting Activities on Nutrition and Physical Activity at Regional Level

None reported

Institutions Involved in Health Reporting Activities

The Norwegian Institute for Public Health (NIPH)
The Norwegian Board of Health

Examples of Health Reporting Activities

A large number of regional health studies, which involve both nutrition and physical activity as health determinants, have been carried out. Examples of the NIPH's national and regional health studies are:

Youth 2004
The Tromsø Health Study (Tromsø IV and V)
The Troms and Finnmark Health Study (TROFINN)
The Nord-Trøndelag Health Study (HUNT 2 and 3)
The Oslo Health Study (HUBRO, The health survey of immigrants, The Health Study of Romsås and Furuset (MoRo), Oslo II)
The Oppland and Hedmark Health Study (OPPHED)
The Hordaland Health Study (HUSK)
The Oslo Study I and II

Changes in the Health Reporting System Between 1990 and 2006

None reported

Poland

General overview of health reporting activities

Since 1990 several institutions in Poland have been engaged in reporting health behaviors among adults and children. The number and quality of data concerning nutrition in Poland is much better than information related to physical activity.

Health Reporting Activities on Nutrition and Physical Activity at National Level

Several institutions provide information about the nutrition of the Polish population. The National Food and Nutrition Institute in Warsaw (Instytut Żywienia i Żywności) is responsible for nutrition monitoring and dietary surveys in the general population and in specific groups (e.g., in children and adolescents) on a national and international level. The Institute works together with European institutions dealing with nutrition monitoring, such as WHO, FAO, and the European Commission. For nutrition monitoring, the Institute use their own epidemiological studies performed in national population samples (e.g., 2000/2001) or use data gathered by the Central Statistical Office (GUS). Every year GUS publish the report "Living Conditions of the Population" including data concerning consumption of various nutrition products.

Universities also contribute data to health reporting in numerous research projects on a national and international level. Some large studies on health and health indicators are performed by the local medical universities or national health institutes in Warszawa, Katowice, Krakow, Gdansk, Lodz. The WHO POLMONICA Study is a good example.

Health Reporting Activities on Nutrition and Physical Activity at Regional Level

However, none reported that results obtained in the frame of the WOBASZ Study allow to analyze and to compare health determinants (nutrition, physical activity) at municipal (voievodship) level as well as to compare health behaviors and risk factors in small, medium-size, large, and voievodships capital cities.

The WHO CINDI Poland Programme is responsible for regular monitoring of risk factors and health behaviors including detailed nutrition and physical activity analysis in several regions (so called demonstration areas), e.g., in Lodz, Torun, Ostrow, Chorzow as well as for international comparisons of health behaviors in selected CINDI countries. The Department of Social and Preventive Medicine, Medical University, Lodz is coordinating center for the CINDI Poland Programme.

Institutions Involved in Health Reporting Activities

The National Food and Nutrition Institute in Warsaw (Instytut Żywienia i Żywności).

Examples of Health Reporting Activities

"2004 GUS Health Status of the Polish Population" included a small set of questions related to physical activity in leisure time and changes in nutrition habits.

The WOBASZ Study is a national representative multicenter project on health behaviors and risk factors performed 2003–2005 under auspices of the Ministry of Health. This recently published (2005–2006) study coordinated by the National Institute of Cardiology in Warsaw together with the medical universities in Gdansk, Katowice, Krakow, Lodz, Poznan allows for detailed analysis of nutrition habits and physical activity in the representative sample of more than 14,000 men and women aged 18–74.

The Mother and Child Institute (Instytut Matki i Dziecka, Warszawa) is responsible for broader health reporting analyses in children and adolescents including some questions on nutrition habits and physical activity. The MCI performed in the frame of the international WHO HBSC Study regular surveys (e.g., 1990,1994, 1998) in representative samples of school children aged 11–15.

Changes in the Health Reporting System Between 1990 and 2006

None reported

Portugal

General Overview of Health Reporting Activities

Health reporting activities in Portugal are the responsibility of the Ministry of Health in collaboration with other institutions such as the Institute of Preventive Medicine at the University of Lisboa, the National School of Public Health and National Observatory of Health.

Health Reporting Activities on Nutrition and Physical Activity at National Level

The National Health Survey-Portugal is a health measurement instrument that gathers information on the health condition of the Portuguese population. Three surveys have been conducted so far in 1987, 1996, and 1999 collecting information at household level on a national random sample of households. Information includes self reported body weight, height, alcohol consumption, and limited information regarding food habits and physical activity. The fourth National Health Survey (Inquérito Nacional de Saúde) is currently under preparation and will collect specific data regarding migrant population.

The Continued Household Budgetary Survey is a continuous survey providing information on family expenditures run by the National Institute of Statistics. According to a standardized protocol, this information is regularly fed into the DAFNE database.

Data quality refers to food availability at the household level. Socio-demographics of each household are provided. Data are provided at national, regional, and provincial level.

The National Observatory of Health was developed in 1998 to provide health-related information regularly on the basis of a panel of households. One of the reports produced is related to Physical Activity of the Portuguese population.

The Prevalence of Obesity in Portuguese Children is a cross-sectional study including individual body measurements on a national random sample of Portuguese children aged 7–9 years; Data collection in 2002–2003. Study conducted by the University of Coimbra and University of Porto.

Health Reporting Activities on Nutrition and Physical Activity at Regional Level

None reported

Institutions Involved in Health Reporting Activities

The Ministry of Health
The Institute of Preventive Medicine
The National School of Public Health

The National Observatory of Health

Examples of Health Reporting Activities

The Prevalence of Obesity in Portuguese Children

Changes in the Health Reporting System Between 1990 and 2006

None reported

Romania

General Overview on Health Reporting Activities

The health information system in Romania relies on the following structures:

The National Institute of Statistics and the National Center for Health Information System Organization and Management, former National Centre for Health Statistics (NCHS) under the Ministry of Public Health is representing the official system for health statistics.

The National Health Insurance House, focusing on amounts paid to providers for their health services, monitoring information channels related to national health programs, coordinated by different institutions or facilities, according to main health priorities (topics).

Health Reporting Activities on Nutrition and Physical Activity at National Level

Indicators related to population health status, nutrition, and physical activity are not nationally released and reported on a regular basis. Health reporting activities in this area are mainly related to health programs and needs assessment studies. Examples would be population subgroups as pregnant women, children aged 0–1, and children aged 1–5.

Health Reporting Activities on Nutrition and Physical Activity at Regional Level

None reported

Institutions Involved in Health Reporting Activities

Within the Ministry of Public Health:

The National Center for Health Information System Organization and Management, former National Centre for Health Statistics (NCHS), District Public Health Authority (DPHA) in 41 districts and of Bucharest, Institutes and Centers of Public Health, Medical Health Care Institutes, National Health Insurance House (NHIH), District Health Insurance House (DHIH), National Institutes of Research-Development.

Outside the Ministry of Health:

The National Institute of Statistics (NIS) is a specialized institution for central public administration, under direct subordination of the government with public financing.

The Quality of Life Institute performs various studies and research in the field of social sciences.

The Ministry of Education and Research with its department for extra curricular activities in schools.

Examples of Health Reporting Activities

There were three studies conducted in partnerships between Romania and the Center for Diseases Control (USA), USAID, UNFPA, and UNICEF regarding the reproductive health survey, i.e., the national survey on reproductive health (1993, 1999, and 2004) and the study on reproductive health in adolescents (1996). Aspects of nutrition as breastfeeding, pregnancy, and motherhood behaviors were slightly touched.

The Ministry of Health has conducted health status surveys on the basis of representative samples in general population as well as at the level of historical and geographical regions in 1959, 1964, 1977, 1983, 1989, and 1997 through the National Center for Health Statistics. Surveys collected and provided information on prevalence regarding some chronic diseases and symptoms in the population by combining interviews with clinical examination performed by family physicians, anthropometric, and laboratory measurements.

Changes within the Health Reporting System Between 1990 and 2006

Since 1990 new information more relevant to national programs indicators were added to the Health Information System (HIS) because the basic reporting process was almost unchanged for the last 15 years. HIS aspects being changed after 1990 are issuing new information and reporting flows managed by the National Health Insurance House and national health programs; standardized formats of main demographic and health indicators, allowing comparability over time and space. Some changes have been done mostly to the process as electronic data collection as opposed to the old paper version.

The Slovak Republic

General Overview of Health Reporting Activities

Collection and analysis of data on the public's health is realized by few approaches in the Slovak Republic. The National Center of Health Information collects and publishes data regularly and annually at national level. These data are published in the Statistic Annual Report. The aim of detection is mainly demographic evolution, public health status, economic development, and international comparison. The Public Health Authority of the Slovak Republic elaborate the report on the health status of citizens of the Slovak Republic regularly every 2 years with respect to inform the Government of the Slovak Republic about public health status and about the perspectives of development. This report includes, except demographic trends and mortality trends on chosen diseases, particularly information about selected risk factors and determinants of health (including nutrition and physical activity). The last report was presented to the Government of the SR in December 2006. In the Slovak Republic among standardized types of assessment, it is possible to categorize data collection on health and lifestyle, which have already been performed for 10 years by the CINDI programme. Additionally to this, there are local studies with the aim to investigate the health status and occurrence of some risk factors on the regional and district level.

Health Reporting Activities on Nutrition and Physical Activity at National Level

- Statistical Office of the Slovak Republic
- Field of whole state statistics in the Slovak Republic
- Development of analyses about selected parameters of socio-economic and ecological trends as a unit or specific parts

- National Center of Health Information
- Statistical survey
- Electronic collection of data
- National health registers
- Standards for health informatics and statistics
- e-Health
- International cooperation

- Public Health Authority of the Slovak Republic
- Performs monitoring of relationships between health determinants and the public's health on the national level
- Performs identification of health risks and development of solution in the field of public health
- Responsible for preparation of the Report about the citizens of Slovak Republic

Health Reporting Activities on Nutrition and Physical Activity at Regional Level

Regional Offices of Public Health (36 offices)

These perform monitoring of relationships between health determinants and public health at regional and local level. Collection and analyses of data on lifestyle, nutrition habits, and level of physical activity are focused by counselling centres (36 centers).

Slovenia

Health Reporting Activities with Respect to Nutrition and Physical Activity
at National Level (including examples)

WHO Countrywide Integrated Noncommunicable Diseases Intervention (CINDI) Risk Factor /Process Evaluation Surveys

Three consecutive cross-sectional surveys, all performed from late autumn to early
spring 1990/1991, 1996/1997, and 2002/2003 were carried out in the Ljubljana
demonstrational area. All local communities covered by the Community Health
Center Ljubljana participated (Brezovica, Dobrova-Polhov Gradec, Dol pri
Ljubljani, Grosuplje, Horjul, Ig, Ljubljana, Medvode, Škofljica, Velike Lašče, and
Vodice). The simple random samples were drawn from the Central Population
Registry, slightly corrected in gender and age (men and younger age groups were
slightly overrepresented), to assure that the gender/age distribution of respondents
would be similar to the general population distribution as much as possible. The age
range was 25–64 years. The sample sizes were 2,436, 2,180, and 2,643, respectively. The sampling was performed by the Statistical Office of the Republic of
Slovenia. People were invited to participate in the survey by an invitation letter
explaining its rationale and describing its course. The response rates were in
1990/1991:69.5% (1,692 participants), in 1996/1997:61.6% (1,342 participants),
and in 2002/2003:52.0% (1,375 participants).

The questions on behavioral risk factors included several questions on nutrition
and physical activity.

WHO Countrywide Integrated Noncommunicable Diseases Intervention (CINDI) Health Monitor Surveys

Two consecutive cross-sectional surveys, performed in May–June 2001 and
2004, were carried out at national level. These surveys are conceptually a part
of a wider international project in the frame of the WHO CINDI programme.
A stratified random sample was drawn from the central population registry of
Slovenia. The sampling was performed by the Statistical Office of Slovenia.
A self-administered postal questionnaire was used, on the basis of the CHM
Core Questionnaire. The response rate was increased by reminding nonrespondents twice (the first reminder contained a new questionnaire form whereas
the second was only a new invitation letter) and by a lottery with prizes associated with healthy behavior (visits to health resorts, bicycles, etc.). An extensive
media campaign was also mounted at national and regional levels. The total
sample sizes were about 15,350, and the age range was 25–64 years. The
response rates were 64% (about 9,600 participants) and 58% (about 8,500
participants), respectively.

The questions on behavioral risk factors included several questions on nutrition
and physical activity.

Stating institutions and their activities

- CINDI Risk Factor/Process Evaluation Surveys

Coordination and realization of the surveys: CINDI Slovenia Preventive Unit, Ljubljana Community Health Center

- CINDI Health Monitor Surveys

Coordination of the surveys: University of Ljubljana, Medical Faculty, Department of Public Health; Co-coordination: CINDI Slovenia Preventive Unit, Ljubljana Community Health Centre: Realization: Regional Institutes of Public Health and CINDI Slovenia Preventive Unit, Ljubljana Community Health Center.

Fundamental Changes in the Health Reporting System Between 1990 and 2006

Only one fundamental change in the system took place during the reporting period (1990–2006). It concerns the WHO Countrywide Integrated Noncommunicable Diseases Intervention (CINDI) Risk Factor/Process Evaluation Surveys. In 2002/2003, the survey was carried out not only in the Ljubljana demonstrational area but also in two other areas – one being in the west of Slovenia and one in the East.

Spain

General Overview of Health Reporting Activities

Health reporting activities in Spain are in the responsibility of autonomous regions and the Spanish Ministry of Health and Consumer Affairs.

The autonomous regions publish their own reports but also provide their data on transmittable and nontransmittable diseases to the national registries. The national registries are in the responsibility of the National Institute of Epidemiology, which belongs to the National Institute of Health Carlos III. However, these activities do not include reporting activities related to nutrition and physical activity.

Health Reporting Activities on Nutrition and Physical Activity at National Level

Information on diet and physical activity is collected for monitoring purposes from different sources, namely the National Health Survey, Continued Budgetary Survey, Continued Food Consumption Panel. These are all reported periodically.

Health Reporting Activities on Nutrition and Physical Activity at Regional Level

Population surveys

A number of autonomous regions conducted nutrition surveys between 1990 and 2000, which include body measurements and food consumption assessment using similar procedures. These data were pooled together according to a standardised protocol:

- The SEEDO and DORICA studies: prevalence of obesity on adult population (25–64 years) based on individual body measurements
- eVe study: Food consumption of Spanish adults (25–64 years)

Institutions Involved in Health Reporting Activities

Spanish Ministry of Health and Consumer Affairs
National Institute of Epidemiology
National Institute of Statistics

Examples of health reporting activities

National Health Survey: Cross-sectional survey performed every second year.

The National Health Survey (Encuesta Nacional de Salud (ENS)) is a survey conducted by the National Institute of Statistics in agreement with the Ministry of Health and Consumer Affairs since 2002. The survey collects data on perceived health and wellbeing as well as determinants of health and lifestyles at household level on a national random sample of households. The sample comprises approximately 22,000 households. Results are provided at national level and at regional level (autonomous region). Data are collected every second year. The first survey was conducted in 1987 by the Spanish Ministry of Health and was repeated every fifth year up to 2001. Then it was transferred to the National Institutes of Statistics.

Includes self-reported body weight and height; limited items referred to alcohol consumption, dietary habits (breakfast, 11 item food frequency questionnaire) and physical activity (three general items). Questionnaires are designed for persons aged 0–15 years and for persons 16 years and older.

Continued Household Budgetary Survey (Encuesta Continua de Presupuestos Familiares (ECPF))

It is in the responsibility of the National Institute of Statistics (INE), a continuous survey providing information on family expenditures. The structure and frequency of data collection changed in 1997 and turned into continuous data collection at the household level. About 8,000 families were approximately interviewed, each of them remaining in the sample for 2 years (8 collaborations in whole). Reports related to nutrition based on this information were produced in 1985 and in 1995. According to a standardized protocol, this information is regularly fed into the DAFNE databank.

Data quality refers to food availability at the household level. Socio-demographics of each household are provided. Data are provided at the national, regional, and provincial level.

Continuing Food Consumption Panel (Panel de consumo, Spanish Ministry of Agriculture, Fisheries and Food (MAPA)

It is an ongoing survey on a household panel; Random national sample. Started in 1987 and produces yearly reports and monthly information sheets. Quality of data refers to food purchases to be consumed at home, out of home and at institutions. Demographics and place of purchase information is reported.

Over time, main changes include the reporting of out of home purchases and institutional purchases. The number of food items and groupings change over time.

Changes in the Health Reporting System Between 1990 and 2006

None reported

Sweden

General Overview of Health Reporting Activities

Health reporting in Sweden is carried out by several national institutes. The Swedish National Institute of Public Health plays a central role in Sweden's national public health policy coordinating public health work at the national level. The Institute's principal role is to monitor and advice on the implementation and advancement of Sweden's national public health policy. The Institute actively contributes to international efforts to improve public health in the EU, WHO, and other UN bodies, taking part in joint activities with the Nordic countries and engaging in direct collaboration with other countries.

Health Reporting Activities on Nutrition and Physical Activity at National Level

Information on nutrition and physical activity is provided in several reports. A Public Health Policy Report is submitted every 4 years, which provides a picture of the public health situation in Sweden. Examples of research projects carried out by the Swedish National Institute of Public Health:

– Health Behavior in School-aged children
– Community-based Study of Physical Activity, Lifestyle and Self-esteem in Swedish School Children (COMPASS)
– Sweden on the Move 2001
– Public Health Policy Report

The National Food Administration (NFA), an autonomous government agency reporting to the Ministry of Agriculture, Food, and Fisheries, is the central administrative authority for matters concerning food. The NFA has the task of protecting the interests of the consumer by working for safe food of good quality, fair practices in the food trade, and healthy eating habits. Scientific experts from the NFA take an active part in the work of the Expert Panels of the European Food Safety Authority, the Council of Europe, FAO/WHO and other international organisations. The NFA's interest lies in nutrition and physical activity. The institute has a common role of annual nutrition reporting. Examples of research projects carried out by the National Food Administration:

– National Dietary Survey
– National Dietary Survey – Children
– The Lunch Choices

The National Board of Health and Welfare is the Swedish national expert and supervisory authority for the social services, public health, infectious diseases prevention, and the health services. The institute publishes guidelines, exercises supportive and scrutinising supervision of the health services, and provides reports of various health determinants. Nutrition and physical activity are common topics and health determinants in various reports. The most common public health report, the National Public Health Report, is published every second year.

Health Reporting Activities on Nutrition and Physical Activity at Regional Level

None reported

Institutions Involved in Health Reporting Activities

The Swedish National Institute of Public Health
The National Board of Health and Welfare
The National Food Administration (NFA)

Examples of Health Reporting Activities

National Public Health Report is published every second year.
Public Health Policy Report

Changes in the Health Reporting System Between 1990 and 2006

None reported

Turkey

General Overview of Health Reporting Activities

The health reporting system of Turkey is mainly based on the central reporting system, which lies in the responsibility of the central state, i.e., the "Ministry of Health." Municipally administered health authorities report the data to the "Ministry of Health," who publish fertility and morbidity statistics annually.

Health reporting activities on nutrition and physical activity at national level

There are no national surveys that give information on physical activity at national level but some data are present according to results of some small scale surveys.

The Ministry of Health collect data on nutrition-related parameters on anthropometry and on breast feeding from routine country-wide health records of the children under five; however, these data are not processed and reported.

Data on food availability, which are collected by the Ministry of Agriculture and Rural Affairs (via municipally administered authorities) are published by the Turkish Statistical Institute annually. The responsible institution for controlling food safety was the Ministry of Health until June 1995. After the year 1995, the main responsibility on food safety was gradually given to the Ministry of Agriculture and Rural Affairs. Although the Ministry of Agriculture and Rural Affairs have data on food analyses (via municipally administered authorities), the data are not processed and reported.

The State Planning Organization is the main responsible institution for establishing the national food and nutritional strategy. The national nutritional strategy has been published in eight Five Year Plans and Supplementary Documents (2002–2005) of the State Planning Organization. The report has been prepared by the responsible state authorities such as the Ministry of Agriculture and Rural Affairs, the Ministry of Health, the Turkish Statistical Institute, the Ministry of Education, universities and international organizations such as WHO, UNICEF, FAO.

Health Reporting Activities on Nutrition and Physical Activity at Regional Level

There are no reporting activities for physical activity

Municipally administered authorities in the Ministry of Health and in the Ministry of Agriculture and Rural Affairs collect and report the data to the Ministries, but the data are not processed and reported at municipal level.

Institutions Involved in Health Reporting Activities

The Ministry of Health

The Turkish Statistical Institute.

Examples of Health Reporting Activities

Nutritional data from the health reporting system and from national surveys are summarized in the annual statistical yearbooks of the Turkish Statistical Institute.

Changes in the Health Reporting System Between 1990 and 2006

None reported apart from the migration of food safety from the Ministry of Health to the Ministry of Agriculture and Rural Affairs.

United Kingdom

General Overview of Health Reporting Activities

Officially the United Kingdom is a unitary state, but one that has devolved some powers to Parliaments or Assemblies in three of the four home countries – Northern Ireland, Scotland, and Wales. In order of the level of devolution, these are:

Scottish Parliament: Full devolved powers for domestic affairs, including tax-raising powers.

Welsh Assembly: Devolved administrative powers, but not tax raising – receives national allocation from UK Government.

Northern Ireland Assembly: Similar to Welsh Assembly, but currently suspended due to disputes between the members; currently Direct Rule from Westminster.

Health services, social care, and education are in each case devolved services, and come under the above systems. Particularly in Scotland, the differences are quite considerable. Services in England are governed by the UK Parliament in Westminster. In each of the four countries, health services are a government service through the local version of the National Health Service (NHS), largely controlled from devolved central government. Education and social care are in each country local government run services, except in Northern Ireland where social care comes within an integrated Health and Social Services structure.

Health Reporting Activities on Nutrition and Physical Activity at National Level

There is no single Ministry of Health function for the UK, though it is normally the English Department of Health that attends international meetings, and will give an English viewpoint with a disclaimer for the other three countries. Similarly, it can be hard to obtain total national statistics for the UK, especially where calculation of any rates is involved, as there is normally no ready mechanism or resource for reworking the separate material from the four home countries.

The position regarding the United Kingdom and its constituent countries is complex, confusing, and continually changing in the detail. However, the broad principle is clear but not easy to follow in a practical situation. An underlying problem is that the United Kingdom does not have a written constitution.

Health Reporting Activities on Nutrition and Physical Activity at Regional Level

None reported

Institutions Involved in Health Reporting Activities

Office of National Statistics for England and Wales (ONS)
General Register Office for Scotland
Statistics and Research Agency for Northern Ireland (HISRA)

Examples of Health Reporting Activities

None reported

Changes in the Health Reporting System Between 1990 and 2006

None reported

5.1.3. Database Entries

The database entries that summarize individual Health Information Activities within the included countries serve as *national examples*. It was not the intention of this report to give a complete overview on the initiated health reporting activities in each included county in the defined period. This fact is important and must be kept in mind when analysing the database entries.

Altogether 17 country representatives collected data on 33 countries. Five of 17 countries (Germany, the Netherlands, Spain, Sweden, and the United Kingdom) performed the task of researching the required information for their country and additional countries (see Sect. 4.2 "geographical coverage").

Originally, there were 251 projects entered into the database. Some projects were only entered to check the performance of the database. For a valid entry, the following information had to be provided:

1. The title of the project
2. The project leader *or* contact persons *or* the project leading institution.

Only project entries that met the validity criteria were counted and were finally part of the interpretations. After excluding project entries, which do not meet these criteria, 239 projects – 196 national and 43 European projects – remained in the database.

(a) General Overview
Table 5.1 below represents the absolute frequency of entered national and European projects for each included country. Concerning the absolute frequency of European projects per country, it was sufficient when the country participated as a partner within the project; it did not necessarily have to be the executing country. In fact, Table 5.1 summarizes the number of all entered projects and activities with national or international scope in which the country is or was involved.

Table 5.1 Absolute frequency of entered projects, separated by countries

Country	Number of projects		
	National	European	Total
Austria	34	16	50
Belgium	6	20	26
Bulgaria	4	6	10
Croatia	0	7	7
Cyprus	2	2	4
Czech Republic	0	7	7
Denmark	5	14	19
Estonia	3	6	9
Finland	6	17	23
France	2	21	23
Germany	40	20	60
Greece	8	18	26
Hungary	3	16	19
Iceland	0	7	7
Ireland	1	14	15
Italy	9	21	30
Latvia	1	6	7
Liechtenstein	0	0	0
Lithuania	0	11	11
Luxembourg	3	9	12
Macedonia	7	2	9
Malta	0	6	6
Norway	12	12	24
Poland	0	11	11
Portugal	2	18	20
Romania	7	9	16
Slovakia	0	6	6
Slovenia	2	5	7
Spain	8	23	31
Sweden	6	15	21
The Netherlands	11	16	27
Turkey	9	4	13
United Kingdom	8	23	31

Table 5.1 shows in some cases extensive differences regarding the absolute frequency of projects per country. Because the aim was to collect national examples, these differences do not necessarily reflect actual differences in health reporting activities related to nutrition and physical activity between the countries. How many database entries were conducted for each country by the responsible partners depends on the actual number of health reporting activities in each country, which fits the defined criteria, but was also decided by the project partners themselves. A number of countries do not have any data entries at national level. Of these, one country (Liechtenstein) is also not involved in any European projects, which were entered into the database.

(b) Survey and Data Collection Methods

Table 5.2 provides information about different kinds of methods and their application in the included projects. Altogether there are three categories, which include 32 different methods aimed at measuring nutrition and physical activity. Regarding

Table 5.2 Absolute frequency of used methods in entered Projects

Methods	Number of national projects	Number of european projects	Number of all projects
Methods measuring food consumption/availability	*86*	*27*	*113*
24-h recall nutrition survey	17	8	25
Repeated 24-h recall nutrition survey	6	1	7
Estimated food records	16	1	17
Weighted food records	10	2	12
Diet history survey	17	5	22
Food frequency questionnaire (FFQ)	39	13	52
Food balance sheets	1	3	4
Total diet studies	2	1	3
Universal product codes and electronic scanning device surveys	0	0	0
Food account method	2	0	2
Household food record method	0	1	1
Household 24-h recall method	0	0	0
Mini nutritional assessment (MNA)	2	0	2
Subjective global assessment (SGA)	1	1	2
Household-budget-survey	8	5	13
Methods measuring physical activity	*80*	*22*	*102*
Physical activity questionnaire	30	8	38
Self-completed physical activity questionnaire	20	5	25
Interviewer administered physical activity questionnaire	11	2	13
International physical activity questionnaire (IPAQ)	8	3	11
Global physical activity questionnaire (GPAQ)	0	0	0
EPIC-Norfolk physical activity questionnaire (EPAQ2)	0	0	0
Double-labeled water method (DLW)	3	0	3
Calorimetry	1	0	1
Heart rate monitoring	1	1	2
Motion sensor studies	0	0	0
Pedometery	2	0	2
Accelerometry	3	1	4
Other methods	5	1	6
Anthropometrical measures	39	9	48
Health-related fitness tests	2	0	2
Other methods	*57*	*8*	*65*
Postharmonisation of national survey data	10	1	11
Development of questionnaire	43	7	50

the category *Methods measuring food consumption/availability* 113 projects (86 national projects/27 European projects) are listed. In addition, 102 projects (80 national projects/22 European projects) aimed at using *Methods measuring physical activity*. Finally, there are 65 projects (57 national projects/8 European projects) listed that covered *Other methods*. In most cases, one project applied different kinds of methods (e.g., a *24-Hour Recall Nutrition Survey*, *Weighted food records* as well as a *Self-Completed Physical Activity Questionnaire*). 69 (of 239) entered projects do not give further details regarding their methods.

Frequently used methods for *measuring food consumption/availability* are the *Food Frequency Questionnaire* (FFQ), which was used in 52 of the entered projects as well as the *24-Hour-Recall Nutrition Survey*, which was used in 25 projects. None of the projects within the database used *Universal product codes and electronic scanning device surveys* and the *Household 24-h recall method* for measuring food consumption and availability.

Frequently used methods within the category *Methods measuring physical activity* are *Anthropometrical measures* (48 projects), the *Physical Activity Questionnaire* (38 projects) as well as the *Self-Completed Physical Activity Questionnaire*, which was used in 25 projects. The *Global Physical Activity Questionnaire (GPAQ)* and the *EPIC-Norfolk Physical Activity Questionnaire (EPAQ2)* are methods, which were not applied in any of the entered projects. Also none of the studies included in the database are *Motion sensor Studies*.

Table 5.3 gives information about the use of each method related to nutrition or physical activity in countries covered in this report. The *Food Frequency Questionnaire (FFQ)*, the *Self-Completed Physical Activity Questionnaire*, and *Anthropometrical measures* for example are methods that are used in every participating country. Additionally, many countries used *24-Hour Recall Nutrition Surveys* (used in 28 countries), *Food balance sheets* (26 countries), and *Household-Budget-Surveys* (28 countries) to measure food consumption and food availability. The *Physical Activity Questionnaire* as well as the *International Physical Activity Questionnaire* (IPAQ) was also used in 31 and 17 countries.

Further information regarding the application of these different kinds of methods, separated by countries can be taken from Table B.1 in appendix B.

(c) Indicators

Table 5.4 provides different indicator categories and their application in the projects entered into the database. The absolute frequencies of used indicator categories are separated by national and European projects. There are 14 categories, which include 122 indicators. As it was in the case of giving details about the applied methods, there are some projects (34), which provide no information about the used indicators, too. Consequently, only projects that provide details regarding their indicators could be considered. Within these projects, frequently used indicators are those that can be categorised into *Indicators on Food and Nutrient Intake in general*, *Indicators on Physical Activity levels and patterns in general*, *Indicators on Socio-demographic factors in general,* and into the category *Further Indicators*. Otherwise, less used indicators are those that can be classified into *Indicators on*

Table 5.3 Absolute frequency of used methods in entered projects by number of countries

Methods	Number of countries		
	National projects	European projects	All projects
Methods measuring food consumption/availability	*21*	*32*	*32*
24-h recall nutrition survey	9	28	28
Repeated 24-h recall nutrition survey	4	14	15
Estimated food records	10	1	11
Weighted food records	3	16	16
Diet history survey	10	13	17
Food frequency questionnaire (FFQ)	17	30	32
Food balance sheets	1	26	26
Total diet studies	2	12	14
Universal product codes and electronic scanning device surveys	0	0	0
Food account method	2	0	2
Household food record method	0	1	1
Household 24-h recall method	0	0	0
Mini nutritional assessment (MNA)	1	0	1
Subjective global assessment (SGA)	1	1	1
Household-budget-survey	6	27	28
Methods measuring physical activity	*22*	*32*	*32*
Physical activity questionnaire	14	30	31
Self-completed physical activity questionnaire	11	32	32
Interviewer administered physical activity questionnaire	8	2	8
International physical activity questionnaire (IPAQ)	5	14	17
Global physical activity questionnaire (GPAQ)	0	0	0
EPIC-Norfolk physical activity questionnaire (EPAQ2)	0	0	0
Double-labeled water method (DLW)	1	0	1
Calorimetry	1	0	1
Heart rate monitoring	1	9	10
Motion sensor studies	0	0	0
Pedometery	2	0	2
Accelerometry	2	9	11
Other methods	4	1	4
Anthropometrical measures	14	30	32
Health-related fitness tests	2	0	2
Other Methods	*9*	*5*	*10*
Postharmonisation of national survey data	3	1	3
Development of questionnaire	7	5	8

Table 5.4 Absolute frequency of used indicator categories in entered projects

Indicator category	Number of national projects	Number of European projects	Number of all projects
Indicators on food and nutrient Intake in general	108	28	136
Vitamins	33	7	40
Mineral content	30	6	36
Energy	61	13	74
Indicators on alcohol in general	101	24	125
Indicators on breastfeeding in general	9	1	10
Indicators on nutritional status in general	32	7	39
Indicators on anthropometry/ body composition in general	90	16	106
Indicators on physical activity levels and patterns in general	118	22	140
Indicators on health-related fitness in general	5	1	6
Indicators on socio-demographic factors in general	124	15	139
Indicators on inequality in general	6	2	8
Indicators on health promotion in general	26	0	26
Further Indicators	112	23	135

Health Related Fitness in general, Indicators on Inequality in general, and into *Indicators on Breastfeeding in general.*

The absolute frequencies of used indicators in the entered projects, separated by the different indicator categories, are shown in Table B.2 in the appendix.

Table 5.5 gives information about the application of the different indicator categories in the included countries. Indicator categories that were used in all covered countries are *Indicators on Food and Nutrient Intake in general, Indicators on Alcohol in general, Indicators on Physical Activity levels, and patterns in general* and indicators, which are subsumed into *Further Indicators.*

Further information regarding the application of each indicator category in the entered projects within the different countries is shown in Table B.3 in Appendix B. Furthermore, in Table B.4 in the appendix, the use of selected indicators in the report covered countries that are separated by indicator categories are shown.

(d) Details for Project Description

The database also includes information about the data collection period and the project period of the entered projects. Only 131 of the 239 projects provide complete details about the start and the end of both periods. 142 of all entered projects specify at least dates of the start and the end of the project period. 166 of the entered projects give at least details regarding the start and the end of the data collection.

Finally, Table 5.6 below provides details about frequently used keywords for project descriptions. Only keywords that were mentioned at least four times are listed. Keywords that were names of a country (e.g., Spain or Federal Republic of Germany) were excluded.

Table 5.5 Absolute frequency of used indicator categories in entered projects by number of countries

	Number of countries		
Indicator category	National projects	European projects	all projects
Indicators on food and nutrient Intake in general	24	32	32
Vitamins	11	23	24
Mineral content	9	23	24
Energy	15	29	29
Indicators on alcohol in general	21	32	32
Indicators on breastfeeding in general	6	1	7
Indicators on nutritional status in general	13	19	21
Indicators on anthropometry/body composition in general	21	30	31
Indicators on physical activity levels and patterns in general	22	31	32
Indicators on health-related fitness in general	5	9	12
Indicators on socio-demographic factors in general	22	31	31
Indicators on inequality in general	3	1	3
Indicators on health promotion in general	7	0	7
Further indicators	21	32	32

Table 5.6 Absolute frequency of used keywords for project description (only keywords that are mentioned at least four times)

Keyword	Frequency
Physical activity	13
Health	11
Obesity	11
Nutrition	9
Health behavior	8
Health survey	8
Diet	7
Food consumption	7
Children	6
Household	5
Lifestyle	5
Official statistics	5
Youth	5
Behavior	4
CINDI	4
Epidemiology	4
Europe	4
Health promotion	4
Nutrition questions	4
Nutrition survey	4
Population	4
Public health	4
Risk factors	4
Survey	4

6
Analysis and Report on Health Information Activities on Nutrition and Physical Activity: The European Commission (DG SANCO) (by M. Sjöström)

6.1. Introduction

This chapter summarises the process through which the European Union (EU) Commission, within the current programme of Community action in the field of public health, adopted by the EU Parliament and the Council, initiates and supports activities surrounding the collection and organisation of information on health within the EU, and the dissemination of the information to a large number of stakeholders.

Throughout this process, which has developed during the last 12–15 years, i.e., since the European Community (EC) was first given the mandate to act in the field of public health, a series of developmental projects have been financially supported. Most of these projects are presented in this book, and also briefly listed in this chapter, and one project is commented on further.

Article 152 of the EC Treaty (Maastricht 1992) states that the Community shall ensure that protection of human health is given high priority in the definition and implementation of all its policies and activities. As nutrition and physical activity are determinants of health, it is essential that the nutrition and activity-related components of all Community policies contribute to ensuring a high level of human health protection.

Nutrition and Physical Activity are both Member State and Community issues. To facilitate and optimise policy formulation, greater and better dissemination of health information at all levels of the EC is needed. A health information system is needed to provide quality, relevant and timely data, information, and knowledge to support such policy-making.

6.2. A Health Information System

For the majority of adults in the EU, who do not smoke or drink excessively, what they eat and their level of physical activity are the most significant controllable risk factors affecting their long-term health. Lifestyle-related diseases, such as overweight,

N. Wolfram et al. (eds.) *Nutrition and Physical Activity*,
© Springer Science+Business Media, LLC 2008

diabetes, cardiovascular, gastro-intestinal diseases, some forms of cancer, osteoporosis, and depression, are now the leading causes of disability-adjusted life-years (DALYs) lost in Europe.

Diet and physical activity work together to influence health. The insight into the underlying mechanisms of this combined effect is relatively meagre. The rapidly growing prevalence of obesity and diabetes Type II, and our inability to prevent and to tackle these major diseases, exemplify the consequences of this dilemma. There is a need for a much better understanding of the basic biological and underlying patho-physiological processes, as well as more relevant baseline data describing food intakes and physical activity habits amongst the general population in order for public health work to be more efficient.

Dietary habits and the everyday physical activity of the EU member state populations depend on individual choices (cultural influences, food preferences) as well as on socioeconomic and environmental factors (affordability and availability of food products and facilities for exercise, quality, safety of products, etc). Socioeconomic and environmental factors are, in turn, shaped by policies that are the responsibility of Member States and the European Community (EC).

This means that a health information system must also take into consideration a broad range of areas and activities.

The range of areas and activities

The Council Resolution on "Health and Nutrition" exemplifies this. The French Presidency of the EU in 2000 chose to highlight nutrition. This activity led to a Council Resolution of December 2000 on "Health and Nutrition" (2001/C 20/01), which invited both the Commission and the Member States to undertake a range of activities on food, diet, and health policies.

In the Resolution, the EU Council invited Member States, within the context of their national nutritional health policy, to:

1. Set the population, from early childhood, in better stead to make informed food choices by promoting healthy attitudes and eating and dietary habits and by providing relevant information.
2. Involve all parties concerned in the discussion and promotion of nutritional health.
3. Continue to develop the production, dissemination, and implementation of nutritional health.
4. Improve the nutritional knowledge of health professionals and those working in the field of foods and nutrition.
5. Participate actively in the data collection networks in Community activities, and in particular to produce scientific evidence.
6. Encourage national experts to participate in Community activities, and in particular to produce scientific evidence.

Similarly, the Council invited the Commission to study ways of promoting better nutrition within the EU, if necessary presenting appropriate proposals to that end and particularly to:

1. Allow for nutritional health to be taken into account when drawing up and implementing any relevant community policies and develop tools for assessing the impact of other community policies on nutritional health.
2. Continue to develop tools to monitor nutritional health and its determinants, drawing on existing tools in use by Member States, to obtain comparable data, and ensure regular assessment of this data, complementing work by Member States.
3. Support and promote regular exchanges of experience in the area of health and nutrition.
4. Facilitate the development of scientific evidence in this field, in particular to provide backing for and to update national or local dietary guidelines and the information given to consumers.
5. Support research into the links between health and nutrition, into diet-related diseases, into an understanding of eating and dietary habits and into the impact of policies on health and nutrition.
6. Facilitate the exchange of information on nutrition-related training courses and professions.
7. Develop the use of nutritional labeling, by adapting it to the needs of consumers, and of other means of providing nutritional information.
8. Examine the possibility of conducting projects to promote diets, which could include subjects as diverse as fruit and vegetable consumption and breastfeeding.
9. Consider the use of new information technologies to improve the information available to those involved in this sector, and also to the public.
10. Plan follow-up to nutrition activities.

The Need

A European Union health monitoring and information system is thus needed, which provides quality, relevant and timely data, knowledge and information, to support public health decision-making at European, national, subnational, and local level.

The Community Public Health programme (2003–2008) (see later) sets down the objective of establishing and operating a sustainable health monitoring and information system. The system aims to produce comparable information on the health and health-related behavior of the population, on diseases and health systems. It will be based on indicators whose definition, methods of collection, and use have been commonly agreed on built upon the work of previous Community health programmes, such as Community action on health monitoring 1997–2001 (see later), and should be complementary to the activities of the Community Statistical Programme (EUROSTAT) and to work currently underway in Community agencies, such as DG Communication, DG RESEARCH, and in international organisations such as the World Health Organisation (WHO) and OECD (Organisation for Economic Co-operation and Development). It will not only provide regular reports on health status in general, but will generate a flow of information, analysis, and exchange of best practice in the public health field at European level. The other activities also report their information to the Health Information System.

6.3. Community Action in the Field of Public Health

The Community has a clear competence or mandate in many areas. A set of programmes adopted by the European Parliament and the Council in the field of public health defines in detail the objectives and the actions. Relevant to this are:

(a) Community action on health promotion, information, education, and training 1996–2000
(b) Community action on health monitoring 1997–2001
(c) Community action in the field of public health 2003–2008

Legally speaking, the public health programmes are based on Article 152 of the Treaty establishing the European Community (Treaty of Maastricht, 1992). The programmes are "incentive measures designed to protect and improve human health," "excluding any harmonisation of the laws and regulations of the Member States."

(a) Community action on health promotion, information, education, and training 1996–2000

The European Parliament and the Council adopted a programme of Community action on health promotion, information, education, and training, for the period of 1996–2000 (later on extended to 2002), within the framework for action in the field of public health. The objective of the programme was to contribute toward ensuring a high level of health protection and should comprise actions aimed at:

1. Encouraging the "health promotion" approach in Member States' health policies by lending support to various cooperation measures (exchanges of experience, pilot projects, networks, etc).
2. Encouraging the adoption of healthy lifestyles and behavior.
3. Promotion awareness of risk factors and health-enhancing aspects.
4. Encouraging intersectoral and multidisciplinary approaches to health promotion, taking account of the socio-economic factors and the physical environment necessary for the health of the individual and the community, especially for disadvantaged groups.

The actions to be implemented under the programme and their specific objectives were set out under the following headings:

A. Health promotion strategies and structures
B. Specific prevention and health promotion measures
C. Health information
D. Health education
E. Vocational training on public health and health promotion

(b) Community action on health monitoring 1997–2001

The European Parliament and the Council adopted a programme of Community action on health monitoring within the framework for action in the field of public health, for the period of 1997–2001. The objective of the programme was to contribute to the establishment of a Community health monitoring system, which made it possible to:

(a) Measure health status, trends, and determinants throughout the Community
(b) Facilitate the planning, monitoring, and evaluation of Community programmes and actions
(c) Provide Member States with appropriate health information to make comparisons and to support their national health policies, by encouraging cooperation between Member States and, if necessary, by supporting their action through promoting coordination of their policies and programmes in this field and encouraging cooperation with nonmember countries and the competent international organisations.

The actions to be implemented under the programme and their specific objectives were set out under the following headings:

A. Establishment of Community health indicators
B. Development of a Community-wide network for sharing health data
C. Analyses and reporting

Establishment of Community Health Indicators

In the area of health indicators, a first set of European Community Health Indicators (ECHI) was produced by the ECHI project and widely disseminated. The objective is to complete the European Community Health Indicators list that will serve as a basis for the European health information and knowledge system including their operational definitions. The ECHI-1 and ECHI-2 projects under the Health Monitoring Programme have developed a comprehensive list of indicators, in close cooperation with many of the other projects run under the programme. The list included approximately 400 items per indicators.

There was a strong wish from the European Commission to extract a shortlist, to prioritize the work for harmonisation of EU Member State's data collection. ECHI undertook the work to select the indicators for the shortlist in close collaboration with the concerned project leaders, Working Parties, and Commission services.

Nutrition and Physical activity-related projects

The two programmes, the Community action on health promotion, information, education, and training and the Community action on health monitoring, existed for a number of years in parallel in the field of public health, and included funding for nutrition and physical activity related projects. The projects are summarized in this book and briefly listed below.

The Programme on health promotion, information, education, and training supported projects, such as the

- EURODIET project (1998–2000) on nutrition and healthy lifestyles
- EPIC, the European Prospective Investigation into Cancer and Nutrition
- European Masters Programme in Public Health Nutrition

Projects specifically concerned with physical activity were also supported by the promotion programme (1996–2000), such as the

- Pan-European surveys on attitudes to nutrition, diet, and lifestyles
- European Network for the promotion of Health Enhancing Physical Activity (HEPA Europe)

The Programme on Community action on health monitoring gave support, above all, to

- DAFNE European Food Availability Databank based on Household Budget Surveys (DAFNE III, IV, V)
- EUPASS, European Physical Activity Surveillance System
- EFCOSUM, European Food Consumption Survey Method
- Monitoring Public Health Nutrition in Europe
- CHILD, Child Health Indicators of Life and Development
- European Nutrition and Health Report, 2004

The EURODIET Project: An Example

The Eurodiet project was initiated in October 1998 with the aim of contributing towards a coordinated European Union (EU) and member state health promotion program on nutrition, diet, and healthy lifestyles, by establishing a network, strategy, and action plan for the development of European Food-Based Dietary guidelines.

The project was supported by the European Commission (DG SANCO) and coordinated by the University of Crete (Greece). Realisation of the project by the Eurodiet Steering Committee entailed a 2-year process (1998–2000) of scientific evaluation, consultation, and debate.

Four Working Parties composed of distinguished European academics analysed and evaluated the scientific evidence (1) on the links between health and nutrients, (2) on the translation of nutrients to food-based guidelines, (3) on the effective promotion of these foods and healthy lifestyles, and (4) on the opportunities and barriers posed by the broader policy framework. Throughout this process expert representatives from the spectrum of interests involved in this important area of public health were invited to participate as observers in the meetings of the Steering Committee and of the Working Parties. This consultative base and the associated debate widened with the posting of the Working Party draft reports on the Eurodiet web site (http://eurodiet.med.uoc.gr), and culminated with the European Conference held in Crete 18–20 May 2000 on "Nutrition and Diet for Healthy Lifestyles in Europe: Science and Policy Implications."

The Core Report presented, in brief, the outcomes of the process. It was designed to give an overview to decision makers. The evidence and reference base for this core report are presented in two parts, published in Public Health Nutrition 2001, Vol 4 (2A) and Vol 4 (2B):

- The Eurodiet proceedings, comprising the final reports of the Working Parties and the proceedings of the Eurodiet Conference
- The scientific papers commissioned for the Eurodiet Working Party reports

These are designed for public policy advisers and others who wish to follow-up either general issues or specific topics in greater depth.

A strong theme of the Eurodiet project was the potentially enormous social and economic benefits to be gained from reducing the burden of nutritionally related morbidity and mortality in Europe. The Eurodiet reports, which were concerned fundamentally with the realisation of these benefits, offered a significant contribution to the emergent debate on nutrition policy in Europe. Unfortunately, however, political and other obstacles and circumstances at late stages diminished the usefulness of the report. It ended as a Status Report with low or very limited implications on policy making.

However, the conclusions were used as a discussion platform in the production of the EU Council Resolution of 14 December 2000 on Health and Nutrition, as well as documents produced by the FAO and WHO.

(c) Community action in the field of public health 2003–2008

The two Programmes were integrated into one in 2002, when the European Parliament and the Council adopted a programme of Community action in the field of public health, for the period of 2003–2008.

The overall aim and general objectives were expressed as follows:

1. The programme, which shall complement national policies, shall aim to protect human health and improve public health.
2. The general objectives of the programme shall be to:

   - Improve information and knowledge for the development of public health (Strand I)
   - Enhance the capability of responding rapidly and in a coordinated fashion to threats to health (Strand II)
   - Promote health and prevent disease through addressing health determinants across all policies and activities (Strand III)

3. The programme shall thereby contribute to:

(a) Ensuring a high level of human health protection in the definition and imple-
    mentation of all Community policies and activities, through the promotion
    of an integrated and intersectoral health strategy.
(b) Tackling inequalities in health
(c) Encouraging cooperation between Member States in the areas covered by
    Article 152 of the Treaty

Community actions and activities shall be implemented in close cooperation with
Member States through support of activities of a transversal nature, which may be
used to implement all or part of the actions and which may, where appropriate,
be combined. These activities are the following:

1. Activities related to the monitoring and rapid reaction systems
2. Network activities operated through structures designated by Member States and
   other activities of Community interest for the purposes of public health monitoring and providing national information, as well as data at Community level, in
   furtherance of the objectives of the programme
3. Activities to counter health threats, including major diseases, and react to
   unforeseen events, enable investigations, and coordinate response
4. Preparation, establishment, and operation of appropriate structural arrangements
   coordinating and integrating networks for health monitoring and for rapid reaction
   to health threats
5. Development of appropriate links between the actions concerning the monitoring
   and rapid reaction systems

The Health Information System

The purpose of the European Union Health Information System is, as discussed
earlier, to provide quality, relevant and timely data, information, and knowledge to
support public health decision-making at European, national, subnational, and local
level. Within each geographical area, the Health Information System is a tool necessary
to make decisions at strategic, control, and operational level, to set directions, to
monitor their implementation, and to evaluate their impact.

Health information represents the main basis for health decision-making processes,
which, in turn, make political decisions possible. Managing a Health Information
System means designing organizations capable of running the Health Information
System processes in an orderly way. Choosing the most relevant set of data and indicators,
up-to-date information technology and relevant statistical analyses, are some of the
essential steps needed to ensure a functional Health Information System.

Working Parties

The Community Public Health Programme aims to produce comparable information
on health and health-related behavior of populations (e.g., data on lifestyles and

other health determinants); on diseases (e.g., incidence and ways to monitor chronic, major, and rare diseases); and on health systems (e.g., indicators on access to care for everyone, on quality of care provided, on health professional resources, and on financial viability of health care systems).

Most of the health information actions supported by the programmes of Community action on Public Health are in relation to the development of indicators and the improvement of the methodology of collection of data and preparation of reports and analysis.

The work on health indicators and data collection is further developed. The work is led by the Unit within the Commission's DG SANCO, which is responsible for the Health Information Strand. The fieldwork is coordinated by advisory Working Parties that are creating the prototype for the health monitoring system. The Working Party on the area of lifestyle is such an example.

The Working Party on Information on Lifestyle and Specific Subpopulations

The Working Party contributes to the improvement of information and knowledge on the lifestyle-related aspects of public health, and to the promotion of healthy lifestyles, as well as dealing with information and knowledge on other health determinants. It shall contribute to the compilation and development of a sustainable health monitoring system in the field of lifestyles, to the collection, the sharing and diffusion of lifestyle-related data. This includes going beyond individual lifestyles to health determinants also related to general living conditions.

The Working Party considers the need to reduce economic and social inequalities by ensuring that its activities take into account those economic and social groups, which are at particular risk (according to the Council Conclusions "Healthy Lifestyles").

More detailed information is available in the Draft Mandate, March 2004; however, it should be noted that the mandate is continuously under development, as well as the Position Paper, which describes in greater detail the visions of the Working Party and identifies the topics for action. The activity field of the Working Party encompasses all the aspects of "lifestyle." Among these are tobacco abuse, alcohol consumption, nutrition, physical activity, and living conditions. In addition, the Working Party considers the influence of different socio-economic and cultural factors in aspects of child health, gender-specific health, health of the elderly, migrant health, and the health of the deprived subpopulations (the poor, homeless, unemployed, and the disabled).

In its activity field, the Working Party will above all:

(a) Contribute lifestyles, living conditions, and determinants indicators to the short list of European health indicators.
(b) Coordinate in this respect with other priority areas of the information and knowledge system.

(c) Advise on the creation of an EU strategy to address positive lifestyle determinants, and healthy living conditions, through improved information and make peer-reviewed information publicly available.
(d) Contribute to the annual work plans of the Public Health Programme 2003–2008.
(e) Examine lifestyles, determinants, and living conditions-related issues as well as issues related to the health of specific and deprived subpopulations in other Community policies and coordinate its own activities with those of related European and international institutions and organisations, such as the WHO, the Council of Europe, and OECD.
(f) Advise on the development of a strategy for the diffusion of MS best practices in healthy improvement and the improvement of the health specific and deprived population groups.

6.4. Summary

- A European Union health information system is needed, which provides quality, relevant and timely data, information, and knowledge, to support public health decision-making at European, national, subnational, and local level.
- A set of programmes in the field of public health define in more detail the objectives and the actions of such a system.
- The objective of one of these programmes, Community action on health monitoring 1997–2001, has been to contribute to the establishment of a Community health monitoring system.
- This task has been fulfilled by encouraging, through above all project funding, cooperation between Member States. Where necessary, by supporting their action through promoting coordination of their policies and programmes in this field and by encouraging cooperation with nonmember countries and competent international organisations.
- By this, it will be possible to (a) measure health status, trends, and determinants throughout the Community; (b) facilitate the planning, monitoring, and evaluation of Community programmes and actions; and (c) provide Member States with appropriate health information to make comparisons and to support their national health policies.
- In the area of health indicators, a first set of European Community Health Indicators (ECHI) has been produced by the ECHI project and widely disseminated. The objective is to complete the European Community Health Indicators list that will serve as a basis for the European health information and knowledge system including their operational definitions.
- Under the current EU public health programme, the work on health indicators and data collection is being further developed. The work is led by the Unit within the Commission DG SANCO, responsible for the Health Information Strand. The fieldwork is coordinated by advisory Working Parties, such as the

Working Party focussed on lifestyle, who are creating the prototype for the health monitoring system.

- The Working Party on Information on Lifestyle and Specific Subpopulations, aims to contribute to the improvement of information and knowledge on the lifestyle-related aspects of public health, and to the promotion of positive life-styles, as well as dealing with information and knowledge on other health determinants. It aims to contribute to the annual work plans of the Public Health Programme 2003–2008, in which topics for project funding are identified.

7
World Health Organisation (Europe) Position and Activities on Measurement of Nutrition and Physical Exercise (by M. Rigby)

7.1. Introduction: The Respective Roles of the WHO and the EC in Europe

By definition of having global responsibility for matters appertaining to health, the World Health Organization (WHO) has an expert body role, which inter alia covers all the Member States of the European Union and those seeking membership. However, its nature and function is distinctly different from the European Commission (EC). It is therefore important to seek maximum synergy and cohesion between the health-related activities and initiatives of the two bodies, while recognising the distinction and respective autonomies of the two.

The WHO is an expert technical agency of the United Nations. Its role is strictly apolitical, and it must strive to develop principles and policies that are without political bias, and that are acceptable to any political philosophy and to any style of government. The WHO has no executive authority or sanctions over national governments, but must lead by weight of evidence. This means that the work of the WHO must be strongly evidence based, though at the same time the WHO does not have the resources itself to undertake or commission major research.

The mission of the WHO is to maximise health, according to the definition within its constitution, namely that health is a "state of complete physical, mental, and social wellbeing, and not merely the absence of disease or infirmity." This is an aspiration supported by virtually all states globally.

The headquarters of the WHO are located in Geneva. The role is to identify global priorities and major initiatives, formulated in a way that accommodates the full range of levels of development, and of cultural and political diversity, of the globe. However, many of the more active interventions are undertaken through the WHO's Regional Offices. The European Region comprises the 53 states within the geographical region of Europe. This WHO region extends from Ireland in the west and Iceland in the North to the states bordering Asia in the East, and the Mediterranean in the South, and also includes Israel. Thus the Member States of the European Union and the Applicant States form something over half of the total nations under the responsibility of WHO Regional Office for Europe.

N. Wolfram et al. (eds.) *Nutrition and Physical Activity*,
© Springer Science+Business Media, LLC 2008

In many parts of the world, the WHO has a local office within each country. Within Europe, country offices were established in those countries being not an EU Member State in the early days of the EC. The WHO Regional Office for Europe is located in Copenhagen. It has also out-posted centers specialising in particular activities located in Rome (primarily covering environment and health – with a particular focus on transport – and physical activity); in Bonn (environment and health, with a particular focus on housing and air pollution, amongst other topics); and Venice (economic development and health). Together, the Rome and Bonn offices are part of WHO Europe's Special Programme on Health and Environment. All other functions – including Nutrition and food security – are handled in the WHO Regional Office in Copenhagen.

Thus the WHO as a technical agency is significantly different from the European Commission, which is a governmental body driven by democratic election processes to develop policies founded not only on evidence but also cognisant of political principles as determined by a democratic parliamentary procedure. The European Commission has developed executive policies, which apply across all Member States, and which in some cases are binding upon Member States. The Commission has fund-raising powers and thus the ability to allocate budgetary support both for policy development and for research, which contrasts with WHO's dependence upon an international subvention. Most significantly, the European Commission has responsibility for a full range of policies similar to any national Government, compared with WHO's responsibility solely for health and health matters.

Thus the WHO and the European Commission share a top-level common concern to ensure the maximization of the health and development of the citizens in all the states under their overview, but approach this through very different mandates, resources, and approaches. It is highly desirable that there is consensus on interpretation of the scientific evidence as to both priorities and methods, while synergy and complementarity on particular programmes is clearly also to be sought. Apart from officer coordination, one potential unifying factor is that both the European Commission and WHO host Ministerial Conferences of health ministers.

Development of shared action programmes between the two bodies is by definition difficult, as WHO must seek a broad equity according to need across all the states in the geographical region. The most fruitful area for collaboration and coordination is on technical matters including identification of societal priorities in health, the main challenges and compromises to health, the technical content of the most appropriate health enhancing programmes, and aspects of definition and measurement. Thus with regard to the core objective of this specific study – the measurement of nutrition and of physical activity – harmonisation of data definitions, survey tools, and population-level analysis is desirable and is in part in sight of being achieved.

7.2. The WHO and the Rising Challenge of Overweight and Obesity

In its role of monitoring health and health status, WHO has identified clearly the growing challenge and future burden of overweight and obesity, both at global level [28] and at European level [38]. In particular, in the WHO European Region calculates that obesity consumes between 2% and 8% of healthcare costs, and causes between 10% and 13% of deaths according to locality. This, therefore, has become an important concern and focus of action for the WHO, not least in its Regional Office for Europe. In January 2007, a search under "obesity" produced 15,700 hits on the WHO Web site.

Of late, WHO has sought to develop policies that actively address specific aspects that contribute to the obesity problem, mandated by the WHO Global Strategy on Diet, Physical Activity, and Health [35]. Some of these are focussed on nutrition and food security [39], others on physical activity [40, 3]. In general, these programmes are focussed on the overall population, but they fall outside of this commissioned study, with its specific focus on the measurement of the determinants of obesity, and thus of nutrition and physical activity.

However, a specific and effective method of the WHO is the ability to present an integrated analysis and recommended approach to meetings of Health Ministers. To this effect, and particularly pertinent for the timing of this project, the WHO Regional Office for Europe organised a "WHO European Ministerial Conference on Counteracting Obesity – Diet and Physical Activity for Health" in Istanbul in mid-November 2006 [41]. Key elements of the briefing papers and the subsequent adoption of a European Charter are covered in a specific later section of this chapter.

7.3. The Total Population, Adults, and Children and Adolescents

The general problems with regard to the rising levels of obesity and overweight are affecting all age groups in the population, but differently. There are also differences in specific issues and methodologies.

In general, this specific information mapping study looks at the total population, but with a focus on adults not least because it is the adult members of society who are the targets of the general measurement tools described. The issues with regard to children are distinct, and in many ways more challenging. They are also more important, not only because the incidence of obesity in children is increasing rapidly and also will have the greatest life long consequences, but also because the specifics both of nutrition and physical activity, and of measurement, are different. For instance, a prime issue is the importance of breastfeeding, then for younger children arise the issues of parental provision of a healthy diet and also the opportunities for safe play and other exercise. In school children come the issues of both parental and self-determination of dietary habits, and the emergence of patterns of activity chosen between physical activity and more sedentary interests. Older children through to adolescents move toward full determination and also necessary discovery and experimentation, while in this period general approaches to physical activity as well as diet become established for adulthood. This not only is a dynamic period in terms of development of behavior, but also at the same time methods of measurement are particularly challenging. It is for this reason that measurement of nutrition and physical activity in children is the subject of the separate second study in this project, and therefore the specific issues of children will not be covered in depth in this review of WHO activities, as they will appear in a separate later volume.

7.4. The WHO and Measurement of Nutrition

As with other agencies, WHO recognises the difference of approach between measurement of food availability and a measurement of dietary intake. These are significantly different in purpose and methodology, but in effect are complimentary. Linked in many ways to food availability is food security, namely ensuring that

- All people at all times have both physical and economic access to enough food for an active, healthy life
- The ways in which food is produced and distributed are respectful of the natural processes of the earth and thus sustainable
- The ability to acquire food is ensured
- The food itself is nutritionally adequate and personally and culturally acceptable

These latter issues, though important, are not in the focus of this particular analysis of population dietary behavior, even though in the longer term they may influence behavior if not addressed adequately. Nutrition, food security, and food safety consequently are a major work area for the WHO Regional Office for Europe, with a dedicated work stream [39], core action commitments [48], annual work plan [42], and extensive publications list [43]. These are too dynamic to record in detail here, but currently cover nutrition policy, food security, infant feeding, child nutrition, and micronutrient deficiencies.

At population level, the measurement of food availability is an important prerequisite, in that without an adequate balance of food availability the opportunity for appropriate dietary behavior is reduced. This specific area is a positive example of collaboration between WHO and the European Commission, as the WHO recognises the importance of and collaborates with the Data Food Networking (DAFNE) project of the Commission [4].

However, at either community or at household level, food availability is not a specific indicator of nutritional behavior and dietary intake of individuals. Thus, in particular, measures of food availability only provide a very broad and indirect measure of changes in nutritional behavior, particularly by age group. Therefore, the WHO Regional Office for Europe in terms of measurement of dietary behavior also recommends the conduct of individual dietary intake studies. The WHO Countrywide Integrated Noncommunicable Diseases Intervention (CINDI) Programme [44] recommends the use of a food-frequency questionnaire to monitor changes in dietary habits. This proposed method is based on standardized definitions of generic foods from which the major food components of interest may be derived. However, there is not yet a recognised standardised tool for the measurement of dietary intake by adults capable of being used generically across different states within Europe, since food habits, the availability of foodstuffs and food composition vary widely from one country to another. Given the interests of the European Commission in developing Health Examination surveys and health interview surveys, this would seem to be a potential area of future collaboration.

7.5. The WHO and Measurement of Physical Activity

At first approach, measurement of effective and physical activity would appear more challenging, because of the need to define physical activity not only by type, but also by effect upon physiology. However, this is an area to which the WHO has devoted considerable attention, and in particular, it has supported the development of specific survey tools. The principal WHO tool is the Global Physical Activity Questionnaire (GPAQ) [29]. This is developed from IPAQ (see later) and operated within the Global Physical Activity Surveillance Programme of WHO Headquarters [30]. However, this is primarily aimed at the developing world.

More specific for developed and European countries is the International Physical Activity Questionnaire (IPAQ). This emerged from a concept developed at a consensus meeting held in the WHO Geneva office (1998), and it is now maintained and developed by a core group of independent scientists across the world and administered by the Unit for Preventive Nutrition at the Karolinska Institute, Sweden [17]. It has both a long and a short version, and has been widely implemented, including being built into a number of national survey tools. Among the major surveys are the Eurobarometers (1992 and 1995) and the World Health Survey (2002).

In the WHO European Region, 32 countries have been implementing the CINDI programme [14], involving the use of the CINDI Health Monitor questionnaire (based on the questionnaire used in the FINBALT project [19]) to monitor physical activity (the original questionnaire including the IPAQ questionnaire to measure physical activity). However, this questionnaire will be recommended for the future surveys only as an optional instrument, and the set of questions used in the FINBALT project will be the core instrument to measure physical activity.

7.6. The WHO and Major Noncommunicable Disease Risk-Factors

While the nature of this project has raised separately the challenges of measuring dietary intake and measuring physical activity, the World Health Organization has moved toward a more integrated analysis of at risk factors for health. This has resulted in the WHO global InfoBase, which is a powerful on-line comparison tool on the basis of extensive data on noncommunicable disease risk factors [31].

It holds data for almost every country worldwide, covering a number of risk factors including tobacco use, alcohol abuse, physical inactivity, raised blood pressure, cholesterol levels, and fruit and vegetable intake. The Internet-based presentation enables three types of user-driven analysis to be calculated on line: in-depth analysis of risk factors within country, comparison between countries, and access to source data for any country.

A related programme is the surveillance of chronic disease risk factors (SuRF) [32]. This provides full methodology and technical publications. The availability of source data by European country appears as a regional page in a data availability page [33]. Thus, as the InfoBase is a global WHO activity, it provides within it a full analysis provision for Europe.

This WHO approach of addressing analysis of chronic risk factors might be seen as an integrated approach. Rather than giving comprehensive analysis of either nutrition or physical activity, it does outline at national population level the proportion of the population who have increased risks of chronic disease. The WHO Health Report 2002 [36] and the European Health Report 2005 [34] estimate the burden of disease in Disability Adjusted Life Years (DALYs) of each of the leading noncommunicable conditions and the leading individual risk factors including overweight, low fruit and vegetable intake, and physical inactivity. As obesity is one of the targeted noncommunicable diseases, the published data specifically identify increased population risk of obesity because of the consumption of either too many energy-dense, nutrient-poor foods and drinks or not enough fruits and vegetables or because of low physical activity. It thus enables consideration of the greatest and most pressing issues to be addressed in any particular setting.

7.7. Health Behavior of School Children

Though for reasons as explained earlier, this chapter will not cover in any depth issues related to the measurement of nutritional or exercise behavior of the children, and it is important to make reference to the major international study on the Health Behaviour in School-aged Children (HBSC) [16]. This study commenced with collaboration between researchers in the three countries of Finland, Norway, and England in 1982; the WHO Regional Office for Europe became a collaborative partner soon afterwards. The HBSC is now a cross-national research study conducted by an international network of research teams. Its aim is to gain new insight into, and to increase understanding of, young people's health, well-being, health behavior, and social context. A growing number of countries and regions have joined the study network, including Canada and USA. The study is also slightly unusual among international activities in addressing the problem of the United Kingdom data by treating the four constituent quasi-autonomous home counties of UK individually. The results of each HBSC survey are made available through publications; neither data nor analyses are available on-line, but there is a data request mechanism well-publicised on the site.

The HBSC approach applies a standardised questionnaire to a structured sample of school children aged 11, 13, and 15 years of age in each participating country, and is repeated every 4 years. The study now includes a high proportion of European Member States. The need for a standardised questionnaire spanning such a wide area and with stability to enable trend analysis, combined with the four-year interval, does create essential limitations to frequent changes or local customisation. However, the scientific rigour and overall stability have made the strength of this study significant. The HBSC International Coordinating Center study is now based at the Child and Adolescent Health Research Unit (CAHRU) at the University of Edinburgh, and the International Database is based at Bergen University.

7.8. The WHO European Childhood Obesity Surveillance Initiative

At the first Member States' consultation (Copenhagen, October 2005) in the process leading to the WHO European Ministerial Conference on Counteracting Obesity (see later), the need was recognised for standardised childhood surveillance systems on which policy development within the WHO European Region could be based. However, a world-wide survey on child growth monitoring practices carried out in 1998–1999 [21] demonstrated that less than one third of the countries expand growth monitoring practices beyond the 6 years of age and that only a few countries have in place surveillance monitoring systems that study the weight and height distribution of children at regular intervals of time.

As a follow-up to this recommendation, the WHO Regional Office for Europe is planning to establish a European childhood obesity surveillance initiative in some countries in the Region. The objective of this initiative will be to design, pilot, and establish a simple sustainable system for the monitoring of the nutritional status of children in primary-school resulting in a correct understanding of the progress of the obesity epidemic but also allowing comparisons among European countries.

7.9. The WHO European Ministerial Conference 2006

As indicated earlier, a major event for the WHO Regional Office for Europe in 2006 was the European Ministerial Conference on Counteracting Obesity [41]. A significant range of briefing papers was prepared, and these are available at this WHO Internet address. One of these included, inter alia, a comparative analysis of the development and implementation of national food and nutrition policies, including an audit of what national level activity countries reported [45]. This concluded by all member states (thus including all EU Member States) agreeing and endorsing a European Charter on Counteracting Obesity [46], which promotes putting the action high on the political agenda in the European Region, commits Member

States to focus efforts on addressing obesity in key areas identified in the Charter and provides political guidance to strengthen action in the Region.

Of particular importance for this EU study is not just the resultant outline for a second European action plan for food and nutrition policy [47], but more so the inbuilt commitment to monitor the resultant action plan (to be finalised in early 2007). This outline for the action plan makes significant references to monitoring, and has a specific section on Monitoring and Evaluation. Given that both the policy declaration and outline for the action plan were endorsed unanimously by all the health ministers of geographical Europe, thereby by definition including all the health ministers of the European Union countries, this should give a firm mandate for further development of indicators and monitoring tool within the Commission area in a way which is also harmonised with WHO objectives.

7.10. Summary

The core functions of the World Health Organization as an expert agency are: providing leadership on matters critical to health and engaging partnerships where joint action is needed; shaping the research agenda and stimulating the generation, translation, and dissemination of valuable knowledge; setting norms and standards, and promoting and monitoring their implementation, articulating ethical and evidence-based policies and scientific tools; providing technical support, catalysing change, and building sustainable institutional capacity; and monitoring the health situation and assessing health trends. It is thus a different role from that of the European Commission, but should be complementary to it, and in harmony with it. WHO has been a leading exponent of the challenges to health of the growing problem of obesity, and recognises the need not only for further policies, but also for programmes of monitoring to ascertain how the behavior of the public is changing. There are opportunities for the European Community countries to benefit from the WHO programme, and also opportunities for the Commission and member states to develop tools that will support those shared objectives.

8
European Networks (by P. Di Mattia)

The aim of the project was also to identify those activities run by European Networks, other than those coordinated by EU Commissions and the WHO, to enter them in the database.

Following the above approach, a search was done. Some networks were identified, though none of them promotes health activities as required by the inventory. Nevertheless, as all named networks are involved in projects that are linked to nutrition and physical activity (congresses, publications, promotions, Web sites, etc.), which may be of interest to the reader, they are listed below in the following format:

ACRONYM: complete name
Web site
Further information

European Networks

EPOMM: European Platform on Mobility Management
http://www.epomm.org [12]
EPOMM is an international partnership aiming to:

- Promote and further develop Mobility Management in Europe
- Fine tune the implementation of Mobility Management between the EPOMM member states and other countries in Europe

EPOMM provides a forum for all those interested in Mobility Management: representatives from EU member governments, local and regional authorities, researchers, major employers, transport operators and other, and interest groups.

EPOMM is the platform where knowledge, research, and other institutes meet. EPOMM stimulates them to cooperate and meet, take initiatives, set up, formulate, and participate in international projects and European R&D projects.

EPOMM disseminates knowledge and organises international expert workshops, seminars, and conferences on mobility management themes. The European Conference on Mobility Management (ECOMM) is held each year in a different

N. Wolfram et al. (eds.) *Nutrition and Physical Activity*,
© Springer Science+Business Media, LLC 2008

country; this conference is one of the major events in Mobility Management and EPOMM is strongly involved in its organisation.

EPOMM also takes part in the structuring of the European Research Area agenda on mobility management and prepares to be a network of excellence on mobility management.

EPOMM stimulates and facilitates a climate of innovation, strategies, and new concepts.

EPOMM is a platform where training and courses on specific mobility management issues are organised and training material on mobility management is developed.

ASPHER: Association of Schools of Public Health in the European Region

http://www.aspher.org [1]

ASPHER is the key independent organisation in Europe dedicated to strengthening the role of public health through the training of public health professionals for both practice and research.

Founded in 1966, ASPHER has over 72 institutional members. These are located throughout the Member States of the European Union (EU), the Council of Europe (CE), and the European Region of the World Health Organisation (WHO).

ESSOP: European Society for Social Paediatrics and Child Health

http://www.essop.org [14]

ESSOP believes in working together to use skills, resources, and knowledge to develop local and global strategies to improve the health and well being of children and young people. Methods include improving communication between all those involved in child and adolescent health and well being, bringing in the latest relevant research world wide, developing tools for advocacy, for teaching, involving children and young people themselves and by providing information about effectiveness and efficacy of interventions, meeting together at conferences, maximising individual and group effectiveness.

ESSOP works with national social/community paediatric organisations, NGOs working in the same field, child advocacy groups, health professionals involved with child health, governments, economists, sociologists, lawyers, and others with the same interests and aspirations.

EANS: European Academy of Nutritional Sciences

http://www.eans.net [5]

EANS is an association of individual nutritional scientists and has the following aims:

- To be the custodian of the quality of the European nutritional science
- To support the high quality education of young nutritional scientists
- To create a platform for discussing, summarizing, and communicating important nutritional issues

To achieve these aims EANS will:

- Encourage and support the organization of high quality symposia and workshops within Europe

- Encourage and support its members to play an active role in public debates on nutrition
- Encourage its members to be active in training programmes for young scientists, both in scientific and communicative fields

EUPHA: European Public Health Association
http://www.eupha.org [13]

The European Public Health Association or EUPHA in short is an umbrella organisation for public health associations in Europe. EUPHA was founded in 1992. EUPHA is an international, multidisciplinary, scientific organisation, bringing together around 12,000 public health experts for professional exchange and collaboration throughout Europe.

Objectives/aims:

- To promote and strengthen public health research and practice in Europe
- To improve communication between policymakers, researchers, and practitioners
- To provide a platform for the exchange of information, experience, and research
- To encourage and promote effective European joint research and other activities in the field of public health research and health services research in Europe

EUPHA publishes a scientific journal six times a year entitled European Journal of Public Health and convenes a scientific conference every year.

EUPHA encourages the creation of sections for specific public health themes, which are international and open to all regular EUPHA members. The goal is to bring together researchers and public health professionals working in the same field for the exchange of information and the setting up of joint policies, reports, and research.

Among other sections are:

- Health promotion
- Food and nutrition

FENS: Federation of European Nutrition Societies
http://www.fensweb.org [15]

MISSION: To conjoint efforts for nutritional development in Europe for health global promotion

VISION: To maintain a permanent bridge for exchanges between European nutritionists with basic and applied perspective

SPECIFIC AIMS:

1. To promote nutrition knowledge and dissemination as a healthy tool
2. To organize a congress every 4 years
3. To facilitate nutrition formation and training as well as scientific exchanges across Europe.

The Federation of European Nutrition Societies (FENS) is a federation consisting of 25 European nutrition societies, each representing one country. The main FENS event is the European Nutrition Conference, arranged every fourth year.

According to the FENS statutes, the Federation is established for public benefit to advance research and education in the science of nutrition. It will promote learning among nutritionists generally, and European nutritionists in particular, by the holding of meetings, discussions, exchange of information and by other appropriate means.

ISBNPA: International Society for Behavioral Nutrition and Physical Activity
http://www.isbnpa.org [18]

The International Society of Behavioral Nutrition and Physical Activity was deliberately formed to be International and to combine interests in diet and physical activity.

ISBNPA has an international presence with nearly 400 members representing 29 countries. Members come together from more than 40 government agencies, industry, and professional organizations as well as close to 150 academic and medical institutions. Members bring to this organization a diversity of experience and expertise, with professional credentials.

ISBNPA purposes are:

- Conduct scientific meetings, congresses, and symposia in which current research on behavior issues in nutrition and physical activity will be discussed by researchers in related fields
- Disseminate information on research being done on behavior issues in nutrition and physical activity through newsletters and other communications
- Provide information to and encourage continued support by public and private bodies that support research in issues of behavior issues in nutrition and physical activity
- Promote and facilitate the dissemination of knowledge of issues of behavior issues in nutrition and physical activity to the public and to educators, scholars, and health professionals through any lawful means
- Promote and assist communication between researchers on issues of nutrition and physical activity behavior with and members of scientific and scholarly organizations whose members do research in other related health and medical fields. This will be done through joint meetings, shared membership lists, joint publications, and any other lawful means.

EUFIC: European Food Information Council
http://www.eufic.org [10]

The European Food Information Council (EUFIC) is a nonprofit organisation, which provides science-based information on food safety, quality, health and nutrition to the media. It also provides information on health and nutrition to professionals, educators, and opinion leaders in a manner that consumers can understand.

In response to the public's increasing need for credible, science-based information on the nutritional quality and safety of foods, EUFIC's mission is to enhance the public's understanding of such issues and to raise the consumers' awareness of the active role they play in safe food handling and choosing a well-balanced and healthy diet.

All information that EUFIC publishes has been subject to a review process by members of its Scientific Advisory Board (SAB). The SAB comprises a group of renowned experts from across Europe, who advise EUFIC on its information and communication programmes, ensuring that all information is based on scientific evidence, relevance and is factually correct.

EUFIC actively participates in European initiatives together with the European Commission Directorate Generals for Research and for Health and Consumer Protection, where it contributes to a number of projects as dissemination partner.

EUFIC is cofinanced by the European Commission and the European food and drink industry.

NS: The Nutrition Society
http://www.nutritionsociety.org [26]

The Nutrition Society was established in 1941 "to advance the scientific study of nutrition and its application to the maintenance of human and animal health."

The Nutrition society is highly regarded by the scientific community, the Society is the largest learned society for nutrition in Europe. Membership is worldwide but most members live in Europe.

Membership is open to those with a genuine interest in the science of human or animal nutrition. The Nutrition Society does

- Publications
- Conferences
- Promoting Nutritional Science
- Professional Study

HEPA: European network for the promotion of health-enhancing physical activity
http://www.euro.who.int/hepa/ [11]

The European network for the promotion of health-enhancing physical activity, HEPA Europe, is a collaborative project, which works for better health through physical activity among all people in the WHO European Region. It does this by strengthening and supporting efforts to increase participation and improve the conditions for healthy lifestyles.

The objectives of HEPA Europe are as follows:

- To contribute to the development and implementation of policies and strategies for health-enhancing physical activity
- To develop, support, and disseminate effective strategies, programmes, approaches, and other examples of good practice
- To support and facilitate multisector approaches

Network activities support cooperation, partnerships, and collaboration with other related sectors, networks, and approaches.

WHO/Europe closely collaborate with the network to achieve consistency with the goals of its programme on transport and health, which include the promotion of physical activity as a healthy means for sustainable transport. The activities of the network are based on policy statements such as the WHO Global Strategy for Diet, Physical Activity and Health and on corresponding statements from the European Commission, as well as on the best available evidence for population-based approaches to promote health-enhancing physical activity.

THE PEP: "Transport-Related Health Impacts, Costs, and Benefits with a Particular Focus on Children" within the context of the UNECE–WHO Pan-European Programme for Transport, Health, and Environment

    http://www.thepep.org/en/welcome.htm [27]

9
Conclusions and Recommendations

The present project was accomplished in the context of the development of a European Health Monitoring System. The main objective of this report was to build up a picture of data availability from routinely repeated or repeatable sources in European countries, which could inform policy makers. It was the intention of this report to provide a coordinated framework for Health Information Activities related to nutrition and physical activity, which were initiated between 1990 and 2006.

Determinants that influence a healthy lifestyle are various. The nutritional behavior and the physical activity of a person are two important aspects, which have to be taken into account in the prevention of nutrition-related diseases. An enormous number and variety of projects, scopes and actions started during the past years, which mainly aimed at assessing a population's health status and health-related aspects.

With respect to this overall objective, the broad collection of nutrition and physical activity-related projects was put together in a comprehensive, precise, and clear manner. First, Health Information Activities are characterized by a variety of scopes and methodologies and second were realised by various institutions and European networks. These circumstances made it necessary to provide a coordinated framework.

The results of this report show the great importance and the need for such an inventory. A multitude of Health Information Activities related to nutrition and physical activity have been entered into the database. The number of entered projects per country differs. Few national project entries were done by new European Union Member States as well as by candidate countries up to 2006. They were predominantly involved in European projects.

Furthermore, the analysis shows that in the majority of projects nearly the same standardised and well-established methods were applied, e.g., *Food Frequency Questionnaire* (FFQ), *24-Hour-Recall Nutrition Survey* for measuring nutritional aspects or *Anthropometrical measures* as well as the *Physical Activity Questionnaire* for the measurement of physical activity-related issues. Thus, further work should include the usability of these different methods to work with them in future health-related projects and to be sure concerning their validity and reliability. In addition, more detailed work is necessary on other methods. This approach could be helpful

N. Wolfram et al. (eds.) *Nutrition and Physical Activity*,
© Springer Science+Business Media, LLC 2008

with regard to the planning and structuring national as well as European projects in the future.

In general, it must be emphasised that the overall aim of the report was not to concentrate on criteria for evaluation and to identify models of best practise. It was intended to give an overview about existing Health Information Activities related to nutrition and physical activity covering actions in all countries belonging to the European Union up to 2006, the European Economic Areas (EEA) and all Candidate countries and including all age groups.

The conceived database provided a helping instrument putting all necessary information together and to ensure simple handling and easy understanding for each involved partner.

Altogether strategic national as well as European guidelines and recommendations have to be considered and should be well established to make sure that consistent data collection takes place within Health Information Activities. To provide for comparable data at national as well as European level, the further development of indicators related to nutrition and physical activity is of crucial importance. The following aspects should be taken into consideration:

- Cultural diversity as well as norms and patterns
- Gender issues
- Ethnic factors
- Health service infrastructure
- Food trends
- Food safety
- Economic factors
- Social determinants
- Marketing of food and beverages
- Physical activity facilities
- Use of media and communication channels

Common data reporting guidelines and standardized methods, which encompass public and private-sector Health Information Activities, should be developed. Regular revision and adaptation concerning developed strategies, policies, and practices as needed for health and population health dimensions have to be realised. These issues should be linked to continuous partnerships and by the cooperation and encouraging with main national and international stakeholders, collaborating partners, agencies, and organisations in the field of health and health-related aspects.

References

[1] Association of Schools of Public Health in the European Region (ASPHER), http://www.aspher.org (accessed 3 February 2007)

[2] Casperson CJ, Powell KE, Christensen GM: Physical activity, exercise, and physical fitness. Public Health Reports 1985, 100, 125–131(the original reference); and Pate PR, Pratt M, Blair SN, et al. Physical Activity and Public Health: A recommendation from the Centre for Disease Control and Prevention and the American College of Sports Medicine. JAMA 1995, 273, 402–407.

[3] Cavill N, Kahlmeier S, Racioppi F: Physical activity and health in Europe: Evidence for action; World Health Organization, Copenhagen, 2006, (available online at http://www.euro.who.int/document/e89490.pdf, accessed 1 February 2007)

[4] Data Food Networking (DAFNE), http://www.nut.uoa.gr/english/dafne/DafneEN.htm (accessed 1 February 2007)

[5] European Academy of Nutritional Sciences (EANS), http://www.eans.net (accessed 3 February 2007)

[6] European Commission (EC), http://ec.europa.eu/health/ph_information/reporting/analysing_reporting_en.htm (accessed 22 January 2007)

[7] European Commission (EC), http://ec.europa.eu/health/ph_programme/programme_en.htm (accessed 22 January 2007)

[8] European Commission (EC), http://ec.europa.eu/health/ph_overview/overview_en.htm (accessed 22 January 2007)

[9] European Commission (EC), http://ec.europa.eu/health/ph_information/information_en.htm (accessed 22 January 2007)

[10] European Food Information Council (EUFIC), http://www.eufic.org (accessed 3 February 2007)

[11] European network for the promotion of health-enhancing physical activity (HEPA), http://www.euro.who.int/hepa/ (accessed 3 February 2007)

[12] European Platform on Mobility Management (EPOMM), http://www.epomm.org (accessed 3 February 2007)

[13] European Public Health Association (EUPHA), http://www.eupha.org (accessed 3 February 2007)

[14] European Society for Social Paediatrics and Child Health (ESSOP), http://www.essop.org (accessed 3 February 2007)

[15] Federation of European Nutrition Societies (FENS), http://www.fensweb.org (accessed 3 February 2007)

[16] Health Behaviour in school-aged children (HBSC), http://www.hbsc.org (accessed 1 February 2007)

[17] International Physical Activity Questionaire (IPAQ), http://www.ipaq.ki.se/ (accessed 1 February 2007)

[18] International Society for Behavioral Nutrition and Physical Activity (ISBNPA), http://www.isbnpa.org (accessed 3 February 2007)

[19] National Public Health Institute, http://www.ktl.fi/portal/english/osiot/research,_people_programs/health_promotion_and_chronic_disease_prevention/projects/finbalt/roskaa/finbalt_health_monitor/ (accessed 1 February 2007)

[20] Oja P, Borms J (eds.): Health Enhancing Physical Activity. In Perspectives. The Multidisciplinary Series of Physical Education and Sport Science, Vol. 6, 2004.

[21] de Onis M, Wijnhoven TMA, Onyango AW: Worldwide practices in child growth monitoring. Journal of Paediatrics, 2004, 144, 461–465.

[22] Rigby M: Principles and challenges of child health and safety indicators; International Journal of Injury Control and Safety Promotion 2005, 12, 2; 71–78.

[23] Sjöström M, Yngve A, Poortvliet E, Warm D, Ekelund U: Diet and physical actitvity – interactions for health; Public Health Nutrition in the European Perspective. Public Health Nutrition 1999, 2, 453–459

[24] Sjöström M, et al.: Making way for a healthier lifestyle in Europe. Monitoring Public Health Nutrition in Europe. List of Indicators. Summary Report – final version. European Commission, 2003

[25] Smolin LA, Grosvenor MB: Nutrition: Science & Applications, Third Edition, 2000.

[26] The Nutrition Society (NS), http://www.nutritionsociety.org (accessed 3 February 2007)

[27] Transport, Health and Environment Pan-European Programme (THE PEP), http://www. thepep.org/en/welcome.htm (accessed 3 February 2007)

[28] World Health Organization (WHO), http://www.who.int/mediacentre/factsheets/fs311/en/ (accessed 1 February 2007)

[29] World Health Organization (WHO), http://www.who.int/chp/steps/GPAQ%20Instrument%2 0and%20Analysis%20Guide%20v2. pdf (accessed 1 February 2007)

[30] World Health Organization (WHO), http://www.who.int/chp/steps/GPAQ/en/index.html (accessed 1 February 2007)

[31] World Health Organization (WHO), http://www.who.int/ncd_surveillance/infobase/web/ InfoBaseCommon/ (accessed 1 February 2007)

[32] World Health Organization (WHO), http://www.who.int/ncd_surveillance/infobase/web/ surf2/start.html (accessed 1 February 2007)

[33] World Health Organization (WHO), http://www.who.int/ncd_surveillance/infobase/web/ surf2/reg_tables.pdf (accessed 1 February 2007)

[34] World Health Organization (WHO): The European health report 2005. Public health action for healthier children and populations. World Health Organization, 2005

[35] World Health Organization (WHO): Global Strategy on Diet, Physical Activity and Health; World Health Organization, Geneva, 2004 (available online at http://www.who.int/dietphysi-calactivity/strategy/eb11344/strategy_english_web.pdf, accessed 1 February 2007)

[36] World Health Organization (WHO): The World Health Report 2002. Reducing Risks, Promoting Healthy Life. World Health Organization, 2002

[37] World Health Organization (WHO): Development of Indicators for Monitoring Progress towards Health for All by the Year 2000. World Health Organization, Geneva, 1981

[38] World Health Organization, Regional Office for Europe (WHO Europe), http://www.euro. who.int/obesity (accessed 1 February 2007)

[39] World Health Organization, Regional Office for Europe (WHO Europe), http://www.euro. who.int/Nutrition (accessed 1 February 2007)

[40] World Health Organization, Regional Office for Europe (WHO Europe), http://www.euro. who.int/healthtopics/HT2ndLvlPage?HTCode=physical_activity (accessed 1 February 2007)

[41] World Health Organization, Regional Office for Europe (WHO Europe), http://www.euro. who.int/obesity/conference2006 (accessed 1 February 2007)

[42] World Health Organization, Regional Office for Europe (WHO Europe), http://www.euro. who.int/nutrition/20060612_3 (accessed 1 February 2007)

[43] World Health Organization, Regional Office for Europe (WHO Europe), http://www.euro. who.int/nutrition/Publications/NutPolicyWho (accessed 1 February 2007)

[44] World Health Organization, Regional Office for Europe (WHO Europe), http://www.euro. who.int/CINDI (accessed 1 February 2007)

[45] World Health Organization, Regional Office for Europe (WHO Europe), http://www.euro. who.int/Document/NUT/Instanbul_conf_%20ebd02.pdf (accessed 1 February 2007)

[46] World Health Organization, Regional Office for Europe (WHO Europe), http://www.euro. who.int/Document/E89567.pdf (accessed 1 February 2007)

[47] World Health Organization, Regional Office for Europe (WHO Europe), http://www.euro. who.int/Document/NUT/Instanbul_conf_edoc09.pdf (accessed 1 February 2007)

[48] World Health Organization, Regional Office for Europe (WHO Europe): Food and Health in Europe: a New Basis for Action; World Health Organization, Copenhagen, 2002

10
Appendix

10.1. Database for Collecting Health Information Activities

Project Description Database:

This database serves project work. In order to work with the database, you need a partner number. Please enter the partner number to access the database.

Please enter your partner number:

[ ]

Start >

For any querries, comments or suggestions please contact:

Resaerch Association Public Health
Medical Faculty
Technische Universität Dresden
Fiedlerstrasse 33
D-01307 Dresden

Germany

Step 1: General Information

Title:

Acronym:

Project Leader:
Name of Project Leader:

Name of Project Leading Institution:

Contact Person in Institution for this Project

Address of Project Leading Institution:

Project Leader's E-Mail:

Project Leader's Phone:

Project Leader's Fax:

Project Partners:
Number of Project Partners:

Scope:

  ⦿ More than 1 country involved

  ○ National

Information about the Project:
Funding Agency (or Agencies):

Start and End of Project:

Start of Project:	End of Project:
09.02.2007	09.02.2007

Date for Start of Project is available Date for End of Project is available

  ⦿ Yes, Date is available   ⦿ Yes, Date is available

  ○ No, Date is not available   ○ No, Date is not available

< Back   **Next >**

N. Wolfram et al. (eds.) *Nutrition and Physical Activity,*
© Springer Science + Business Media, LLC 2008

Step 1.2: Methods and Literature

Title:

Acronym:

Method:

Summary of the methods
employed in this study:

If the study carried out fieldwork,
what was the <u>Sample Size</u> of the
study?

Sample Size

Is Information on Sample Size available?

⦿ Yes, Information is available

◯ No, Information is not available

Start and End of <u>Data Collection</u>:

Start of Data Collection:

09.02.2007

End of Data Collection:

09.02.2007

Date for Start of Data Collection is
available

⦿ Yes, Date is available

◯ No, Date is not available

Date for End of Data Collection is
available

⦿ Yes, Date is available

◯ No, Date is not available

Published Literature

Which scientific journal articles,
books, and conference abstracts
have been published based on this
Health Information Activity?

(Please refer to the Style Guide
about how to format this list)

Click here to assess the
StyleGuide

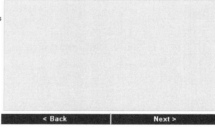

< Back   Next >

Step 1.3: Methodological Categorisation

Title:
Acronym:

How can the methodology
employed in this Health
Information Activity best be
described? Please tick all that
applies!

☐ **Methods measuring food consumption/availability**

☐ 24-Hour Recall Nutrition Survey

☐ Repeated 24-h Recall Nutrition Survey

☐ Estimated food records

☐ Weighed food records

☐ Diet History Survey

☐ Food Frequency Questionnaire (FFQ)

☐ Food balance sheets

☐ Total diet studies

☐ Universal product codes and electronic scanning device surveys

☐ Food account method

☐ Household food record method

☐ Household 24-h recall method

☐ Mini Nutritional Assessment (MNA)

☐ Subjective Global Assessment (SGA)

☐ Household-Budget-Survey

☐ **Methods measuring physical activity**

☐ Physical Activity Questionnaire

☐ Self-Completed Physical Activity Questionnaire

☐ Interviewer Administered Physical Activity Questionnaire

☐ International Physical Activity Questionnaire (IPAQ)

☐ Global Physical Activity Questionnaire (GPAQ)

☐ EPIC-Norfolk Physical Activity Questionnaire (EPAQ2)

☐ Double Labelled Water Method (DLW)

☐ Calorimetry

☐ Heart Rate Monitoring

☐ Motion sensor Studies

☐ Pedometery

☐ Accelerometry

☐ Other Methods

☐ Antropometrical measures

☐ Health related Fitness tests

☐ **Other Methods**

☐ Postharmonisation of national survey data

☐ Development of Questionnaire

< Back   Next >

Step 2: Geographical Coverage

Title:
Acronym:

Which countries are covered by the
data generated during this health
information activity?

- ☐ Austria
- ☐ Belgium
- ☐ Bulgaria
- ☐ Croatia
- ☐ Cyprus
- ☐ Czech Republic
- ☐ Denmark
- ☐ Estonia
- ☐ Finland
- ☐ France
- ☑ Germany
- ☐ Greece
- ☐ Hungary
- ☐ Iceland
- ☐ Ireland
- ☐ Italy
- ☐ Latvia
- ☐ Liechtenstein
- ☐ Lithuania
- ☑ Luxembourg
- ☐ Macedonia
- ☐ Malta
- ☐ Norway
- ☐ Poland
- ☐ Portugal
- ☐ Romania
- ☐ Slovakia
- ☐ Slovenia
- ☐ Spain
- ☐ Sweden
- ☐ The Netherlands
- ☐ Turkey
- ☑ UK

< Back   Next >

Step 2.1: Regional Geographical Coverage

Title:
Acronym:

Which regions are covered by the
data generated during this health
information activity?

- [ ] England (Königreich)
- [ ] Wales (Fürstentum)
- [ ] Schottland (Königreich)
- [ ] Nordirland (Provinz).
- [ ] Grevenmacher
- [ ] Luxemburg
- [ ] Diekirch
- [ ] Bayern
- [ ] Berlin
- [ ] Brandenburg
- [ ] Bremen
- [ ] Hamburg
- [ ] Hessen
- [ ] Mecklenburg-Vorpommern
- [ ] Niedersachsen
- [ ] Nordrhein-Westfalen
- [ ] Rheinland-Pfalz
- [ ] Saarland
- [ ] Sachsen
- [ ] Sachsen-Anhalt
- [ ] Schleswig-Holstein
- [ ] Thüringen
- [ ] Baden-Württemberg

< Back	Next >

Step 3: Towards which indicators does the activity provide data?

Title:
Acronym:

Towards which indicators does
the activity provide data?

☐ **Indicators on Food and Nutrient Intake in general**

☐ Consumption of vegetables

☐ Consumption of vegetables; average per capita adult intake of less than 300g/day

☐ Availability of vegetables

☐ Consumption of potatoes

☐ Availability of potatoes

☐ Consumption of vegetable juice

☐ Availability of vegetable juice

☐ Consumption of fruit

☐ Consumption of fruit; average per capita adult intake of less than 100g/ day

☐ Availability of fruit

☐ Consumption of fruit juice

☐ Availability of fruit juice

☐ Consumption of drinks

☐ Availability of drinks

☐ Consumption of meat and meat products

☐ Consumption of meat and meat products; average per capita adult intake of more than 80g red meat/ day

☐ Availability of meat and meat products

☐ Consumption of fish

☐ Consumption of fish; average per capita adult intake of more than 80g fish/ day

☐ Availability of fish

☐ Consumption of carbohydrates

☐ Availability of carbohydrates

☐ Non-starch polysaccharides (nsp) content of the typical diet

☐ Non-starch polysaccharides (nsp) content of the typical diet; average diet with less than 25g/d

☐ Consumption of milk

☐ Availability of milk

☐ Consumption of milk products

☐ Availability of milk products

☐ Consumption of salt

☐ Availability of salt

☐ Consumption of sweets (incl. fast food and chips)

☐ Availability of sweets (incl. fast food and chips)

☐ Saturated fatty acids content of the typical diet

☐ Saturated fatty acids content of the typical diet; average diet with saturated fatty acid content of more than 10% of energy intake

☐ Mono-unsaturated fatty acids content of the typical diet

☐ Mono-unsaturated fatty acids content of the typical diet; average diet with low MUFA

☐ Polyunsaturated fatty acids content of the typical diet

☐ Polyunsaturated fatty acids content of the typical diet; average diet with less than 7-8% of energy from PUFA

☐ **Vitamins**
☐ Vitamin content of the typical diet: vitamin C
☐ Vitamin content of the typical diet: vitamin D
☐ Vitamin content of the typical diet: vitamin E
☐ Vitamin content of the typical diet: folate
☐ Vitamin content of the typical diet: carotenoids
☐ **Mineral Content**
☐ Mineral content of the typical diet: Fe
☐ Mineral content of the typical diet: I
☐ Mineral content of the typical diet: Ca
☐ Mineral content of the typical diet: Se
☐ **Energy**
☐ Energy intake
☐ Food frequency
☐ Energy density
☐ **Indicators on Alcohol in general**
☐ Total alcohol consumption
☐ The share of abstainers
☐ The frequency of heavy drinking occassions (binge drinking)
☐ The share of total alcohol consumption consumed with meals
☐ The contribution of alcohol to energy intake
☐ **Indicators on Breastfeeding in general**
☐ Initiation breastfeeding and Exclusive breastfeeding rates through out the first 48 hours of life
☐ Duration of breastfeeding at birth
☐ Duration of breastfeeding at 6 months of age
☐ Duration of breastfeeding at 12 months of age
☐ Duration of breastfeeding at 18 months of age
☐ Duration of breastfeeding at 24 months of age
☐ Quality of breastfeeding exclusive breastfeeding rates at birth
☐ Quality of breastfeeding exclusive breastfeeding rates at 6 or more months of age
☐ **Indicators on Nutritional Status in general**
☐ Retinol levels
☐ Total plasma carotenoid levels
☐ Blood lipid pattern hdl
☐ Blood lipid pattern ldl
☐ Blood lipid pattern triacyl glycerides
☐ Haemoglobin level
☐ Serum ferritin level
☐ Serum transferrin receptor level
☐ Folic acid status
☐ Selenium status
☐ Serum 25-hydroxy vitamin d3 status
☐ **Indicators on Anthropometry/ Body Composition in general**
☐ Body mass index (bmi)
☐ Waist circumfence
☐ Waist-to-hip ratio (whr)
☐ Sagittal abdominal diameter (sad)

☐ **Indicators on Physical Activity levels and patterns in general**

☐ Total amount of activity expressed as activity energy expenditure (kcal, joules, met mins, etc.)

☐ Total amount of activity expressed as physical activicty level (pal)

☐ Time (mins/ day or week) spent at health enhancing physical activity, i.e. at moderate intensity levels

☐ Time (mins/ day or week) spent at health enhancing physical activity, i.e. at vigorous intensity levels

☐ Sedentary behaviour

☐ Environmental determinants for physical activity

☐ **Indicators on Health Related Fitness in general**

☐ Maximal aerobic power

☐ Walk test, 2 km

☐ Bodily control

☐ Muscular strength

☐ Joint mobility

☐ **Indicators on Socio-demografic factors in general**

☐ Educational level, population by educational class: elementary

☐ Educational level, population by educational class: lower secondary

☐ Educational level, population by educational class: upper secondary

☐ Educational level, population by educational class: tertiary

☐ Occupation; population by occupational class: upper non-manual

☐ Occupation; population by occupational class: lower non-manual

☐ Occupation; population by occupational class: skilled manual

☐ Occupation; population by occupational class: unskilled manual

☐ Occupation; population by occupational class: self employed

☐ Occupation; population by occupational class: farmer

☐ Total unemployed

☐ The percentage of population long term unemployed, more than 12 month

☐ Population below poverty line (with income below 60% of the national median)

☐ Household income as the percentage of households with a total income below 50% of the median income of the country

☐ Household income as the number of households with income in the lowest 5%

☐ The percentage of households with income below budget standards

☐ **Indicators on Inequality in general**

☐ **Indicators on Health Promotion in general**

☐ Nutritional policy

☐ Nutritional statutory legislation

☐ Nutrional intervention: fortification

☐ **Further Indicators**

☐ Consumption of Water/ Beverages

☐ Fast Food

☐ Leisure Activity

☐ Workplace Activity

☐ Dietetic Education

☐ Sleep

☐ TV/PC Consumption

☐ Weight Reduction

☐ Ethnicity

☐ Medication

☐ Obesity related metabolic disorders

☐ Eating disorders

☐ Eating behaviour

☐ Malnutrition

< Back   Next >

Step 4: Age Groups

Title:

Acronym:

Age Groups used

Please specify the age groups that are assessed during data collection

	Group ranges from age ...	... to age ...
01	0	0
02	0	0
03	0	0
04	0	0
05	0	0
06	0	0
07	0	0
08	0	0
09	0	0
10	0	0
11	0	0
12	0	0
13	0	0
14	0	0
15	0	0
16	0	0
17	0	0
18	0	0
19	0	0
20	0	0
21	0	0
22	0	0
23	0	0
24	0	0
25	0	0

< Back   Next >

Step 4.1: Age Groups Freetext

Title:

Acronym:

Age Groups used

If you could not describe the age
groups used in the Project by using
the previous screen, please
describe the age groups with free
text here

(e.g. if studies involved mother and
child)

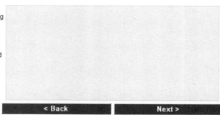

Step 5: Problem Description

Title:

Acronym:

Data entry finished

Did you finished describing this
project?

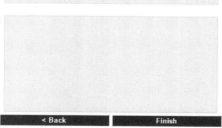

○ Yes, I filled in all available information that describes this
project.

◉ No, I will come back to fill more fields for this project next
time.

Problem Description

Did you face difficulties while filling
out the form for this particular
study? If yes, which were the
problems?

10.2. Database Entries: Methods and Indicators

Table 7 Absolute frequency of used methods in entered Projects, separated by countries

Methods	National Projects	European Projects	Total
Austria			
Methods measuring food consumption/availability	**5**	**10**	**15**
24-Hour Recall Nutrition Survey	0	5	5
Repeated 24-h Recall Nutrition Survey	0	1	1
Weighted food records	0	1	1
Food Frequency Questionnaire (FFQ)	1	4	5
Food balance sheets	0	2	2
Household-Budget-Survey	1	3	4
Methods measuring physical activity	**4**	**7**	**11**
Physical Activity Questionnaire	1	3	4
Self-Completed Physical Activity Questionnaire	0	2	2
International Physical Activity Questionnaire (IPAQ)	0	2	2
Heart Rate Monitoring	0	1	1
Accelerometry	0	1	1
Anthropometrical measures	0	3	3

Methods	National Projects	European Projects	Total
Belgium			
Methods measuring food consumption/availability	**3**	**14**	**17**
24-Hour Recall Nutrition Survey	0	4	4
Repeated 24-h Recall Nutrition Survey	1	1	2
Estimated food records	1	0	1
Weighted food records	0	2	2
Diet History Survey	1	2	3
Food Frequency Questionnaire (FFQ)	2	4	6
Food balance sheets	0	2	2
Total diet studies	0	1	1
Household-Budget-Survey	0	4	4
Methods measuring physical activity	**3**	**11**	**14**
Physical Activity Questionnaire	1	5	6
Self-Completed Physical Activity Questionnaire	1	3	4
International Physical Activity Questionnaire (IPAQ)	1	3	4
Heart Rate Monitoring	2	1	3
Accelerometry	0	1	1
Other Methods	1	0	1

(continued)

Table 7 (continued)

Methods	National Projects	European Projects	Total
Belgium			
Anthropometrical measures	1	4	5
Health related Fitness tests	1	0	1
Other Methods	**3**	**0**	**3**
Development of Questionnaire	3	0	3

Methods	National Projects	European Projects	Total
Bulgaria			
Methods measuring food consumption/availability	**4**	**6**	**10**
24-Hour Recall Nutrition Survey	3	1	4
Estimated food records	1	0	1
Diet History Survey	2	0	2
Food Frequency Questionnaire (FFQ)	2	2	4
Food balance sheets	1	1	2
Total diet studies	1	0	1
Food account method	1	0	1
Household-Budget-Survey	0	1	1
Methods measuring physical activity	**1**	**5**	**6**
Physical Activity Questionnaire	0	2	2
Self-Completed Physical Activity Questionnaire	0	3	3
Anthropometrical measures	1	2	3

Methods	National Projects	European Projects	Total
Croatia			
Methods measuring food consumption/availability	**0**	**7**	**7**
24-Hour Recall Nutrition Survey	0	2	2
Food Frequency Questionnaire (FFQ)	0	2	2
Food balance sheets	0	1	1
Household-Budget-Survey	0	2	2
Methods measuring physical activity	**0**	**4**	**4**
Physical Activity Questionnaire	0	2	2
Self-Completed Physical Activity Questionnaire	0	2	2
Anthropometrical measures	0	2	2

(continued)

Table 7 (continued)

Methods	National Projects	European Projects	Total
Cyprus			
Methods measuring food consumption/availability	**2**	**2**	**4**
24-Hour Recall Nutrition Survey	0	1	1
Diet History Survey	1	0	1
Food Frequency Questionnaire (FFQ)	1	0	1
Food balance sheets	0	1	1
Household-Budget-Survey	0	1	1
Methods measuring physical activity	**2**	**1**	**3**
Physical Activity Questionnaire	2	0	2
Self-Completed Physical Activity Questionnaire	0	1	1
Anthropometrical measures	2	0	2

Methods	National Projects	European Projects	Total
Czech Republic			
Methods measuring food consumption/availability	**0**	**6**	**6**
24-Hour Recall Nutrition Survey	0	2	2
Food Frequency Questionnaire (FFQ)	0	2	2
Food balance sheets	0	1	1
Household-Budget-Survey	0	1	1
Methods measuring physical activity	**0**	**4**	**4**
Physical Activity Questionnaire	0	2	2
Self-Completed Physical Activity Questionnaire	0	2	2
Anthropometrical measures	0	2	2

Methods	National Projects	European Projects	Total
Denmark			
Methods measuring food consumption/availability	**0**	**9**	**9**
24-Hour Recall Nutrition Survey	0	3	3
Repeated 24-Hour Recall Nutrition Survey	0	1	1
Weighted food records	0	2	2
Diet History Survey	0	1	1
Food Frequency Questionnaire (FFQ)	0	4	4
Food balance sheets	0	1	1
Total diet studies	0	1	1
Household-Budget-Survey	0	1	1
Methods measuring physical activity	**0**	**8**	**8**
Physical Activity Questionnaire	0	5	5
Self-Completed Physical Activity Questionnaire	0	2	2
International Physical Activity Questionnaire (IPAQ)	0	1	1
Anthropometrical measures	0	4	4

(continued)

Table 7 (continued)

Methods	National Projects	European Projects	Total
Estonia			
Methods measuring food consumption/availability	**2**	**4**	**6**
Estimated food records	2	0	2
Food Frequency Questionnaire (FFQ)	0	2	2
Methods measuring physical activity	**2**	**4**	**6**
Physical Activity Questionnaire	1	2	3
Self-Completed Physical Activity Questionnaire	1	2	3
Anthropometrical measures	1	2	3

Methods	National Projects	European Projects	Total
Finland			
Methods measuring food consumption/availability	**2**	**9**	**11**
24-Hour Recall Nutrition Survey	0	3	3
Repeated 24-h Recall Nutrition Survey	0	1	1
Estimated food records	1	0	1
Weighted food records	0	1	1
Food Frequency Questionnaire (FFQ)	1	3	4
Food balance sheets	0	2	2
Household-Budget-Survey	0	3	3
Methods measuring physical activity	**2**	**8**	**10**
Physical Activity Questionnaire	1	3	4
Self-Completed Physical Activity Questionnaire	1	3	4
International Physical Activity Questionnaire (IPAQ)	0	2	2
Anthropometrical measures	0	3	3

Methods	National Projects	European Projects	Total
France			
Methods measuring food consumption/availability	**2**	**14**	**16**
24-Hour Recall Nutrition Survey	0	3	3
Repeated 24-h Recall Nutrition Survey	2	1	3
Weighted food records	0	2	2
Diet History Survey	0	2	2
Food Frequency Questionnaire (FFQ)	2	4	6
Food balance sheets	0	2	2

(continued)

Table 7 (continued)

Methods	National Projects	European Projects	Total
France			
Total diet studies	0	1	1
Household-Budget-Survey	0	4	4
Methods measuring physical activity	**2**	**11**	**13**
Physical Activity Questionnaire	1	5	6
Self-Completed Physical Activity Questionnaire	0	3	3
International Physical Activity Questionnaire (IPAQ)	0	2	2
Heart Rate Monitoring	2	1	3
Accelerometry	0	1	1
Anthropometrical measures	0	5	5

Methods	National Projects	European Projects	Total
Germany			
Methods measuring food consumption/availability	**22**	**11**	**33**
24-Hour Recall Nutrition Survey	2	4	6
Repeated 24-h Recall Nutrition Survey	0	1	1
Estimated food records	8	0	8
Weighted food records	5	1	6
Diet History Survey	5	0	5
Food Frequency Questionnaire (FFQ)	9	4	13
Food balance sheets	0	1	1
Household-Budget-Survey	3	3	6
Methods measuring physical activity	**12**	**10**	**22**
Physical Activity Questionnaire	1	3	4
Self-Completed Physical Activity Questionnaire	6	3	9
Interviewer Administered Physical Activity Questionnaire	1	1	2
International Physical Activity Questionnaire (IPAQ)	0	3	3
Calorimetry	1	0	1
Heart Rate Monitoring	0	1	1
Accelerometry	0	1	1
Anthropometrical measures	10	4	14
Other Methods	**30**	**2**	**32**
Postharmonisation of national survey data	6	1	7
Development of Questionnaire	24	1	25

(continued)

Table 7 (continued)

Methods	National Projects	European Projects	Total
Greece			
Methods measuring food consumption/availability	**2**	**12**	**14**
24-Hour Recall Nutrition Survey	0	3	3
Repeated 24-h Recall Nutrition Survey	0	1	1
Weighted food records	0	2	2
Diet History Survey	1	1	2
Food Frequency Questionnaire (FFQ)	1	3	4
Food balance sheets	0	2	2
Total diet studies	0	1	1
Household-Budget-Survey	1	4	5
Methods measuring physical activity	**2**	**9**	**11**
Physical Activity Questionnaire	2	4	6
Self-Completed Physical Activity Questionnaire	0	3	3
International Physical Activity Questionnaire (IPAQ)	0	2	2
Heart Rate Monitoring	0	1	1
Accelerometry	0	1	1
Anthropometrical measures	0	4	4
Other Methods	**7**	**0**	**7**
Development of Questionnaire	7	0	7

Methods	National Projects	European Projects	Total
Hungary			
Methods measuring food consumption/availability	**3**	**14**	**17**
24-Hour Recall Nutrition Survey	1	4	5
Repeated 24-h Recall Nutrition Survey	1	1	2
Estimated food records	1	0	1
Weighted food records	0	2	2
Diet History Survey	1	0	1
Food Frequency Questionnaire (FFQ)	0	3	3
Food balance sheets	0	2	2
Total diet studies	0	1	1
Household-Budget-Survey	0	4	4
Methods measuring physical activity	**3**	**10**	**13**
Physical Activity Questionnaire	0	3	3
Self-Completed Physical Activity Questionnaire	0	3	3
Interviewer Administered Physical Activity Questionnaire	1	0	1
International Physical Activity Questionnaire (IPAQ)	0	2	2
Heart Rate Monitoring	0	1	1
Accelerometry	0	1	1
Other Methods	1	1	2
Anthropometrical measures	0	3	3
Other Methods	**3**	**2**	**5**
Development of Questionnaire	3	2	5

(continued)

Table 7 (continued)

Methods	National Projects	European Projects	Total
Iceland			
Methods measuring food consumption/availability	**0**	**6**	**6**
24-Hour Recall Nutrition Survey	0	2	2
Food Frequency Questionnaire (FFQ)	0	3	3
Methods measuring physical activity	**0**	**4**	**4**
Physical Activity Questionnaire	0	2	2
Self-Completed Physical Activity Questionnaire	0	2	2
Anthropometrical measures	0	2	2

Methods	National Projects	European Projects	Total
Ireland			
Methods measuring food consumption/availability	**1**	**9**	**10**
24-Hour Recall Nutrition Survey	1	1	2
Diet History Survey	0	1	1
Food Frequency Questionnaire (FFQ)	1	2	3
Food balance sheets	0	1	1
Household-Budget-Survey	0	3	3
Methods measuring physical activity	**1**	**6**	**7**
Physical Activity Questionnaire	0	3	3
Self-Completed Physical Activity Questionnaire	1	3	4
Anthropometrical measures	0	3	3

Methods	National Projects	European Projects	Total
Italy			
Methods measuring food consumption/availability	**6**	**15**	**21**
24-Hour Recall Nutrition Survey	2	4	6
Repeated 24-h Recall Nutrition Survey	0	1	1
Weighted food records	0	2	2
Diet History Survey	3	2	5
Food Frequency Questionnaire (FFQ)	3	4	7
Food balance sheets	0	3	3
Total diet studies	0	1	1
Household-Budget-Survey	0	5	5
Methods measuring physical activity	**6**	**11**	**17**
Physical Activity Questionnaire	5	5	10
Self-Completed Physical Activity Questionnaire	0	3	3
International Physical Activity Questionnaire (IPAQ)	0	2	2
Heart Rate Monitoring	0	1	1
Accelerometry	0	1	1
Anthropometrical measures	1	5	6
Other Methods	**2**	**0**	**2**
Development of Questionnaire	2	0	2

(continued)

Table 7 (continued)

Methods	National Projects	European Projects	Total
Latvia			
Methods measuring food consumption/availability	**1**	**5**	**6**
24-Hour Recall Nutrition Survey	0	1	1
Estimated food records	1	0	1
Food Frequency Questionnaire (FFQ)	0	2	2
Food balance sheets	0	1	1
Household-Budget-Survey	0	1	1
Methods measuring physical activity	**1**	**4**	**5**
Physical Activity Questionnaire	0	2	2
Self-Completed Physical Activity Questionnaire	1	2	3
Anthropometrical measures	0	2	2

Methods	National Projects	European Projects	Total
Lithuania			
Methods measuring food consumption/availability	**2**	**10**	**12**
24-Hour Recall Nutrition Survey	1	3	4
Estimated food records	1	0	1
Food Frequency Questionnaire (FFQ)	0	6	6
Food balance sheets	0	1	1
Household-Budget-Survey	0	1	1
Methods measuring physical activity	**2**	**7**	**9**
Physical Activity Questionnaire	1	3	4
Self-Completed Physical Activity Questionnaire	0	4	4
International Physical Activity Questionnaire (IPAQ)	1	0	1
Anthropometrical measures	0	3	3

Methods	National Projects	European Projects	Total
Luxembourg			
Methods measuring food consumption/availability	**0**	**5**	**5**
Food Frequency Questionnaire (FFQ)	0	2	2
Household-Budget-Survey	0	2	2
Methods measuring physical activity	**0**	**4**	**4**
Physical Activity Questionnaire	0	3	3
Self-Completed Physical Activity Questionnaire	0	1	1
Anthropometrical measures	0	3	3

(continued)

Table 7 (continued)

Methods	National Projects	European Projects	Total
Macedonia			
Methods measuring food consumption/availability	**4**	**1**	**5**
Food Frequency Questionnaire (FFQ)	1	0	1
Mini Nutritional Assessment (MNA)	2	0	2
Household-Budget-Survey	1	0	1
Methods measuring physical activity	**3**	**1**	**4**
Self-Completed Physical Activity Questionnaire	0	1	1
Accelerometry	1	0	1
Anthropometrical measures	2	0	2
Other Methods	**1**	**1**	**2**
Development of Questionnaire	1	1	2

Methods	National Projects	European Projects	Total
Malta			
Methods measuring food consumption/availability	**0**	**6**	**6**
24-Hour Recall Nutrition Survey	0	1	1
Food Frequency Questionnaire (FFQ)	0	2	2
Food balance sheets	0	1	1
Household-Budget-Survey	0	2	2
Methods measuring physical activity	**0**	**4**	**4**
Physical Activity Questionnaire	0	2	2
Self-Completed Physical Activity Questionnaire	0	2	2
Anthropometrical measures	0	2	2

Methods	National Projects	European Projects	Total
Norway			
Methods measuring food consumption/availability	**0**	**11**	**11**
24-Hour Recall Nutrition Survey	0	3	3
Repeated 24-h Recall Nutrition Survey	0	1	1
Weighted food records	0	2	2
Diet History Survey	0	1	1
Food Frequency Questionnaire (FFQ)	0	4	4
Food balance sheets	0	2	2
Total diet studies	0	1	1
Household-Budget-Survey	0	4	4
Methods measuring physical activity	**0**	**6**	**6**
Physical Activity Questionnaire	0	3	3
Self-Completed Physical Activity Questionnaire	0	2	2
International Physical Activity Questionnaire (IPAQ)	0	1	1
Anthropometrical measures	0	3	3

(continued)

Table 7 (continued)

Methods	National Projects	European Projects	Total
Poland			
Methods measuring food consumption/availability	**0**	**10**	**10**
24-Hour Recall Nutrition Survey	0	2	2
Weighted food records	0	1	1
Diet History Survey	0	1	1
Food Frequency Questionnaire (FFQ)	0	2	2
Food balance sheets	0	1	1
Total diet studies	0	1	1
Household-Budget-Survey	0	3	3
Methods measuring physical activity	**0**	**6**	**6**
Physical Activity Questionnaire	0	4	4
Self-Completed Physical Activity Questionnaire	0	2	2
Anthropometrical measures	0	3	3

Methods	National Projects	European Projects	Total
Portugal			
Methods measuring food consumption/availability	**1**	**13**	**14**
24-Hour Recall Nutrition Survey	0	3	3
Repeated 24-h Recall Nutrition Survey	0	1	1
Weighted food records	0	2	2
Diet History Survey	0	2	2
Food Frequency Questionnaire (FFQ)	1	4	5
Food balance sheets	0	3	3
Total diet studies	0	1	1
Household-Budget-Survey	0	5	5
Methods measuring physical activity	**2**	**9**	**11**
Physical Activity Questionnaire	1	5	6
Self-Completed Physical Activity Questionnaire	0	3	3
Interviewer Administered Physical Activity Questionnaire	1	0	1
International Physical Activity Questionnaire (IPAQ)	0	1	1
Anthropometrical measures	1	4	5

(continued)

Table 7 (continued)

Methods	National Projects	European Projects	Total
Romania			
Methods measuring food consumption/availability	**5**	**8**	**13**
24-Hour Recall Nutrition Survey	1	1	2
Estimated food records	1	0	1
Diet History Survey	1	2	3
Food Frequency Questionnaire (FFQ)	3	4	7
Food balance sheets	0	1	1
Total diet studies	1	0	1
Food account method	1	0	1
Household food record method	0	1	1
Subjective Global Assessment (SGA)	1	1	2
Household-Budget-Survey	1	1	2
Methods measuring physical activity	**6**	**7**	**13**
Physical Activity Questionnaire	1	2	3
Self-Completed Physical Activity Questionnaire	3	3	6
Interviewer Administered Physical Activity Questionnaire	2	0	2
International Physical Activity Questionnaire (IPAQ)	1	0	1
Pedometery	1	0	1
Other Methods	1	0	1
Anthropometrical measures	4	4	8
Other Methods	**5**	**2**	**7**
Postharmonisation of national survey data	1	0	1
Development of Questionnaire	3	2	5

Methods	National Projects	European Projects	Total
Slovakia			
Methods measuring food consumption/availability	**0**	**6**	**6**
24-Hour Recall Nutrition Survey	0	2	2
Food Frequency Questionnaire (FFQ)	0	2	2
Food balance sheets	0	1	1
Household-Budget-Survey	0	1	1
Methods measuring physical activity	**0**	**4**	**4**
Physical Activity Questionnaire	0	2	2
Self-Completed Physical Activity Questionnaire	0	2	2
Anthropometrical measures	0	2	2

(continued)

Table 7 (continued)

Methods	National Projects	European Projects	Total
Slovenia			
Methods measuring food consumption/availability	**2**	**5**	**7**
24-Hour Recall Nutrition Survey	0	1	1
Food Frequency Questionnaire (FFQ)	2	2	4
Food balance sheets	0	1	1
Household-Budget-Survey	0	1	1
Methods measuring physical activity	**2**	**4**	**6**
Physical Activity Questionnaire	0	2	2
Self-Completed Physical Activity Questionnaire	1	2	3
Interviewer Administered Physical Activity Questionnaire	1	0	1
International Physical Activity Questionnaire (IPAQ)	2	0	2
Heart Rate Monitoring	1	0	1
Anthropometrical measures	1	2	3
Health related Fitness tests	1	0	1

Methods	National Projects	European Projects	Total
Spain			
Methods measuring food consumption/availability	**6**	**15**	**21**
24-Hour Recall Nutrition Survey	3	5	8
Repeated 24-h Recall Nutrition Survey	0	1	1
Weighted food records	1	2	3
Diet History Survey	1	2	3
Food Frequency Questionnaire (FFQ)	3	5	8
Food balance sheets	0	3	3
Total diet studies	0	1	1
Household-Budget-Survey	1	5	6
Methods measuring physical activity	**6**	**11**	**17**
Physical Activity Questionnaire	5	5	10
Self-Completed Physical Activity Questionnaire	0	2	2
International Physical Activity Questionnaire (IPAQ)	0	3	3
Heart Rate Monitoring	0	1	1
Accelerometry	0	1	1
Anthropometrical measures	5	5	10
Other Methods	**1**	**0**	**1**

(continued)

Table 7 (continued)

Methods	National Projects	European Projects	Total
Sweden			
Methods measuring food consumption/availability	**0**	**8**	**8**
24-Hour Recall Nutrition Survey	0	3	3
Repeated 24-h Recall Nutrition Survey	0	1	1
Weighted food records	0	1	1
Food Frequency Questionnaire (FFQ)	0	4	4
Food balance sheets	0	1	1
Household-Budget-Survey	0	2	2
Methods measuring physical activity	**0**	**6**	**6**
Physical Activity Questionnaire	0	3	3
Self-Completed Physical Activity Questionnaire	0	2	2
International Physical Activity Questionnaire (IPAQ)	0	1	1
Anthropometrical measures	0	3	3

Methods	National Projects	European Projects	Total
The Netherlands			
Methods measuring food consumption/availability	**7**	**9**	**16**
24-Hour Recall Nutrition Survey	0	2	2
Repeated 24-h Recall Nutrition Survey	2	0	2
Estimated food records	2	0	2
Weighted food records	0	1	1
Diet History Survey	0	1	1
Food Frequency Questionnaire (FFQ)	5	4	9
Total diet studies	0	1	1
Methods measuring physical activity	**9**	**8**	**17**
Physical Activity Questionnaire	4	5	9
Self-Completed Physical Activity Questionnaire	4	2	6
Interviewer Administered Physical Activity Questionnaire	2	0	2
Pedometery	1	0	1
Accelerometry	2	0	2
Other Methods	2	0	2
Anthropometrical measures	2	5	7

(continued)

Table 7 (continued)

Methods	National Projects	European Projects	Total
Turkey			
Methods measuring food consumption/availability	0	4	4
Food Frequency Questionnaire (FFQ)	0	2	2
Methods measuring physical activity	4	4	8
Physical Activity Questionnaire	0	2	2
Self-Completed Physical Activity Questionnaire	0	2	2
Anthropometrical measures	4	2	6
Other Methods	5	0	5
Postharmonisation of national survey data	3	0	3

Methods	National Projects	European Projects	Total
United Kingdom			
Methods measuring food consumption/availability	7	16	23
24-Hour Recall Nutrition Survey	3	5	8
Repeated 24-h Recall Nutrition Survey	0	1	1
Estimated food records	0	1	1
Weighted food records	4	2	6
Diet History Survey	1	2	3
Food Frequency Questionnaire (FFQ)	1	5	6
Food balance sheets	0	3	3
Total diet studies	0	1	1
Household-Budget-Survey	0	5	5
Methods measuring physical activity	8	13	21
Physical Activity Questionnaire	4	6	10
Self-Completed Physical Activity Questionnaire	3	3	6
Interviewer Administered Physical Activity Questionnaire	2	1	3
International Physical Activity Questionnaire (IPAQ)	0	3	3
Double Labelled Water Method (DLW)	3	0	3
Heart Rate Monitoring	0	1	1
Accelerometry	0	1	1
Anthropometrical measures	4	5	9
Other Methods	0	1	1
Development of Questionnaire	0	1	1

Table 8 Absolute frequency of used indicators in entered Projects, separated by indicator categories

Indicator	Number of National Projects	Number of European Projects	Number of all Projects
Indicators on Food and Nutrient Intake in general	**108**	**28**	**136**
Consumption of vegetables	74	27	101
Availability of vegetables	6	3	9
Consumption of potatoes	57	12	69
Availability of potatoes	6	3	9
Consumption of vegetable juice	45	13	58
Availability of vegetable juice	2	3	5
Consumption of fruit	73	25	98
Availability of fruit	5	3	8
Consumption of fruit juice	48	15	63
Availability of fruit juice	3	3	6
Consumption of drinks	51	14	65
Availability of drinks	5	3	8
Consumption of meat and meat products	65	18	83
Availability of meat and meat products	6	3	9
Consumption of fish	66	18	84
Availability of fish	5	3	8
Consumption of carbohydrates	48	12	60
Availability of carbohydrates	1	2	3
Non-starch polysaccharides (nsp) content of the typical diet	11	3	14
Consumption of milk	57	16	73
Availability of milk	4	3	7
Consumption of milk products	53	11	64
Availability of milk products	3	3	6
Consumption of salt	35	10	45
Availability of salt	0	3	3
Consumption of sweets (incl. fast food and chips)	61	15	76
Availability of sweets (incl. fast food and chips)	3	2	5
Saturated fatty acids content of the typical diet	39	11	50
Mono-unsaturated fatty acids content of the typical diet	37	9	46
Polyunsaturated fatty acids content of the typical diet	36	8	44

(continued)

Table 8 (continued)

Indicator	Number of National Projects	Number of European Projects	Number of all Projects
Vitamins	**33**	**7**	**40**
Vitamin content of the typical diet: vitamin C	25	5	30
Vitamin content of the typical diet: vitamin D	22	5	27
Vitamin content of the typical diet: vitamin E	24	4	28
Vitamin content of the typical diet: folate	22	6	28
Vitamin content of the typical diet: carotenoids	18	5	23

Indicator	Number of National Projects	Number of European Projects	Number of all Projects
Mineral Content	**30**	**6**	**36**
Mineral content of the typical diet: Fe	22	5	27
Mineral content of the typical diet: I	18	5	23
Mineral content of the typical diet: Ca	22	4	26
Mineral content of the typical diet: Se	12	2	14

Indicator	Number of National Projects	Number of European Projects	Number of all Projects
Energy	**61**	**13**	**74**
Energy intake	27	8	35
Food frequency	44	5	49
Energy density	10	1	11

Indicator	Number of National Projects	Number of European Projects	Number of all Projects
Indicators on Alcohol in general	**101**	**24**	**125**
Total alcohol consumption	90	17	107
The share of total alcohol consumption consumed with meals	5	0	5
The contribution of alcohol to energy intake	6	2	8

Indicator	Number of National Projects	Number of European Projects	Number of all Projects
Indicators on Breastfeeding in general	**9**	**1**	**10**
Duration of breastfeeding at 6 months of age	6	1	7
Quality of breastfeeding exclusive breastfeeding rates at 6 or more months of age	3	0	3

(continued)

Table 8 (continued)

Indicator	Number of National Projects	Number of European Projects	Number of all Projects
Indicators on Anthropometry/ Body Composition in general	**90**	**16**	**106**
Body mass index (bmi)	77	14	91
Waist circumfence	23	2	25
Waist-to-hip ratio (whr)	19	2	21

Indicator	Number of National Projects	Number of European Projects	Number of all Projects
Indicators on Physical Activity levels and patterns in general	**118**	**22**	**140**
Time (mins/ day or week) spent at health enhancing physical activity, i.e. at moderate intensity levels	56	12	68
Time (mins/ day or week) spent at health enhancing physical activity, i.e. at vigorous intensity levels	54	13	67
Sedentary behaviour	25	12	37

Indicator	Number of National Projects	Number of European Projects	Number of all Projects
Indicators on Socio-demographic factors in general	**124**	**15**	**139**
Educational level, population by educational class: elementary	83	11	94
Educational level, population by educational class: lower secondary	83	10	93
Educational level, population by educational class: upper secondary	82	10	92
Educational level, population by educational class: tertiary	82	10	92
Occupation; population by occupational class: upper non-manual	50	5	55
Occupation; population by occupational class: lower non-manual	50	5	55
Occupation; population by occupational class: skilled manual	51	5	56
Occupation; population by occupational class: unskilled manual	51	6	57
Occupation; population by occupational class: self employed	49	6	55
Occupation; population by occupational class: farmer	49	6	55
Total unemployed	40	5	45
The percentage of population long term unemployed, more than 12 month	10	0	10

(continued)

Table 8 (continued)

Indicator	Number of National Projects	Number of European Projects	Number of all Projects
Population below poverty line (with income below 60% of the national median)	25	0	25
Household income as the percentage of households with a total income below 50% of the median income of the country	22	1	23
Household income as the number of households with income in the lowest 5%	21	1	22
The percentage of households with income below budget standards	28	1	29

Indicator	Number of National Projects	Number of European Projects	Number of all Projects
Further Indicators	**112**	**23**	**135**
Fast Food	33	5	38
Leisure Activity	30	13	43
Workplace Activity	20	3	23
Sleep	23	4	27
TV/PC Consumption	11	9	20
Ethnicity	34	7	41
Medication	38	6	44
Obesity related metabolic disorders	20	1	21
Eating disorders	11	0	11
Eating behaviour	58	5	63
Malnutrition	6	1	7

Table 9 Absolute frequency of used indicator categories in entered Projects, separated by countries

Indicator category	National Projects	European Projects	Total
Austria			
Indicators on Food and Nutrient Intake in general	14	9	23
Vitamins	5	3	8
Mineral Content	5	3	8
Energy	6	4	10
Indicators on Alcohol in general	24	9	33
Indicators on Breastfeeding in general	1	0	1
Indicators on Nutritional Status in general	2	1	3
Indicators on Anthropometry/ Body Composition in general	13	5	18
Indicators on Physical Activity levels and patterns in general	21	7	28
Indicators on Health Related Fitness in general	1	1	2
Indicators on Socio-demographic factors in general	28	4	32
Indicators on Health Promotion in general	12	0	12
Further Indicators	20	7	27

(continued)

Table 9 (continued)

Indicator category	National Projects	European Projects	Total
Belgium			
Indicators on Food and Nutrient Intake in general	5	12	17
Vitamins	1	4	5
Mineral Content	1	3	4
Energy	1	4	5
Indicators on Alcohol in general	2	12	14
Indicators on Nutritional Status in general	0	2	2
Indicators on Anthropometry/ Body Composition in general	3	6	9
Indicators on Physical Activity levels and patterns in general	3	10	13
Indicators on Health Related Fitness in general	1	1	2
Indicators on Socio-demographic factors in general	4	7	11
Indicators on Health Promotion in general	2	0	2
Further Indicators	2	11	13

Indicator category	National Projects	European Projects	Total
Bulgaria			
Indicators on Food and Nutrient Intake in general	4	5	9
Vitamins	4	0	4
Mineral Content	4	0	4
Energy	4	1	5
Indicators on Alcohol in general	1	6	7
Indicators on Anthropometry/ Body Composition in general	4	2	6
Indicators on Physical Activity levels and patterns in general	4	3	7
Indicators on Socio-demographic factors in general	1	2	3
Indicators on Health Promotion in general	3	0	3
Further Indicators	0	5	5

Indicator category	National Projects	European Projects	Total
Croatia			
Indicators on Food and Nutrient Intake in general	0	5	5
Vitamins	0	1	1
Mineral Content	0	1	1
Energy	0	2	2
Indicators on Alcohol in general	0	6	6
Indicators on Anthropometry/ Body Composition in general	0	2	2
Indicators on Physical Activity levels and patterns in general	0	3	3
Indicators on Socio-demographic factors in general	0	1	1
Further Indicators	0	4	4

(continued)

Table 9 (continued)

Indicator category	National Projects	European Projects	Total
Cyprus			
Indicators on Food and Nutrient Intake in general	0	1	1
Energy	0	1	1
Indicators on Alcohol in general	0	2	2
Indicators on Physical Activity levels and patterns in general	0	1	1
Further Indicators	0	1	1

Indicator category	National Projects	European Projects	Total
Czech Republic			
Indicators on Food and Nutrient Intake in general	0	5	5
Vitamins	0	1	1
Mineral Content	0	1	1
Energy	0	2	2
Indicators on Alcohol in general	0	6	6
Indicators on Anthropometry/ Body Composition in general	0	2	2
Indicators on Physical Activity levels and patterns in general	0	3	3
Indicators on Socio-demographic factors in general	0	1	1
Further Indicators	0	4	4

Indicator category	National Projects	European Projects	Total
Denmark			
Indicators on Food and Nutrient Intake in general	2	8	10
Vitamins	0	3	3
Mineral Content	0	2	2
Energy	2	3	5
Indicators on Alcohol in general	0	8	8
Indicators on Nutritional Status in general	0	2	2
Indicators on Anthropometry/ Body Composition in general	0	5	5
Body mass index (bmi)	0	5	5
Indicators on Physical Activity levels and patterns in general	1	8	9
Indicators on Socio-demographic factors in general	1	4	5
Further Indicators	2	8	10

(continued)

Table 9 (continued)

Indicator category	National Projects	European Projects	Total
Estonia			
Indicators on Food and Nutrient Intake in general	2	4	6
Energy	0	1	1
Indicators on Alcohol in general	2	5	7
Indicators on Breastfeeding in general	1	0	1
Indicators on Anthropometry/ Body Composition in general	3	2	5
Indicators on Physical Activity levels and patterns in general	3	4	7
Indicators on Socio-demographic factors in general	3	1	4
Further Indicators	2	5	7

Indicator category	National Projects	European Projects	Total
Finland			
Indicators on Food and Nutrient Intake in general	5	9	14
Vitamins	2	2	4
Mineral Content	2	2	4
Energy	4	4	8
Indicators on Alcohol in general	5	10	15
Indicators on Nutritional Status in general	1	1	2
Indicators on Anthropometry/ Body Composition in general	3	4	7
Indicators on Physical Activity levels and patterns in general	4	7	11
Indicators on Socio-demographic factors in general	4	4	8
Further Indicators	5	8	13

Indicator category	National Projects	European Projects	Total
France			
Indicators on Food and Nutrient Intake in general	1	12	13
Vitamins	0	4	4
Mineral Content	0	3	3
Energy	0	5	5
Indicators on Alcohol in general	0	12	12
Indicators on Nutritional Status in general	0	2	2
Indicators on Anthropometry/ Body Composition in general	0	7	7
Indicators on Physical Activity levels and patterns in general	0	9	9
Indicators on Health Related Fitness in general	0	1	1
Indicators on Socio-demographic factors in general	0	6	6
Further Indicators	0	10	10

(continued)

Table 9 (continued)

Indicator category	National Projects	European Projects	Total
Germany			
Indicators on Food and Nutrient Intake in general	22	11	33
Vitamins	11	4	15
Mineral Content	12	4	16
Energy	15	5	21
Indicators on Alcohol in general	18	12	30
Indicators on Breastfeeding in general	3	0	3
Indicators on Nutritional Status in general	9	2	11
Indicators on Anthropometry/ Body Composition in general	18	8	26
Indicators on Physical Activity levels and patterns in general	21	10	31
Indicators on Health Related Fitness in general	0	1	1
Indicators on Socio-demographic factors in general	26	6	32
Indicators on Health Promotion in general	6	0	6
Further Indicators	24	9	33

Indicator category	National Projects	European Projects	Total
Greece			
Indicators on Food and Nutrient Intake in general	5	10	15
Vitamins	0	4	4
Mineral Content	0	3	3
Energy	0	4	4
Indicators on Alcohol in general	2	11	13
Indicators on Nutritional Status in general	1	2	3
Indicators on Anthropometry/ Body Composition in general	3	6	9
Indicators on Physical Activity levels and patterns in general	5	7	12
Indicators on Health Related Fitness in general	0	1	1
Indicators on Socio-demographic factors in general	4	6	10
Further Indicators	3	9	12

Indicator category	National Projects	European Projects	Total
Hungary			
Indicators on Food and Nutrient Intake in general	3	11	14
Vitamins	0	4	4
Mineral Content	0	3	3
Energy	1	5	6
Indicators on Alcohol in general	3	13	16
Indicators on Nutritional Status in general	0	2	2
Indicators on Anthropometry/ Body Composition in general	2	7	9
Indicators on Physical Activity levels and patterns in general	3	8	11
Indicators on Health Related Fitness in general	0	1	1
Indicators on Socio-demographic factors in general	3	5	8
Indicators on Inequality in general	3	2	5
Further Indicators	2	9	11

(continued)

Table 9 (continued)

Indicator category	National Projects	European Projects	Total
Iceland			
Indicators on Food and Nutrient Intake in general	0	5	5
Vitamins	0	1	1
Mineral Content	0	1	1
Energy	0	1	1
Indicators on Alcohol in general	0	5	5
Indicators on Anthropometry/ Body Composition in general	0	2	2
Indicators on Physical Activity levels and patterns in general	0	4	4
Indicators on Socio-demographic factors in general	0	2	2
Further Indicators	0	5	5

Indicator category	National Projects	European Projects	Total
Ireland			
Indicators on Food and Nutrient Intake in general	1	7	8
Vitamins	0	1	1
Mineral Content	0	1	1
Energy	0	1	1
Indicators on Alcohol in general	1	8	9
Indicators on Anthropometry/ Body Composition in general	0	3	3
Indicators on Physical Activity levels and patterns in general	0	4	4
Indicators on Socio-demographic factors in general	0	5	5
Further Indicators	1	8	9

Indicator category	National Projects	European Projects	Total
Italy			
Indicators on Food and Nutrient Intake in general	5	13	18
Vitamins	1	4	5
Mineral Content	0	3	3
Energy	1	6	7
Indicators on Alcohol in general	4	13	17
Indicators on Nutritional Status in general	1	2	3
Indicators on Anthropometry/ Body Composition in general	2	7	9
Indicators on Physical Activity levels and patterns in general	6	9	15
Indicators on Health Related Fitness in general	0	1	1
Indicators on Socio-demographic factors in general	4	6	10
Further Indicators	7	10	17

(continued)

Table 9 (continued)

Indicator category	National Projects	European Projects	Total
Latvia			
Indicators on Food and Nutrient Intake in general	1	5	6
Energy	0	2	2
Indicators on Alcohol in general	1	6	7
Indicators on Anthropometry/ Body Composition in general	1	2	3
Indicators on Physical Activity levels and patterns in general	1	4	5
Indicators on Socio-demographic factors in general	1	1	2
Further Indicators	1	5	6

Indicator category	National Projects	European Projects	Total
Lithuania			
Indicators on Food and Nutrient Intake in general	2	10	12
Vitamins	1	2	3
Mineral Content	1	2	3
Energy	1	5	6
Indicators on Alcohol in general	1	10	11
Indicators on Nutritional Status in general	0	1	1
Indicators on Anthropometry/ Body Composition in general	2	5	7
Indicators on Physical Activity levels and patterns in general	3	7	10
Indicators on Socio-demographic factors in general	2	4	6
Further Indicators	1	8	9

Indicator category	National Projects	European Projects	Total
Luxembourg			
Indicators on Food and Nutrient Intake in general	0	4	4
Indicators on Alcohol in general	0	4	4
Indicators on Anthropometry/ Body Composition in general	0	3	3
Indicators on Physical Activity levels and patterns in general	0	3	3
Indicators on Socio-demographic factors in general	0	3	3
Further Indicators	0	5	5

Indicator category	National Projects	European Projects	Total
Macedonia			
Indicators on Food and Nutrient Intake in general	2	1	3
Indicators on Alcohol in general	0	1	1
Indicators on Nutritional Status in general	2	1	3
Indicators on Anthropometry/ Body Composition in general	4	0	4
Indicators on Physical Activity levels and patterns in general	5	0	5
Indicators on Socio-demographic factors in general	1	1	2
Indicators on Health Promotion in general	1	0	1
Further Indicators	3	1	4

(continued)

Table 9 (continued)

Indicator category	National Projects	European Projects	Total
Malta			
Indicators on Food and Nutrient Intake in general	0	4	4
Energy	0	1	1
Indicators on Alcohol in general	0	5	5
Indicators on Anthropometry/ Body Composition in general	0	2	2
Indicators on Physical Activity levels and patterns in general	0	3	3
Indicators on Socio-demographic factors in general	0	1	1
Further Indicators	0	4	4

Indicator category	National Projects	European Projects	Total
Norway			
Indicators on Food and Nutrient Intake in general	11	9	20
Vitamins	0	3	3
Mineral Content	0	2	2
Energy	10	3	13
Indicators on Alcohol in general	12	9	21
Indicators on Nutritional Status in general	6	2	8
Indicators on Anthropometry/ Body Composition in general	7	4	11
Indicators on Physical Activity levels and patterns in general	11	6	17
Indicators on Socio-demographic factors in general	9	5	14
Further Indicators	12	8	20

Indicator category	National Projects	European Projects	Total
Poland			
Indicators on Food and Nutrient Intake in general	0	8	8
Vitamins	0	2	2
Mineral Content	0	1	1
Energy	0	3	3
Indicators on Alcohol in general	0	9	9
Indicators on Nutritional Status in general	0	1	1
Indicators on Anthropometry/ Body Composition in general	0	3	3
Indicators on Physical Activity levels and patterns in general	0	5	5
Indicators on Socio-demographic factors in general	0	3	3
Further Indicators	0	7	7

(continued)

Table 9 (continued)

Indicator category	National Projects	European Projects	Total
Portugal			
Indicators on Food and Nutrient Intake in general	1	11	12
Vitamins	0	2	2
Mineral Content	0	1	1
Energy	0	3	3
Indicators on Alcohol in general	1	11	12
Indicators on Nutritional Status in general	0	2	2
Indicators on Anthropometry/ Body Composition in general	1	5	6
Indicators on Physical Activity levels and patterns in general	2	8	10
Indicators on Socio-demographic factors in general	2	7	9
Further Indicators	0	11	11

Indicator category	National Projects	European Projects	Total
Romania			
Indicators on Food and Nutrient Intake in general	5	7	12
Vitamins	1	1	2
Mineral Content	0	1	1
Energy	4	2	6
Indicators on Alcohol in general	5	6	11
Indicators on Breastfeeding in general	1	0	1
Indicators on Nutritional Status in general	4	2	6
Indicators on Anthropometry/ Body Composition in general	6	3	9
Indicators on Physical Activity levels and patterns in general	5	3	8
Indicators on Health Related Fitness in general	1	0	1
Indicators on Socio-demographic factors in general	7	4	11
Indicators on Health Promotion in general	1	0	1
Further Indicators	7	7	14

Indicator category	National Projects	European Projects	Total
Slovakia			
Indicators on Food and Nutrient Intake in general	0	5	5
Vitamins	0	1	1
Mineral Content	0	1	1
Energy	0	2	2
Indicators on Alcohol in general	0	6	6
Indicators on Anthropometry/ Body Composition in general	0	2	2
Indicators on Physical Activity levels and patterns in general	0	3	3
Indicators on Socio-demographic factors in general	0	1	1
Further Indicators	0	4	4

(continued)

Table 9 (continued)

Indicator category	National Projects	European Projects	Total
Slovenia			
Indicators on Food and Nutrient Intake in general	2	4	6
Energy	1	1	2
Indicators on Alcohol in general	2	5	7
Indicators on Nutritional Status in general	1	0	1
Indicators on Anthropometry/ Body Composition in general	2	2	4
Indicators on Physical Activity levels and patterns in general	2	3	5
Indicators on Health Related Fitness in general	1	0	1
Indicators on Socio-demographic factors in general	2	1	3
Further Indicators	2	4	6

Indicator category	National Projects	European Projects	Total
Spain			
Indicators on Food and Nutrient Intake in general	5	14	19
Vitamins	3	4	7
Mineral Content	1	3	4
Energy	2	6	8
Indicators on Alcohol in general	5	12	17
Indicators on Nutritional Status in general	1	2	3
Indicators on Anthropometry/ Body Composition in general	5	7	12
Indicators on Physical Activity levels and patterns in general	5	10	15
Indicators on Health Related Fitness in general	0	1	1
Indicators on Socio-demographic factors in general	5	7	12
Further Indicators	5	10	15

Indicator category	National Projects	European Projects	Total
Sweden			
Indicators on Food and Nutrient Intake in general	4	8	12
Vitamins	2	2	4
Mineral Content	2	2	4
Energy	5	3	8
Indicators on Alcohol in general	3	8	11
Indicators on Nutritional Status in general	0	1	1
Indicators on Anthropometry/ Body Composition in general	3	4	7
Indicators on Physical Activity levels and patterns in general	4	7	11
Indicators on Socio-demographic factors in general	5	4	9
Further Indicators	6	8	14

(continued)

Table 9 (continued)

Indicator category	National Projects	European Projects	Total
The Netherlands			
Indicators on Food and Nutrient Intake in general	6	8	14
Vitamins	3	2	5
Mineral Content	3	1	4
Energy	5	3	8
Indicators on Alcohol in general	8	7	15
Indicators on Breastfeeding in general	2	0	2
Indicators on Nutritional Status in general	1	1	2
Indicators on Anthropometry/ Body Composition in general	7	5	12
Indicators on Physical Activity levels and patterns in general	9	8	17
Indicators on Health Related Fitness in general	1	0	1
Indicators on Socio-demographic factors in general	10	4	14
Indicators on Inequality in general	1	0	1
Further Indicators	9	8	17

Indicator category	National Projects	European Projects	Total
Turkey			
Indicators on Food and Nutrient Intake in general	1	3	4
Indicators on Alcohol in general	1	4	5
Indicators on Breastfeeding in general	1	0	1
Indicators on Nutritional Status in general	1	0	1
Indicators on Anthropometry/ Body Composition in general	4	2	6
Indicators on Physical Activity levels and patterns in general	4	3	7
Indicators on Socio-demographic factors in general	4	1	5
Indicators on Inequality in general	2	0	2
Indicators on Health Promotion in general	1	0	1
Further Indicators	2	4	6

Indicator category	National Projects	European Projects	Total
United Kingdom			
Indicators on Food and Nutrient Intake in general	3	14	17
Vitamins	0	4	4
Mineral Content	0	3	3
Energy	0	6	6
Indicators on Alcohol in general	4	13	17
Indicators on Breastfeeding in general	0	1	1
Indicators on Nutritional Status in general	2	2	4
Indicators on Anthropometry/ Body Composition in general	2	7	9
Indicators on Physical Activity levels and patterns in general	2	10	12
Indicators on Health Related Fitness in general	0	1	1
Indicators on Socio-demographic factors in general	3	6	9
Further Indicators	1	10	11

Table 10 Absolute frequency of used indicators in entered Projects by number of countries, separated by indicator categories

Indicator	Number of Countries		
	National Projects	European Projects	all Projects
Indicators on Food and Nutrient Intake in general	**24**	**32**	**32**
Consumption of vegetables	22	32	32
Availability of vegetables	5	15	17
Consumption of potatoes	16	25	29
Availability of potatoes	5	15	17
Consumption of vegetable juice	16	24	27
Availability of vegetable juice	2	15	16
Consumption of fruit	21	32	32
Availability of fruit	4	15	16
Consumption of fruit juice	16	25	27
Availability of fruit juice	2	15	15
Consumption of drinks	17	31	31
Availability of drinks	4	15	16
Consumption of meat and meat products	20	31	31
Availability of meat and meat products	5	15	17
Consumption of fish	19	31	31
Availability of fish	4	15	16
Consumption of carbohydrates	16	30	30
Availability of carbohydrates	1	14	14
Non-starch polysaccharides (nsp) content of the typical diet	7	15	19
Consumption of milk	17	31	31
Availability of milk	3	15	16
Consumption of milk products	16	21	23
Availability of milk products	2	15	15
Consumption of salt	14	20	21
Availability of salt	0	15	15
Consumption of sweets (incl. fast food and chips)	16	30	30
Availability of sweets (incl. fast food and chips)	2	12	12
Saturated fatty acids content of the typical diet	14	30	30
Mono-unsaturated fatty acids content of the typical diet	12	29	29
Polyunsaturated fatty acids content of the typical diet	12	29	29

(continued)

Table 10 (continued)

Indicator	Number of Countries		
	National Projects	European Projects	all Projects
Vitamins	**11**	**23**	**24**
Vitamin content of the typical diet: vitamin C	9	17	18
Vitamin content of the typical diet: vitamin D	7	22	23
Vitamin content of the typical diet: vitamin E	8	15	17
Vitamin content of the typical diet: folate	7	23	24
Vitamin content of the typical diet: carotenoids	7	17	18

Indicator	Number of Countries		
	National Projects	European Projects	all Projects
Mineral Content	**9**	**23**	**24**
Mineral content of the typical diet: Fe	8	22	23
Mineral content of the typical diet: I	6	23	24
Mineral content of the typical diet: Ca	8	15	17
Mineral content of the typical diet: Se	6	14	17

Indicator	Number of Countries		
	National Projects	European Projects	all Projects
Energy	**15**	**29**	**29**
Energy intake	9	28	28
Food frequency	12	6	15
Energy density	4	9	12

Indicator	Number of Countries		
	National Projects	European Projects	all Projects
Indicators on Alcohol in general	**21**	**32**	**32**
Total alcohol consumption	20	31	31
The share of total alcohol consumption consumed with meals	2	0	2
The contribution of alcohol to energy intake	3	14	15

(continued)

Table 10 (continued)

Indicator	Number of Countries		
	National Projects	European Projects	all Projects
Indicators on Breastfeeding in general	**6**	**1**	**7**
Duration of breastfeeding at 6 months of age	4	1	5
Quality of breastfeeding exclusive breastfeeding rates at 6 or more months of age	3	0	3

Indicator	Number of Countries		
	National Projects	European Projects	all Projects
Indicators on Anthropometry/ Body Composition in general	**21**	**30**	**31**
Body mass index (bmi)	20	30	31
Waist circumfence	11	10	17
Waist-to-hip ratio (whr)	7	10	15

Indicator	Number of Countries		
	National Projects	European Projects	all Projects
Indicators on Physical Activity levels and patterns in general	**22**	**31**	**32**
Time (mins/ day or week) spent at health enhancing physical activity, i.e. at moderate intensity levels	15	30	30
Time (mins/ day or week) spent at health enhancing physical activity, i.e. at vigorous intensity levels	15	30	30
Sedentary behaviour	14	30	30

Indicator	Number of Countries		
	National Projects	European Projects	all Projects
Indicators on Socio-demographic factors in general	**22**	**31**	**31**
Educational level, population by educational class: elementary	19	21	25
Educational level, population by educational class: lower secondary	19	20	24
Educational level, population by educational class: upper secondary	19	20	24
Educational level, population by educational class: tertiary	19	20	24

(continued)

Table 10 (continued)

Indicator	Number of Countries		
	National Projects	European Projects	all Projects
Occupation; population by occupational class: upper non-manual	14	18	22
Occupation; population by occupational class: lower non-manual	14	18	22
Occupation; population by occupational class: skilled manual	15	18	23
Occupation; population by occupational class: unskilled manual	15	19	24
Occupation; population by occupational class: self employed	14	19	23
Occupation; population by occupational class: farmer	14	19	23
Total unemployed	12	19	23
The percentage of population long term unemployed, more than 12 month	5	0	5
Population below poverty line (with income below 60% of the national median)	7	0	7
Household income as the percentage of households with a total income below 50% of the median income of the country	5	16	19
Household income as the number of households with income in the lowest 5%	5	16	19
The percentage of households with income below budget standards	12	16	22

Indicator	Number of Countries		
	National Projects	European Projects	all Projects
Further Indicators	**21**	**32**	**32**
Fast Food	9	7	14
Leisure Activity	14	32	32
Workplace Activity	8	16	18
Sleep	7	13	15
TV/PC Consumption	6	30	30
Ethnicity	8	17	19
Obesity related metabolic disorders	8	1	9
Eating disorders	4	0	4
Eating behaviour	13	6	13
Malnutrition	5	1	6

10.3. Project Identity Cards: European Projects

European Nutrition and Health Report

Project Leader

Project Leader	Ibrahim Elmadfa
Address	Althanstraße14
	AT - 1090 Vienna
Executing Institution	Institute of Nutritional Sciences,
	University of Vienna
Funding Agency	European Commission

Project Information

Start of Project	01/10/2002
End of Project	01/10/2004
Start of Data Collection	01/10/2002
End of Data Collection	01/10/2004
URL	
Scope	European

Keywords[1]

Abstract (English) Nutrition reports are the most important tool for the accurate documentation of population's nutritional status, the identification of groups at risk for developing nutrition-related disorders, and the longitudinal monitoring of nutrition-related factors. Several European countries are issuing national nutrition reports. The European Nutrition and Health Report will collect all relevant data, which is available from the participating countries and convert them when necessary to a consolidated European Report as a basis for future activities on the field of public health and nutrition.

The report will deliver information on the development of food consumption during the past decades and nutrient intake on population group level, and – where possible – the nutritional status on the individual level. The report will also deal with current food quality/safety issues

Abstract (Original Language)

Age Groups

Vary from country to country. From children aged 2 years to people older than 85 years

---

[1] Sections for which no information was provided by the partner were left blank.

Countrywide Integrated Noncommunicable Disease Intervention

CINDI

Project Leader

Project Leader	Aushra Shatchkute
Address	The CINDI Programme
	WHO Regional Office for Europe
	Scherfigsvej 8
	2100 Copenhagen
	Denmark
Executing Institution	
Funding Agency	WHO

Project Information

Start of Project	07/09/1990
End of Project	07/09/1993
Start of Data Collection	07/09/1990
End of Data Collection	07/09/1990
URL	http://www.euro.who.int/CINDI
Scope	European

Keywords Noncommunicable disease control; Health policy; Health plan implementation; Europe

Abstract (English) The aim of CINDI programme is to support member states in developing integrated policies for noncommunicable disease prevention by combining health promotion and disease prevention through intersectorial collaboration and community involvement, enhancing the role of health professionals, and making better use of existing resources.

Abstract (Original Language)

Age Groups

6	75

Estonian Family and Fertility Survey

Estonian ffs

Project Leader

Project Leader	Kalev Katus
Address	P.O. Box 3012 10504, Tallinn
	Estonia
Executing Institution	Estonian Demographic Association, Estonian
	Demographic Institute
Funding Agency	Coordinated: UN ECE 1990s European FFS, 2000s
	Gender and Generation Survey

Project Information

Start of Project	
End of Project	
Start of Data Collection	24/09/2006
End of Data Collection	24/09/2006
URL	
Scope	European

Keywords

Abstract (English)

Abstract (Original Language)

Age Groups

FINBALT Health Monitor

Finbalt

Project Leader

Project Leader	Ritva Prättälä
Address	National Public Health Institute
	Department of Epidemiology and Health Promotion
	Mannerheimintie 166
	FIN-00300 Helsinki
	Finland
Executing Institution	Department of Epidemiology and Health Promotion, National Public Health Institute
Funding Agency	

Project Information

Start of Project	
End of Project	
Start of Data Collection	
End of Data Collection	
URL	http://www.ktl.fi/portal/english/osiot/research,_people___pro grams/epidemiology_and_health_promotion/projects/finbalt/
Scope	European

Keywords

Abstract (English) Monitoring health and health-related lifestyles is essential for planning and evaluation of health promotion and disease prevention programmes as well as health care reform implementation processes. A decade ago, Lithuania joined international health behavior monitoring project (FINBALT HEALTH MONITOR), which together with other Baltic states was launched as an initiative from National Public Health Institute of Finland. In Lithuania, this project has developed into national health behavior monitoring programme that is a part of the State Public Health Monitoring Programme. In Finland such a system is in operation since 1978. In Estonia, health behavior surveys have been conducted since 1990 and in Latvia since 1998. Common project protocol is strictly followed and standardised questionnaire is used in implementing this international project. Joint database has been established accumulating information collected, the analysis involving all countries is being performed presenting results in joint publications.

The success of and experience gained in FINBALT HEALTH MONITOR was adopted by Countrywide Integrated Noncommunicable Diseases Intervention (CINDI) Programme coordinated by the World Health Organization. In 2001–2002, health behavior surveys were conducted in 26 CINDI countries. This was how FINBALT HEALTH MONITOR developed into CINDI HEALTH MONITOR becoming part of process evaluation of CINDI performance.

Abstract (Original Language)

Age Groups

20	24
25	34
35	44
45	54
55	64

European Prospective Investigation into Cancer and Nutrition

EPIC

Project Leader

Project Leader	Dr. Paul Kleihuues
Address	150, cours Albert Thomas
	FR - 69372 Lyon Cedex 08
Executing Institution	International Agency for Research on Cancer
Funding Agency	EU

Project Information

Start of Project	01/09/2002
End of Project	01/09/2003
Start of Data Collection	01/09/2002
End of Data Collection	01/09/2003
URL	http://www.iarc.fr/epic
Scope	European

Keywords

Abstract (English) EPIC was designed to investigate the relationships between diet, nutritional status, lifestyle, and environmental factors and the incidence of cancer and other chronic diseases. EPIC is the largest study of diet and health ever undertaken, having recruited over half a million (520,000) people in ten European countries: Denmark, France, Germany, Greece, Italy, The Netherlands, Norway, Spain, Sweden, and the United Kingdom.

Within these countries, EPIC research scientists are based in 23 centers: one in France (Paris), Greece (Athens), and Norway (Tromsø), two in Denmark (Aarhus and Copenhagen), Germany (Heidelberg and Potsdam), Sweden (Malmo and Umea), the Netherlands (Bilthoven and Utrecht), and the United Kingdom (Cambridge and Oxford), five in Italy (Florence, Milan, Naples, Ragusa, and Turin) and Spain (Granada, Murcia, Asturias, Pamplona, and San Sebastian with Barcelona the coordination center). Originally, there were seven countries involved but between 1995 and 2000 Sweden, Denmark and Norway, which were already involved in similar studies, joined EPIC and thus broadened the European cohort to include Scandinavian populations.

Recruitment into the study, which was initiated in 1992, was principally from the general population aged 20 years or over, and took place between 1993 and 1999. Detailed information on diet and lifestyle was obtained by questionnaire, and anthropometric measurements and blood samples were taken at recruitment. The blood is stored in liquid nitrogen for future analyses. By studying very many people in different countries with differing diets, using carefully designed and tested questionnaires, EPIC should produce much more specific information about the effect of diet on long-term health than any previous study. The first results were presented in June 2001 at the European Conference on Nutrition and Cancer. It is planned to follow-up the study participants for the next 10 years at least, continuing to study the role of nutrition and lifestyle in cancer development and other chronic diseases.

In September 2001 the 5 A Day Initiative project, under the auspices of the German Cancer Society in Frankfurt, Germany entered into a collaborative research agreement with the EPIC study.

Abstract (Original Language)

Age Groups

Health Indicators in the European Regions

ISARE

Project Leader

Project Leader	André Ochoa
Address	62, Boulevard Garibaldi
	F-75015
	Paris
Executing Institution	FNORS (Fédération Nationale des
	Observatoires Régionauxde la Santé)
Funding Agency	EU

Project Information

Start of Project	15/09/1999
End of Project	15/09/2004
Start of Data Collection	15/09/2006
End of Data Collection	15/09/2006
URL	http://www.isare.org
Scope	European

Keywords Health Monitoring Programme; Health indicators; European Commission; European regions

Abstract (English) The Isare project was carried out on the initiative of the Fédération Nationale des Observatoires Régionaux de Santé (FNORS) within the framework of the Health Monitoring Programme from European Commission. The first phase, Isare I (1999–2001), made it possible to identify for each country, the most appropriate subnational level ("health region") for the exchange of health indicators within the European Union and to assess the extent of data availability at those levels. The second phase, Isare II (2002–2004), made it possible to test the feasibility of collecting regional data in each European country.

Abstract (Original Language)

Age Groups

European Physical Activity Surveillance System

EUPASS

Project Leader

Project Leader	Alfred Rütten
Address	Strasse der Nationen 62
	D-09111 Chemnitz
Executing Institution	Technische Universität Dresden
Funding Agency	EU DG Sanco

Project Information

Start of Project	01/10/1999
End of Project	31/12/2000
Start of Data Collection	01/10/1999
End of Data Collection	31/12/2000
URL	http://www.ipaq.ki.se/IPAQ.asp?mnu_sel=IIA&pg_sel=FFG
Scope	European

Keywords Physical activity; Measurement; Public health; International comparison; Monitoring; Indicator testing

Abstract (English) The purpose of the International Physical Activity Questionnaires (IPAQ) is to provide a set of well-developed instruments that can be used internationally to obtain comparable estimates of physical activity. There are two versions of the questionnaire. The short version is suitable for use in national and regional surveillance systems and the long version provide more detailed information often required in research work or for evaluation purposes.

The public health burden of a sedentary lifestyle has been recognised globally, but until recently, the prevalence and impact of the problem has not been studied in a uniform and systematic fashion. The questionnaire is the most feasible instrument for measuring physical activity in large groups or populations. However, many of the existing instruments are not comparable in the type of activities surveyed (i.e., leisure-time activities only) and format for data collection.

In response to the global demand for comparable and valid measures of physical activity within and between countries, IPAQ was developed for surveillance activities and to guide policy development related to health-enhancing physical activity across various life domains.

Abstract (Original Language)

Age Groups

European Prospective Investigation into Cancer and Nutrition (EPIC)-Potsdam-Studie

EPIC-Potsdam-Studie

Project Leader

Project Leader	Prof. Dr. Heiner Boeing
Address	Deutsches Institut für Ernährungsforschung
	Potsdam-Rehbrücke (DIFE)
	Arthur-Scheunert-Allee 114-116
	14558 Nuthetal
	Deutschland
Executing Institution	Deutsches Institut für Ernährungsforschung
	Potsdam-Rehbrücke (DIfE), Abteilung Epidemiologie
Funding Agency	

Project Information

Start of Project	01/01/1994
End of Project	
Start of Data Collection	01/01/1994
End of Data Collection	01/01/1998
URL	http://www.dife.de/de/index.php?request=/de/forschung/projekte/epic.php
Scope	European

Keywords

Abstract (English) The European Prospective Investigation into Cancer and Nutrition (EPIC)-Potsdam-Study is part of a European cohort study with about 521,000 study participants. The study was designed to investigate the relationships between diet, nutritional status, lifestyle, environmental factors, and the incidence of cancer and other chronic diseases. EPIC was initiated in 1994 and is conducted as a long-term study with an observation period of about 20 years.

Abstract (Original Language) Die European Prospective Investigation into Cancer and Nutrition (EPIC)-Potsdam-Studie ist Teil einer europäischen Kohortenstudie mit insgesamt ca. 521 000 Studienteilnehmern. Ziel ist, den Einfluss der Ernährung auf die Entstehung von Krebs und andere chronische Erkrankungen zu erforschen. Die 1994 begonnene EPIC-Potsdam-Studie ist als Langzeitstudie mit einer Nachbeobachtungszeit von 20 Jahren konzipiert worden.

Age Groups

35	64
40	64

Health Behaviour in School-Aged Children 2001/2002

HBSC 2001/2002

Project Leader

Project Leader	Prof. Klaus Hurrelmann
Address	Universität Bielefeld
	Fakultät für Gesundheitswissenschaften
	WHO Collaborating Centre for Child and Adolescent Health Promotion
	Postfach 10 01 31
	33501 Bielefeld
Executing Institution	Fakultät für Gesundheitswissenschaften, Universität Bielefeld
Funding Agency	

Project Information

Start of Project	01/01/1994
End of Project	
Start of Data Collection	01/02/2002
End of Data Collection	31/05/2002
URL	http://www.hbsc-germany.de/
Scope	European

Keywords Health behavior; Youth; Comparison; International; Prevention; Health promotion; Alcohol consumption; Nutrition questions; Sport; Smoking

Abstract (English) Health Behavior in School-aged Children (HBSC) is a cross-national research study conducted in collaboration with the WHO Regional Office for Europe. The study is carried out at four-year intervals.

There are 35 nations from Europe and North America who participate at the study. In Germany, there are five States who participate.

Using a questionnaire young people attending school, aged 9 till 17-years-old were asked about their health behavior.

The study aims to gain new insight into, and increase our understanding of young people's health and well-being, health behaviors, and their social context.

Furthermore, the study results deliver insight the health situation of children and youth with a view to national as well as international comparison.

Abstract (Original Language) Die Studie ist Teil eines international vergleichenden Forschungsvorhabens "Health Behaviour in School-aged Children (HBSC)", welches alle vier Jahre unter Schirmherrschaft der Weltgesundheitsorganisation (WHO) durchgeführt wird.

An der Studie nehmen 35 Staaten aus Europa und Nordamerika teil. In Deutschland sind insgesamt sechs Bundesländer beteiligt.

Mit Hilfe eines Fragebogens werden Schülerinnen und Schüler im Alter von 9–17 Jahren zum Gesundheitsverhalten im Kindes- und Jugendalter befragt.

Um welche Themen geht es:

- Gesundheitszustand
- Lebenszufriedenheit und Lebensqualität
- Psychisches Wohlbefinden
- Körperliche Aktivität
- Ernährung und Essverhalten
- Schule und Unterricht
- Freizeitverhalten
- Soziale Unterstützung in der Familie und im Freundeskreis
- Unfälle
- Mobbing
- Risikoverhalten (Alkohol, Rauchen, etc.)

Was sind die Ziele?

In der Studie sollen die Beziehungen zwischen dem Gesundheitsverhalten und der subjektiv berichteten Gesundheit von Kindern und Jugendlichen im Alter von 9 bis 17 Jahren untersucht werden. Dabei wird ein besonderer Schwerpunkt auf die Identifikation von Präventionsmöglichkeiten in dieser Altersklasse gelegt.

Weiterhin geben die Ergebnisse Auskunft über die gesundheitliche Lage von Kindern und Jugendlichen im nationalen und internationalen Vergleich.

Age Groups

Adolescents aged 11, 13, and 15

Statistisches Jahrbuch 2006

Project Leader

Project Leader	
Address	Statistisches Bundesamt
	Gustav-Stresemann Ring 11
	65189 Wiesbaden
Executing Institution	Statistisches Bundesamt
Funding Agency	

Project Information

Start of Project	
End of Project	
Start of Data Collection	
End of Data Collection	
URL	http://www.destatis.de/jahrbuch/
Scope	European

Keywords Statistic; Yearbook; Population development; Health care; Education; School; Culture; University; Religion; Judiciary; Occupation; Economy; Professional association; Habitation; Social contribution; Public; Economics; Ecology

Abstract (English) The Statistical Yearbook 2006 consists of two volumes: the Statistical Yearbook 2006 for the Federal Republic of Germany and the International Statistical Yearbook.

The Statistical Yearbook 2006 for the Federal Republic of Germany is the classic among the publications of the Federal Statistical Office. It is the most comprehensive statistical reference book on the German market. Since 55 years, this statistical report of the nation's situation compiled essential data from all spheres of life, work, and business in Germany and abroad.

Abstract (Original Language) Das Statistische Jahrbuch besteht aus zwei Bänden: Dem Statistischen Jahrbuch für die Bundesrepublik Deutschland und dem Statistischen Jahrbuch für das Ausland.

Das Statistische Jahrbuch 2006 für die Bundesrepublik Deutschland ist der "Klassiker" unter den Publikationen des Statistischen Bundesamtes. Es ist das umfassendste statistische Nachschlagewerk auf dem deutschen Markt. Seit nunmehr 55 Jahren enthält dieser "statistische Bericht zur Lage der Nation" einen vollständigen Überblick über die Verhältnisse in Deutschland.

Age Groups

Data Food Networking

DAFNE

Project Leader

Project Leader	Prof. A. Trichopolou (Coordinator)
Address	Mikras Asias 75, Goudi
	Athens, 11527
Executing Institution	Public Health Nutrition and Nutritional Epidemiology Unit,
	Department of Hygiene and Epidemiology, Medical School,
	University of Athens
Funding Agency	European Union

Project Information

Start of Project	01/01/1990
End of Project	31/12/2006
Start of Data Collection	
End of Data Collection	
URL	http://www.nut.uoa.gr/english/
Scope	European

Keywords

Abstract (English) Since 1990, Greece has been coordinating the Data Food Networking (DAFNE) initiative, which refers to a joint effort of European countries to compare the food habits of their populations and monitor overtime trends in food availability, through the creation of a nonstatic, regularly-updated food databank. The overall aim is the development of a nutrition monitoring tool that could assist the formulation, implementation, and evaluation of nutritional policies across Europe. The DAFNE databank is based on information collected in the context of household budget surveys (HBS). HBS are periodically conducted by the National Statistical Offices of most European countries in country-representative samples of households. The DAFNE initiative is already in its fifth stage, which ends at the end of 2006.

Abstract (Original Language) Από τις αρχές της δεκαετίας του 1990, η Ελλάδα συντονίζει το χρηματοδοτούμενο από την Ευρωπαϊκή Ενωση πρόγραμμα, DAFNE (DAta Food NEtworking), που στοχεύει στη διαχρονική παρακολούθηση και σύγκριση των διατροφικών συνηθειών των Ευρωπαϊκών πληθυσμών με τη δημιουργι'α μι'ας δυναμικη'ς και διαρκω'ς εμπλουτιζο'μενης βα' σης δεδομε' νων. Η βάση δεδομένων DAFNE περιλαμβάνει επεξεργασμένα στοιχεία των Ερευνών Οικογενειακών Προϋ πολογισμών (ΕΟΠ). Οι ΕΟΠ διενεργούνται σε τακτά χρονικά διαστήματα από τις Εθνικές Στατιστικές Υπηρεσίες των περισσότερων Ευρωπαϊκών χωρών, με παραπλήσια μεθοδολογία, επιτρέποντας έτσι διακρατικές συγκρίσεις. Οι ΕΟΠ δεν έχουν ως πρωταρχικό στόχο τη συλλογή διατροφικών πληροφοριών, αλλά την καταγραφή των αγαθών και υπηρεσιών, που διατίθενται στα μέλη αντιπροσωπευτικού δείγματος νοικοκυριών κάθε χώρας. Εντούτοις, συλλέγοντας πληροφορίες για τις ποσότητες και αξίες των τροφίμων που είναι διαθέσιμα στο νοικοκυριό, αποτυπώνουν ικανοποιητικά τις διατροφικές επιλογές ενός αντιπροσωπευτικού δείγματος του πληθυσμού. Παράλληλα, η ταυτόχρονη καταγραφή δημογραφικών και κοινωνικο–οικονομικών χαρακτηριστικών επιτρέπει τη συνεκτίμηση της επίδρασης των χαρακτηριστικών αυτών στη διαμόρφωση των διατροφικών επιλογών.

Age Groups

The Household Budget Surveys are completed per family and information is selected for all memebers of the selected family

European Food Availability Databank Based on Household Budget Surveys

DAFNE

Project Leader

Project Leader	Antonia Trichopoulou
Address	University of Athens
	School of Medicine
	Dept.of Hygiene and Epidemiology
	75, M.Asias str., Athens 11527
	Greece
Executing Institution	University of Athens
Funding Agency	EU

Project Information

Start of Project	08/09/1997
End of Project	08/09/2006
Start of Data Collection	08/09/1980
End of Data Collection	08/09/1980
URL	http://www.nut.uoa.gr/dafnesoftweb/
Scope	European

Keywords Socio-economic data; Socio-demographic data; Household Budget Survey Europe

Abstract (English) The DAFNE initiative aims at creating a cost-effective European databank on the basis of the food, socio-economic, and demographic data from nationally representative Household Budget Surveys.

Abstract (Original Language)

Age Groups

The project involves families

Nutrition and Diet for Healthy Lifestyles in Europe

EURODIET

Project Leader

Project Leader	A.G. Kafatos
Address	School of Medicine, Preventive Medicine & Nutrition Unit, Heraklion Greece
Executing Institution	University of Crete
Funding Agency	the European Commission Directorate General for Health & Consumer Protection (Unit F/3), and the Ministry of Health Greece

Project Information

Start of Project	
End of Project	
Start of Data Collection	25/10/2006
End of Data Collection	25/10/2006
URL	http://eurodiet.med.uoc.gr/
Scope	European

Keywords

Abstract (English) The Eurodiet project was initiated in October 1998 with the aim to contribute toward a coordinated European Union (EU) and member state health promotion programme on nutrition, diet, and healthy lifestyles, by establishing a network, strategy, and action plan for the development of European dietary guidelines. The project has been supported by the European Commission (DG SANCO)[*] and coordinated by the University of Crete (Greece). Realisation of the project by the Eurodiet Steering Committee has entailed a two-year process (1998–2000) of scientific evaluation, consultation, and debate:

Four Working Parties composed of distinguished European academics analysed and evaluated the scientific evidence (1) on the links between health and nutrients (2) on the translation of nutrients to food-based guidelines, (3) on effective promotion of these foods and healthy lifestyles, and (4) on the opportunities and barriers posed by the broader policy framework. Throughout this process expert representatives from the spectrum of interests involved in this important area of public health have been invited to participate as observers in the meetings of the Steering Committee and of the Working Parties. This consultative base and the associated debate widened with the posting of the Working Party draft reports on the Eurodiet Web site (http://eurodiet.med.uoc.gr), and culminated with the European Conference held in Crete 18–20 May 2000 on Nutrition and Diet for Healthy Lifestyles in Europe: Science and Policy Implications.

This Core Report presents, in brief, the outcomes of this process. It is designed to give an overview to decision makers. The evidence and reference base for this core report are presented in two parts[**]: The Eurodiet proceedings, comprising the final reports of the Working Parties and the proceedings of the Eurodiet Conference. The scientific papers commissioned for the Eurodiet Working Party reports. These are designed for public policy advisers and others who wish to follow-up either general issues or specific topics in greater depth.

A strong theme of the Eurodiet project is the potentially enormous social and economic benefits to be gained from reducing the burden of nutritionally-related morbidity and mortality in Europe. The Eurodiet reports, which are concerned fundamentally with the realisation of these benefits, offer a significant contribution to the emergent debate on nutrition policy in Europe.

Abstract (Original Language)

Age Groups

The Data Food Networking

DAFNE

Project Leader

Project Leader	Antonia Trichopoulou
Address	Department of Hygiene and Epidemiology, School of Medicine, University of Athens, 75 Mikras Asias Str., GR-115 27 Athens Greece
Executing Institution	
Funding Agency	European Commission

Project Information

Start of Project	
End of Project	
Start of Data Collection	
End of Data Collection	
URL	http://www.nut.uoa.gr/english/dafne/DafneEN.htm
Scope	European

Keywords Household budget surveys; DAFNE; Dietary patterns; Disparities; Diet; Survey

Abstract (English) DAFNE is the acronym for Data Food Networking and aims at the creation of a pan-European food data bank on the basis of household budget surveys. The project was conceived in the early 1980s. On the one hand, it had long been recognised that the FAO food balance sheets data are a valuable resource for ascertaining trends of food availability over time, but are less satisfactory for intercountry comparisons. On the other hand, individual nutrition surveys, apart from being expensive and labor intensive, are frequently implemented with different methodologies and are regularly undertaken in a minority of the European countries. In 1987, a WHO workshop took place in Athens, Greece, and the proceedings were published in the European Journal of Clinical Nutrition. The participating scientists examined the possibilities offered by the household budget surveys (HBS) for the development of harmonised and comparable data between the European countries.

The DAFNE I project was supported by the European Commission's "Cooperation in Science and Technology with Central and Eastern European Countries" programme and by the COST 99 programme on Food Consumption and Composition Data. In the context of this project, raw nutritional data from HBS undertaken in comparable time periods were utilised. These data refer to households as the statistical unit and originally covered five European countries, namely Belgium, Germany, Greece, Hungary, and Poland. The methodology followed to derive comparable nutritional data for individuals, rather than households, as well as the results obtained through this process are presented in this Compendium as a show piece of the importance of this data source. DAFNE I documented the feasibility of the proposed approach and generated some important results that are briefly considered further on.

The DAFNE I data firmly document the remarkable disparity of food habits among European countries. The disparity has both qualitative and quantitative elements. In addition, there are important nutritional disparities among socioeconomic groups as defined by their educational level and permanent residence. Indeed, the distribution patterns of food availability provide new insight into the socioeconomic determinants of food preferences as conditioned by market forces. From the abundant information available in the DAFNE data bank, we have chosen – for the purposes of this publication – to concentrate on nine principal food groups: meat; fish, and seafood; total added lipids; fresh vegetables; total vegetables; fresh fruits; total fruits; alcoholic beverages; and nonalcoholic beverages. Average meat consumption exceeds 140 g per person per day and decreases as the level of education gets higher or one moves from the rural to the urban areas. Fish and seafood consumption is higher in Greece (39 g/person/day), followed by Belgium (27 g/person/day), whereas it is minimal in Hungary (5 g/person/day). In Belgium, more educated and urban residents have generally higher fish consumption. In Greece, there is no educational gradient; however, rural residents consume more fish and seafood, probably because of immediate availability in the costal areas and in the islands. Total added lipids cover both liquid oils, generally of vegetable origin, and solid or semisolid fat, either from animal sources or following industrial processing of vegetable oils (margarine). The distinction between the terms *fat* and *lipid* is particularly important for the olive oil consuming countries, because although olive oil is included in the total lipids, it is not a fat, which usually implies saturated fat. Thus, consumption of total added lipids is 90 g/person/day in Greece, 59 g/person/day in Poland, 53 g/person/day in Hungary, 45 g/person/day in Belgium, and 40 g/person/day in Germany. In all countries, however, there is a remarkable decrease in lipid consumption as the education level gets higher or one moves from the rural to the urban areas (a decrease that should have beneficial health effects for northern and central Europeans, but detrimental effects for the olive oil consumers). Segregation of total lipids into specific fats and oils is revealing. Butter availability is 26 g/person/day in Poland, 15 g/person/day in Germany, 3 g/person/day in Belgium, 3.5 g/person/day in Hungary, and 1.3 g/person/day only in Greece. Availability of other types of animal fat (e.g., lard) follows a different pattern: it is very high in Hungary (27 g/person/day), followed by Poland (16 g/personlday), Germany (1.6 g/person/day), Belgium (1.2 g/person/day), and Greece (0.1 g/person/day). Analysis of the data for vegetable oils reveals a striking peak for Greece at 82 ml/person/day, essentially from olive oil, with Hungary a distant second at 14 ml/person/day mostly from seed oils. The consumption of vegetable fat (mainly margarine) is higher in Belgium (22 g/person/day), followed by Germany (18 g/person/day), Poland (12 g/person/day), Hungary (7.5 g/person/day), and Greece (6.6 g/person/day). Vegetable fat consumption in Belgium shows a clear differentiation among the different socioeconomic groups, being high among the less educated (22 g/person/day) and lower among the more educated (16 g/person/day). For eggs, consumption varies little between and within countries and is about one egg every other day. For vegetables, consumption is highest in Greece with 268 g/person/day. Next come Poland with 202 g/person/day, Hungary with 201 g/person/day, Belgium with 162 g/person/day, and Germany with 143 g/person/day. However, the proportion of vegetables consumed fresh is 94% in Greece, 93% in Hungary, 87% in Poland, 64% in Belgium, and only 58% in Germany. This is interesting because it indicates that total vegetable consumption in a country does not necessarily represent the desirable intake of fresh vegetables. There are also subtle disparities by educational level and degree of urbanisation, reflecting different agroeconomic systems in different countries. For fruit availability, the pattern is similar to that for vegetables, with Greece having an overall fruit availability of 341 g/person/day (100% fresh), followed by Germany (236 g/person/day – 69% fresh), Belgium (198 g/person/day – 76% fresh), Hungary (159 g/person/day – 94% fresh), and Poland (100 g/person/day – 95% fresh). The higher availability of fruits among the urban households in all countries could be accounted for by market dynamics, good transportation systems, and, to some extent, under-reporting of fruit consumption at source by the rural population.

Consumption of alcoholic beverages reveals interesting patterns, although data were not available for Poland. Beer intake is very high in Germany (146 ml/person/day), followed by Belgium (82 ml/person/day), Hungary (43 ml/person/day), and Greece (18 ml/person/day), whereas intake of spirits is highest in Belgium (13 ml/person/day), followed by Germany (8 ml/person/day), Greece (5.8 ml/person/day), and Hungary (4.8 ml/person/day). Wine consumption is higher in German households (42 ml/person/day) and lower in Greek households (13 ml/person/day). However, it should be noted that in the Greek culture, wine is usually drank in taverns with friends rather than at home. The consumption of commercially available nonalcoholic beverages is a reflection of market penetration, which in turn depends on disposable income. Thus, consumption is very high in Belgium and Germany, very low in Hungary and Poland, with Greece occupying an intermediate position.

In the context of the DAFNE project, individual consumption estimates (one per family) have been used for the estimation of percentile values for food group distributions. Estimates were calculated for all households and for consuming households only. These quantities along with their corresponding confidence intervals are presented in tables and histograms by country. Thus, in Greece, one half of the population consume more than 258 g/person/day of fruits and one quarter of the population consume more than 469 g/person/day. For Belgium, the corresponding figures are 151 g/person/day and 265 g/person/day; for Germany 129 g/person/day and 259 g/person/day; for Hungary 93 g/person/day and 205 g/person/day; and for Poland 65 g/person/day and 129 g/person/day.

This presentation of the data is useful when the proportion of the population that meets the recommended daily intake needs to be determined. These results, along with others that appear in this compendium, suggest that large variation between countries and various socioeconomic groups within countries do exist. Nutrition is of paramount importance in disease prevention and health promotion. Therefore, these data could be valuable in the identification of groups at higher risk and in the planning of a rational food and nutrition policy.

Abstract (Original Language)

Age Groups

Health Behavior in School-Aged Children (Iskoláskorú gyermekek egészségmagatartása 2002)

HBSC Hungary 2002

Project Leader

Project Leader	Dr. Ágnes Németh
Address	Diószegi u
	1113 Budapest
	Hungary
Executing Institution	National Institute of Child Health
Funding Agency	WHO Collaborative study

Project Information

Start of Project	03/01/2001
End of Project	30/04/2002
Start of Data Collection	03/01/2002
End of Data Collection	30/04/2002
URL	http://www.hbsc.org/countries/hungary.html and www.ogyei.hu
Scope	European

Keywords Health behavior; Health survey

Abstract (English) Hungary joined the HBSC research programme in 1985. Since then there have been five representative data collections in Hungary: in 1985, 1990, 1993, 1997, and 2002. The research is based on data collection using anonymous questionnaires repeated about every four years. Research objectives are to monitor self-reported health, well-being, and health behaviour of adolescents (age 11–15 years, in Hungary 17 years, too). Topics from 2002: Nutrition, meals, diet, body-image; physical activity; time spent in physical inactivity: TV, computer, VCR, studying; Risk behaviour: smoking, alcohol, drugs; sexual behaviour; violence, accidents; Family: relationship, style of upbringing; Peers: relationships, leisure time activities; Health: perception of health, life satisfaction, symptoms of depression; School environment: relationship with school, teachers, peers, school rules; Social inequalities: parents' socio-economic situation.

Abstract (Original Language) Magyarország az Egészségügyi Világszervezet Európai Irodájának (EVSZ/EURO) kérésére 1985-ben csatlakozott a HBSC kutatáshoz. Magyarországon 5 országosan reprezentatív adatfelvétel történt: 1985-ben, 1990-ben, 1993-ban, 1997-ben és 2002-ben.

A kutatás négyévenként megismételt országosan reprezentatív, anonim módon végzett kérdoíves adatfelvételekbol áll. A serdülokorú (11–15 éves, Magyarországon a 17 évesek is) fiatalok önminosített egészségi állapotának, közérzetének és egészségmagatartásának monitorozása, és erre épülve megfelelo intézkedések tervezése és végrehajtása. A 2002-es vizsgálat témakörei: Táplálkozás: étkezési szokások, diéta, testkép; Fizikai aktivitás; Fizikailag passzív szabadidos tevékenységek (televízió, videó, számítógép) és tanulásra fordított ido; Rizikómagatartás: szerhasználat (dohányzás, alkohol, drogok); Szexuális magatartás; Eroszak és balesetek; Család: kapcsolatok és nevelési stílus; Kortársak: kapcsolatok, szabadido eltöltés; Egészség: egészség értékelése, élettel való elégedettség, panaszok, depresszióra jellemzo tünetek; Iskolai környezet: iskolához, tanárokhoz, társakhoz fuzodo kapcsolat, iskolai szabályok; szociális egyenlotlenségek: szülok szocio-ökonómiai helyzete objektív, szubjektív.

Age Groups

11	17

World Health Survey Hungary 2003 (Világ-Egészségfelmérés 2003)

WHS Hungary 2003 (VEF 2003)

Project Leader

Project Leader	Dr. József Vitrai
Address	H 1097 Budapest IX.ker. Gyáli út 2-6; H 1966 Bp. Pf.64
	Tel: (+36-1) 476-1100
	Fax: (+36-1) 476-1226; (+36-1) 476-1223
Executing Institution	National Center for Epidemiology
Funding Agency	WHO, Ministry of Health

Project Information

Start of Project	01/08/2002
End of Project	01/01/2004
Start of Data Collection	09/05/2003
End of Data Collection	15/06/2003
URL	http://www.oek.hu/oek.web?to=978,1109,836,8&nid=29&pid= 1&lang=hun
Scope	European

Keywords Health survey

Abstract (English) The World Health Survey of the WHO is a cross-sectional, multination study that was conducted in approx. 70 countries. In Hungary, the survey was implemented by the National Center for Epidemiology. The survey was implemented on a nation-wide representative sample of the adult (18 years +), noninstitutionalized population. The questionnaire topics included health status and lifestyle (smoking, alcohol, physical activity, and nutrition), determinants of health, health insurance, health expenditures, and other questions related to health care use.

Abstract (Original Language) A WHO körülbelül hetven országban, egységes szerkezetu kérdoív alapján szervezte meg a Világ Egészségfelmérést (WHS). A WHO-val együttmuködve a magyarországi vizsgálatot a Johan Béla Országos Epidemológiai Központ végezte. A felmérés országos reprezentatív mintán történt, a célpopuláció a 18. életévét betöltött, nem intézményben élo felnott magyar lakosság volt. A kérdoív a lakosság egészségérol és életmódjáról (dohányzás, alkohol, testmozgás, táplálkozás), az egészséget befolyásoló tényezokrol, ezen belül az egészségbiztosításról, az egészségügyi kiadásokról és más, az egészségügyi szolgáltatások igénybevételével kapcsolatos kérdésekrol szólt.

Age Groups

Adult population 18 years and over

A pan-EU Survey on Consumer Attitudes to Physical Activity, Body-Weight, and Health

pan-EU

Project Leader

Project Leader	Mike Gibney
Address	Nutrition Unit
	Department of Clinical Medicine
	Trinity College
	Dublin
	Ireland
Executing Institution	
Funding Agency	European Comission

Project Information

Start of Project	07/09/1997
End of Project	07/09/2006
Start of Data Collection	07/02/1997
End of Data Collection	07/02/1997
URL	
Scope	European

Keywords

Abstract (English) A pan-EU consumer attitudinal survey was carried out to describe the attitudes to physical activity, body weight, and health across the 15 member states of the EU to explore the influence of socio-cultural factors, physical activity levels, and body-weight status on these attitudes. Some strategy recommendations to increase levels of physical activity in the EU and to stem the continuing rise in obesity, by means of preventing further weight gain, are proposed based on the data arising from this survey.

Abstract (Original Language)

Age Groups

15	24
25	34
35	44
45	54
55	64
65	and older

Breastfeeding Promotion in Europe

Project Leader

Project Leader	Dr. Adriano Cattaneo
Address	Via dell'Istria 65/1
	IT - 34137 Triestre
Executing Institution	IRCCS Burlo Garofolo
Funding Agency	EU

Project Information

Start of Project	01/06/2002
End of Project	01/06/2004
Start of Data Collection	01/06/2002
End of Data Collection	01/06/2004
URL	
Scope	European

Keywords

Abstract (English) The protection, promotion, and support of breastfeeding are a public health priority throughout Europe. Low rates and early cessation of breastfeeding have important adverse health and social implications for women, children, the community, and the environment result in greater expenditure on national health care provision and increase inequalities in health. The Global Strategy on Infant and Young Child Feeding, adopted by all WHO member states at the 55th World Health Assembly in May 2002, provides a basis for public health initiatives to protect, promote, and support breastfeeding.

Extensive experience clearly shows that breastfeeding can be protected, promoted, and supported only through concerted and coordinated action. This blueprint for action, written by breastfeeding experts representing all EU and associated countries and the relevant stakeholder groups, including mothers, is a model plan that outlines the actions that a national or regional plan should contain and implement. It incorporates specific interventions and sets of interventions for which there is an evidence base of effectiveness. It is hoped that the application of the blueprint will achieve a Europe wide improvement in breastfeeding practices and rates (initiation, exclusivity, and duration); more parents, who are confident, are empowered and satisfied with their breastfeeding experience; and health workers are with improved skills and greater job satisfaction.

Prevailing budgets, structures, human, and organizational resources will have to be considered to develop national and regional action plans on the basis of the blueprint. Action plans should build on clear policies, strong management, and adequate financing. Specific activities for the protection, promotion, and support of breastfeeding should be supported by an effective plan for information, education, and communication, and by appropriate pre and in-service training. Monitoring and evaluation, as well as research on agreed operational priorities, are essential for effective planning. Under six headings, the blueprint recommends objectives for all these actions identifies responsibilities, and indicates possible output and outcome measures.

A comprehensive national policy should be based on the Global Strategy on Infant and Young Child Feeding and integrated into overall health policies. Specific policies for socially disadvantaged groups and children in difficult circumstances may be needed to reduce inequalities. Professional associations should be encouraged to issue recommendations and practice guidelines on the basis of national policies. Long and short-term plans should be developed by relevant ministries and health authorities, which should also designate suitably qualified coordinators and inter-sectoral committees. Adequate human and financial resources are needed for implementation of the plans.

Adequate IEC is crucial for the reestablishment of a breastfeeding culture in countries where artificial feeding has been considered the norm for several years/generations. IEC messages for individuals and communities must be consistent with policies, recommendations, and laws as well as consistent with practices within the health and social services sector. Expectant and new parents have the right to full, correct, and optimal infant feeding information, including guidance on safe, timely, and appropriate complementary feeding, so that they can make informed decisions. Face-to-face counselling needs to be provided by adequately trained health workers, peer counsellors, and mother-to-mother support groups. The particular needs of the women least likely to breastfeed must be identified and actively addressed. The distribution of marketing materials on infant feeding provided by manufacturers and distributors of products under the scope of the International Code of Marketing of Breast-milk Substitutes should be prevented.

Pre and in-service training for all health worker groups needs improvement. Pre- and postgraduate curricula and competency on breastfeeding and lactation management as well as textbooks should be reviewed and developed. Evidence-based in-service courses should be offered to all relevant health care staff, with particular emphasis on staff in frontline maternity and child care areas. Manufacturers and distributors of products under the scope of the International Code should not influence training materials and courses. Relevant health care workers should be encouraged to attend advanced lactation management courses shown to meet best practice criteria for competence.

Protection of breastfeeding is largely based on the full implementation of the International Code, including mechanisms for enforcement and prosecution of violations and a monitoring system that is independent of commercial-vested interests; and on maternity protection legislation that enables all working mothers to exclusively breastfeed their infants for six months and to continue thereafter.

Promotion depends on the implementation of national policies and recommendations at all levels of the health and social services system so that breastfeeding is perceived as the norm. Effective support requires commitment to establish standards for best practice in all maternity and child care institutions/services. At individual level, it means access for all women to breastfeeding supportive services, including assistance provided by appropriately qualified health workers and lactation consultants, peer counsellors, and mother-to-mother support groups. Family and social support through local projects and community programmes, on the basis of collaboration between voluntary and statutory services, should be encouraged. The right of women to breastfeed whenever and wherever they need must be protected.

Monitoring and evaluation procedures are integral to the implementation of an action plan. To ensure comparability, monitoring of breastfeeding initiation, exclusivity, and duration rates should be conducted using standardised indicators, definitions, and methods. These have not been agreed yet in Europe; more work is urgently needed to develop consensus and issue practical instructions.

Monitoring and evaluation of practices of health and social services, of implementation of policies, laws, and codes, of the coverage and effectiveness of IEC activities, and of the coverage and effectiveness of training, using standard criteria, should also be an integral part of action plans.

Research needs to elucidate the effect of marketing practices under the scope of the International Code, of more comprehensive maternity protection legislation, of different IEC approaches and interventions, and in general, of public health initiatives. The cost/benefit, cost/effectiveness, and feasibility of different interventions also need further research. The quality of research methods need to substantially improve, in particular with regards to adequate study design, consistency in the use of standard definitions of feeding categories, and use of appropriate qualitative methods when needed. Ethical guidelines should ensure freedom from all competing and commercial interests; the disclosure and handling of potential conflicts of interest of researchers is of paramount importance.

Abstract (Original Language)

Age Groups

Children Environment and Health Action Plan for Europe

CEHAPE

Project Leader

Project Leader	
Address	via Francesco Crispi, 10
	I-00187 Rome
	Italy
Executing Institution	
Funding Agency	WHO

Project Informatin

Start of Project	08/09/2000
End of Project	08/09/2005
Start of Data Collection	08/09/2006
End of Data Collection	08/09/2006
URL	http://www.euro.who.int/childhealthenv/policy/20020724_2
Scope	European

Keywords Children; Obesity; Overweight; Environment; Health; Indicators

Abstract (English) The project consists in developing a set of Children's Environmental Health Indicators that will be used to monitor the implementation of Regional Plan for Europe. The aim is to reduce the prevalence of overweight and obesity by implementing health promotion activities and promoting the benefits of physical activity in children's daily life providing information and education as well as pursuing opportunities for partnership and synergies with other sectors.

Abstract (Original Language)

Age Groups

The plan involves implementation of policies.

Dietary Surveys within WHO coordinated CINDI Project

CINDI Diet

Project Leader

Project Leader	Prof. Vilius Grabauskas
Address	A.Mickeviciaus 9 LT-44307,Kaunas
	Lithuania
Executing Institution	Kaunas University of Medicine
Funding Agency	

Project Information

Start of Project	01/09/1983
End of Project	
Start of Data Collection	01/09/1983
End of Data Collection	
URL	
Scope	European

Keywords CINDI; Noncommunicable diseases; Risk factors; Diet; Physical activity

Abstract (English) Countrywide Integrated Noncommunicable Disease (CINDI) project aims to reduce mortality and morbidity from noncommunicable diseases by reducing common risk factors. Since 1983, five CINDI random sample surveys were carried out in Kaunas city and five rural regions of Lithuania (last survey in 2006). About 3,000 men and women aged 25–64 participated in every survey. The 24-h recall and Food Frequency Questionnaire were used for dietary assessment.

Abstract (Original Language)

Age Groups

25	64
35	64

Health Behavior Among Lithuanian Adult Population

LHBM

Project Leader

Project Leader	Assoc. Prof. Dr. Jurate Klumbiene
Address	Institute for Biomedical Research
	Eiveniu 4 LT-50009, Kaunas
	Lithuania
Executing Institution	Institute for Biomedical Research of Kaunas University of Medicine
Funding Agency	State budget, WHO

Project Information

Start of Project	01/04/1994
End of Project	
Start of Data Collection	01/14/2006
End of Data Collection	
URL	
Scope	European

Keywords Health behavior; Monitoring; Sociodemographic factors; Nutrition; Physical activity; Obesity

Abstract (English) Lithuanian health behavior monitoring started in 1994 by the initiative of National Public Health Institute in Finland. Four countries – Finland, Estonia, Latvia, and Lithuania – participate in the project. The aim of the project is to assess health behavior including food and physical activity habits of different sociodemographic groups and to monitor the time trends in health behavior. In Lithuania, seven surveys on national samples of adult population have been carried out every two years. For every survey, a national random sample of 3,000 Lithuanians aged 20–64 was taken from National Population Register. These data were collected through postal surveys using the self-administrated questionnaire. The response rate varied between 74% and 62%. The standardized questionnaire contained questions on sociodemographic characteristics, smoking, alcohol consumption, nutrition, and physical activity. The Food Frequency Questionnaire was used for monitoring of food habits. More than 20 items were included. Several questions on physical activity were included.

Abstract (Original Language)

Age Groups

20	24
25	34
35	44
45	54
55	64

Health Behavior Survey among Schoolchildren

LHBSC

Project Leader

Project Leader	Prof. A.Zaborskis
Address	Eiveniu 4, LT-50009, Kaunas
	Lithuania
Executing Institution	Institute for Biomedical Research of Kaunas University
	of Medicine
Funding Agency	

Project Information

Start of Project	01/01/1994
End of Project	
Start of Data Collection	01/04/1994
End of Data Collection	
URL	
Scope	European

Keywords Health behavior; Schoolchildren; Nutrition habits; Physical activity

Abstract (English) The Health Behavior Survey among Lithuanian schoolchildren has been carried out within international HBSC study. Lithuania joined this project in 1994. Four surveys in 4-year intervals were conducted. The target population is schoolchildren 11, 13, and 15 years of age. Clustered sampling design was used. The sampling unit was the class. About 6,000 of children were selected for every study. Response rate was more than 90%. The Food Frequency Questionnaire was used for evaluation of nutrition habits. Several questions on physical activity were included.

Abstract (Original Language)

Age Groups

11	11
13	13
15	15

NORBAGREEN Study

NORBAGREEN

Project Leader

Project Leader	Dr. Janina Petkeviciene
Address	Eiveniu 4 LT-50009, Kaunas
	Lithuania
Executing Institution	Institute for Biomedical Research of Kaunas University of Medicine
Funding Agency	Nordic Council of Ministers

Project Information

Start of Project	01/01/2002
End of Project	01/09/2003
Start of Data Collection	01/04/2002
End of Data Collection	01/05/2002
URL	http://www.norden.org/pub/ebook/2003-556.pdf
Scope	European

Keywords Food frequency questionnaire; Vegetables; Fruits; Fish; Bread; Potatoes; Validation

Abstract (English) In 2002, the study was carried out in five Nordic countries (Finland, Sweden, Norway, Denmark, and Iceland) and in the Baltic countries (Estonia, Latvia, and Lithuania). The aim was to examine the consumption frequency of fruit, vegetables, bread, and fish as well as of potatoes with comparable methods in the Nordic and the Baltic countries and to produce and validate a food frequency questionnaire for this purpose. The Food Frequency Questionnaire contained one global question on total consumption per food group and several questions on the consumption of different preparation forms of vegetables, potatoes, and fruit. In addition, it covered the consumption of individual vegetables and fruits, the consumption of fish as a main dish and as a side dish, and the consumption of breads with different levels of fiber content. The questionnaire was applied using Paper Assisted Personal Interviews (PAPI) in the Baltic countries. In Lithuania, 100 sampling points were used to select the PAPI samples. The sampling points were chosen according to national population-statistical data, taking into consideration the population density in each region. 1,076 interviews were completed (age range 15–74 years). The samples were country representative with respect to sex and age.

Age Groups

15	74

School Workshops on the Issue: Nutrition and Health Possibilities for Preventive Actions

NHPA

Project Leader

Project Leader	Vujovic V, Gerazova V, Ristova
Address	Clinical Center, Department of Psychiatry
	Vodnjanska 17, Skopje
	Macedonia
Executing Institution	Clinical Center, Department of Psychiatry
Funding Agency	

Project Information

Start of Project	
End of Project	
Start of Data Collection	
End of Data Collection	
URL	
Scope	European

Keywords Workshops; Bulimia; Anorexia; Schools

Abstract (English) The goal of the work is to show the possibilities for preventive acting onto adolescents in order to decrease the number of patients with symptoms of bulimia and anorexia. The evaluation questionnaires showed that after holding the workshops in the period of 1 month, the public awareness about bulimia and anorexia has been increased. This survey covered 80 persons in the age group 13–19 in three primary and secondary schools.

Abstract (Original Language)

Age Groups

13	19

Health Behavior in School Children in Portugal

HBSC Portugal

Project Leader

Project Leader	Bente Wold
Address	University of Bergen
	Norway
Executing Institution	Research Center for Health Promotion
Funding Agency	WHO

Project Information

Start of Project	14/09/1982
End of Project	14/09/2006
Start of Data Collection	14/09/2006
End of Data Collection	14/09/2006
URL	http://www.hbsc.org/countries/portugal.html
Scope	European

Keywords Health education; Health promotion; Youth; Children; Portugal

Abstract (English) A major goal of this international approach is to influence health promotion and health education policies and programmes in schools and among young people in general. Data are collected through surveys among 11- to 18-year olds. All participating countries use a common methodology and pool their data to form the cross-national data file. By analysing trends over time, it is possible to show changes in health behaviors in a particular country.

Abstract (Original Language)

Age Groups

11	12
13	14
15	16
17	18

Health Behavior in School Children Spain

HBSC Spain

Project Leader

Project Leader	Bente Wold
Address	University of Bergen
	Norway
Executing Institution	Research Center for Health Promotion
Funding Agency	WHO

Project Information

Start of Project	12/09/1982
End of Project	12/09/2006
Start of Data Collection	12/09/1985
End of Data Collection	12/09/1985
URL	http://www.hbsc.es/
Scope	European

Keywords Health education; Health promotion; Youth; Children; Spain

Abstract (English) A major goal of this international approach is to influence health promotion and health education policies and programs in schools and among young people in general. Data are collected through surveys among 11- to 18-year olds. All participating countries use a common methodology and pool their data to form the cross-national data file. By analysing trends over time, it is possible to show changes in health behaviors in a particular country.

Abstract (Original Language)

Age Groups

11	12
13	14
15	16
17	18

Promoting and Sustaining Health Increased Vegetable and Fruit Consumption Among European Schoolchildren

Pro Children

Project Leader

Project Leader	Knut-Inge Klepp
Address	Department of Nutrition
	University of Oslo
	P.O. Box 1046 Blindern
	N-0316 Oslo
	Norway
Executing Institution	Department of Nutrition, University of Oslo
Funding Agency	the Fifth Framework Programme of the European Commission

Project Information

Start of Project	01/04/2002
End of Project	01/03/2006
Start of Data Collection	25/10/2006
End of Data Collection	25/10/2006
URL	
Scope	European

Keywords

Abstract (English)   Recent research has demonstrated the health benefits of eating a diet rich in fruit and vegetables. In Northern European countries, the consumption of fruit and vegetables tend to be below current recommendations. In several Southern European countries, there is a concern that both the amount and variation in fruit and vegetables eaten may be on decline. Thus, the main objective of this project is to develop effective strategies to promote adequate consumption levels of fruit and vegetables. Young adolescents (11–13 years) and their parents are the main target groups of this project.

Specific objectives include:

Assessing vegetable and fruit consumption and determinants of consumption levels (phase 1)

- To develop valid and reliable instruments for assessing fruits and vegetables consumption among schoolchildren and their parents, and for identifying factors influencing consumption patterns both among schoolchildren and their parents
- To describe:
    1. The consumption levels of fruits and vegetables among schoolchildren and their parents

2. Factors influencing such consumption levels
3. Cross-national differences in consumption patterns and determinants

Design, implementation, and evaluation of an intervention programme (phase 2)

To design, implement, and evaluate the effect of culturally relevant intervention programmes in different European settings. The objective is to produce a 20% increase in the consumption of fruits and vegetables among participating children and parents.

The Pro Children project consists of eight major work packages, aimed at:

- Designing a valid and reliable instrument for assessing intake of fruit and vegetables in European schoolchildren and their parents
- Identifying determinants of young adolescents' fruit and vegetable intake
- Developing a theory-based instrument to assess the psychosocial determinants of this intake
- Conducting cross-sectional survey across all nine European partner countries
- Designing cuturally relevant and theoretically similar intervention strategies to be tested in the Netherlands, Norway, and Spain
- Investigating the process of implementation across the three intervention sites
- Investigating the outcome and its sustainabililty, i.e., change in reported fruit and vegetable intake, change in psychosocial determinants, and change in school and community policy, and availability issues concerning fruit and vegetables
- Designing a joint database and secure high-quality and comparable data across countries

Interpreting collected and pooled data, report and disseminate results to the scientific community, professional organisations, policy makers, and to the general public.

Abstract (Original Language)

Age Groups

Promoting Fruit and Vegetable Consumption in Children across Europe

Pro Children

Project Leader

Project Leader	Knut-Inge Klepp
Address	Department of Nutrition
	Faculty of Medicine
	University of Oslo
	P.O. Box 1046 Blindern
	N-0316 Oslo
	Norway
Executing Institution	
Funding Agency	European Commission

Project Information

Start of Project	07/04/2002
End of Project	07/09/2005
Start of Data Collection	07/10/2003
End of Data Collection	07/10/2003
URL	http://www.univie.ac.at/prochildren/
Scope	European

Keywords

Abstract (English) The Pro Children Project was funded by the European Commission to study fruit and vegetable intakes in 11- to 13-year-old children in nine European countries and their families, and to develop and evaluate school-based interventions to promote fruit and vegetable intake.

Abstract (Original Language)

Age Groups

11	13

Health Behaviour School Children – Romania

WHO/HBSC

Project Leader

Project Leader	Prof. Dr. Adriana Baban
Address	Republicii 37, Cluj-Napoca 400015
	Romania
Executing Institution	Romanian Association of Health Psychology
Funding Agency	

Project Information

Start of Project	31/10/2005
End of Project	31/12/2007
Start of Data Collection	10/03/2006
End of Data Collection	25/04/2006
URL	
Scope	European

Keywords

Abstract (English)

Abstract (Original Language)

Age Groups

11	11
13	13
15	15

Study on NUTRITIONAL STATUS of Pregnant Women

Project Leader

Project Leader	Ecaterina Stativa and Michaela Nanu; Project Director Alin Stanescu
Address	Lacul Tei Boulevard no. 120, 2 district, Bucharest
Executing Institution	A study conducted by "Alfred Rusescu" Institute for Mother and Child Care in cooperation and with the support of the UNICEF Representative Office in Romania
Funding Agency	UNICEF – Romania

Project Information

Start of Project	01/10/2003
End of Project	31/10/2005
Start of Data Collection	11/10/2004
End of Data Collection	21/10/2004
URL	
Scope	European

Keywords

Abstract (English) Pregnant women are considered to be among the high risk groups. The goal of this survey was to assess the nutritional status of pregnant women in general, and particularly the status of iron and iodine micronutrients. Health care services targeting this population group have a major role to play in the early detection of and fight against nutritional disorders; such services should concentrate on monitoring the progress of pregnancy. The overall objectives of the survey were to assess the nutritional status of pregnant women and new born child, to assess some nutritional practices in the surveyed population, to evaluate the contribution of health care services in preventing nutritional deficiencies.
Findings from the study:

General aspects:

- About half of the women who give birth live in the rural area
- Pregnant women cumulating the most significant social risk (poor level of education, large number of births, low socio-economic status of the mother) live in the country side and/or are of Roma origin

Iodine status:

- The iodine deficiency in pregnant women stays within the limits of a mild deficiency, greater in the rural area
- In their first trimester of pregnancy, the iodine deficiency is present
- The iodine deficiency of the newborn baby falls within the limits of a moderate deficiency, being more severe than that of the mother

Iron status:

- High prevalence of anemia in pregnant women
- Higher prevalence in the rural area

Growth status of new born:

- High prevalence of infants with low birth weight

Feeding practices:

- A large proportion of pregnant women have improper diet (low intake of foods rich in proteins, iron, iodine) bottle feeding and weaning occur too early in the infant's life

Promotion of breastfeeding during prenatal care and in maternity hospitals

- Insufficient information regarding the initiation, promotion, and continuation of breastfeeding
- The less informed women are those in the rural area and with a poor education
- Prenatal visits
- 32% of pregnant women had their first prenatal consultation only in the second trimester of pregnancy
- 6% did not have any consultation during their pregnancy, especially women with a poor level of education and living in rural areas

On the basis of this findings were made some recommendations regarding the prevention of iodine deficiency, anemia prevention, the development of social and health care-integrated services, and legislatives aspects.

Abstract (Original Language) Femeile gravide sunt considerate printre grupele cu cel mai inalt grad de risc. Scopul acestei anchete a fost de a evalua statusul nutritional al femeilor gravide in general, si in special statusul nutritional in ceea ce priveste aportul de fier si iod. Serviciile de sanatate care se adreseaza acestui grup populational au un rol major in detectarea precoce si combaterea tulburarilor de nutritie; aceste servicii ar trebui sa se concentreze pe monitorizarea evolutiei sarcinilor. Obiectivele generale ale studiului au fost: sa evalueze statusul nutritional al gravidelor; sa evalueze unele practici alimentare in randul populatiei studiate; sa evalueze contributia serviciilor de sanatate in prevenirea deficientelor nutritionale. Rezultate:

Apecte generale:

- Proape jumatate dintre femeile care au nascut locuiesc in zone rurale
- Femeile gravide cumuleaza un risc social crescut (nivel scazut de educatie, numar mare de nasteri, nivel socio-economic scazut al mamei) in zonele rurale sau in randul etniei Rroma

Satusul nutritional in ceea ce priveste iodul:

- Deficitul de iod la gravide se situeaza in categoria deficit usor, fiind mai crescut in zonele rurale
- In primul trimestru de sarcina deficitul de iod este prezent
- La nou nascut deficitul de iod este moderat, fiind mai sever decat la mama

Satusul nutritional in ceea ce priveste fierul:

- Prevalenta ridicata a anemiei la gravide
- Prevalenta mai mare a anemiei in zonele rurale

Satusul dezvoltarii fizice la nou nascut:

- Prevalenta ridicata a copiilor cu greutate mica la nastere

Pactici alimentare:

- Dieta neadecvata este larg raspandita in randul gravidelor (aport scazut de alimente bogate in proteine, fier, iod)
- Hranirea cu biberonul si intarcarea au loc la o varsta mica a copilului

Promovarea in timpul sarcinii si in maternitati a alaptarii copilului:

- Informare insuficienta referitor la initierea, promovarea si continuarea alaptarii
- Cel mai putin informate sunt gravidele din zonele rurale si cele cu un nivel educational scazut

Vizitele prenatale:

- 32% dintre gravide au facut prima consultatie prenatala abia in cel de al doilea trimestru de sarcina
- 6% nu au mers deloc la medic pe perioada sarcinii, in special femeile cu nivel educational redus si locuind la tara.

Pe baza acestor rezultate s-au formulat o serie de recomandari referitor la prevenirea deficitului de iod, prevenirea anemiei, dezvoltarea serviciilor sociale si de sanatate integrate si aspecte legislative.

Age Groups

13	44	Were included pregnant women of 13- to 44-years old and their new born children of 3- to 5-days old

Study on NUTRITIONAL STATUS of School children Aged 6–7 Years

Project Leader

Project Leader	Ecaterina Stativa and Michaela Nanu; Project Director Alin Stanescu
Address	Lacul Tei Boulevard no. 120, 2 district, Bucharest
Executing Institution	A study conducted by "Alfred Rusescu" Institute for Mother and Child Care in cooperation and with the support of the UNICEF Representative Office in Romania
Funding Agency	

Project Information

Start of Project	01/0/2003
End of Project	31/10/003
Start of Data Collection	01/11/2003
End of Data Collection	29/02/2004
URL	
Scope	European

Keywords

Abstract (English) Schoolchildren in the first grade are considered to be among the high risk groups. The goal of this survey was to assess the nutritional status of children in general, and particularly the status of iron and iodine micronutrients. The survey starts from the assumption that the child's development status, right from the moment of birth, is a very useful indicator for assessing the nutrition status and some specific deficiencies. Health care services targeting this population group have a major role to play in the early detection of and fight against nutritional disorders; such services should concentrate on monitoring the child's physical and mental development. The overall objectives of the survey were to assess the nutritional status of schoolchildren 6- to 7-years old, to assess some nutritional practices in the surveyed population, to evaluate the contribution of health care services in preventing nutritional deficiencies.
Findings from the study:

Iodine status

- Movement of iodine status among schoolchildren from 2002 to 2004
- The positive trend is related to iodised diet salt consumption
- The knowledge level regarding iodised salt consumption: 89.4% of schoolchildren parents know about iodised salt consumption but only 73.9% are using iodised salt.
- 96.3% of the schoolchildren families are using salt with iodine; this fact was tested through iodine determination in household used salt, even sometimes the families were not aware about it.
- 10.1% of schoolchildren received potassium and iodine during the last month.
- 25.8% of schoolchildren received vitamins.

Iron status:

- High prevalence of anemia in schoolchildren
- Higher prevalence in the rural area

Growth status:

- High prevalence of more weight for height because of an imbalanced diet
- The prevalence of less height for age falls within the limits of a mild deficit
- Less obvious signs of a chronic dietary deficiency

Feeding practices

- 12.4% from schoolchildren in urban area and 14.9% in rural area do not eat or eat only occasionally milk or milk product

In rural area, the schoolchildren are eating less meat than those from urban area.

The fish is not included regularly in schoolchildren diet

On the basis of this findings were made some recommendations regarding the prevention of iodine deficiency, anemia prevention, the improvement of anthropometric indicators, the development of social and health care-integrated services, and legislatives aspects.

Abstract (Original Language) Prescolarii, scolarii in clasa intai sunt considerati printre grupele cu inalt grad de risc. Scopul acestei anchete a fost de a evalua statusul nutritional al copiilor in general, si in special statusul nutritional in ceea ce priveste aportul de fier si iod. Studiul a pornit de la premiza ca statusul de dezvoltare a copilului, chiar din momentul nasterii este cel mai util indicator pentru evaluarea statusului de nutritie si a unor deficiente specifice. Serviciile de sanatate care se adreseaza acestor grupe de varsta au un rol major in detectarea precoce si combaterea tulburarilor de nutritie; aceste servicii ar trebui sa se concentreze pe monitorizarea dezvoltarii fizice si psihice a copilului. Obiectivele generale ale studiului au fost: sa evalueze statusul nutritional al copiilor de 6–7 ani; sa evalueze unele practici alimentare in randul populatiei studiate; sa evalueze contributia serviciilor de sanatate in prevenirea deficientelor nutritionale.
Rezultate:
Statusul nutritional in ceea ce priveste iodul:

- Imbunatatirea statusului iodului la scolarii de 6–7 ani, in 2004 fata de 2002
- Evolutia pozitiva este legata de consumul de sare iodata
- Nivelul de cunostinte in ceea ce priveste consumul de sare iodata: 89.4% dintre parintii scolarilor au cunostinte despre consumul de sare iodata, insa numai 73.9% folosesc sarea iodata
- 96.3% dintre familiile scolarilor folosesc sare cu iod: acest fapt a fost dovedit prin determinarea iodului in sarea folosita in gospodarie, chiar daca familiile nu cunosteau acest lucru
- 10.1% dintre scolari au primit Iodura de Potasiu in ultima luna
- 25.8% dintre scolari au primit vitamine

Statusul nutritional in ceea ce priveste fierul:

- Prevalenta ridicata a anemiei la copilul de 6–7 ani
- Prevalenta mai mare in zonele rurale

Statusul dezvoltarii fizice:

- Prevalenta ridicata a greutatii crescute fata de inaltime datorata unei diete dezechilibrate
- Prevalenta inaltimii mici fata de varsta se incadreaza intr-un deficit usor
- Semne mai putin evidente ale unui deficit alimentar cronic

Practici alimentare

- 12.4% dintre copiii de 6–7 ani din urban si 14.9% din rural nu consuma sau consuma ocazional lapte sau produse din lapte

In rural copiii consuma carne mai putin decat cei din urban.

Pestele nu este inclus in mod normal in dieta scolarilor.

Pe baza acestor rezultate s-au formulat o serie de recomandari referitor la prevenirea deficitului de

Age Groups

| 6 | 7 | From 6-years old to 7 years 11 months and 29 days |

Tobacco, Alcohol, and Drug Use among 16-years-old Teenagers (The European School Survey Project on Alcohol and Other Drugs/ESPAD), two Editions in 1999 and 2003

ESPAD

Project Leader

Project Leader	Silvia Florescu in Romania; at European level The Swedish Council for Information on alcohol and Other Drugs (CAN), represented by Björn Hibell
Address	31 Vaselor street, 021253, Bucharest
Executing Institution	National School of Public Health and Health Services Management, former National Institute for Research and Development in Health, former Health Services Management Institute
Funding Agency	Ministry of Public Health

Project Information

Start of Project	01/01/1999
End of Project	31/12/2003
Start of Data Collection	01/05/2003
End of Data Collection	01/05/2003
URL	
Scope	European

Keywords Cross-sectional study; Alcohol use; Tobacco use; Drug use; School survey; Prevalence rates

Abstract (English) *Objectives:* The study collects data regarding the alcohol, tobacco, and drug use among high schools teenagers of 16 in Romania, to participate in European comparison, to describe the temporal change of drug use among the pupils from schools, and to rely the preventive interventions on evidence.

Results: Were assessed the prevalence of drug, alcohol, tobacco use; the level of knowledge, the attitude, the practices concerning the drug, alcohol, tobacco use; the risk perception and the demographical and family features for groups at risk; the patterns of drugs use; the reasons for use and the accessibility to drug, alcohol, and tobacco; the influence, the pressure, and the family, and social environment compliance; the associated effects on health, on social abilities, on school performance at different levels of use.

The report shows how changed over time the phenomena, how appeared and increased over the time the consumer subgroup inside of 1983, 1987 cohort of high schools students, which are the practice patterns changes at individual level, how spread are different practice patterns.

Abstract (Original Language) *Obiective:* Colectarea de date referitor la consumul de alcool, tutun, droguri de catre liceenii de 16 ani din Romania in scopul realizarii unei comparatii la nivel European, pentru a descrie evolutia si modificarile inregistrate in ceea ce priveste consumul acestor substante printre liceeni si pentru a fundamenta interventiile preventive.

Rezultate: Au fost evaluate prevalenta consumului de alcool, tutun, droguri; nivelul de cunostinte, atitudini, practici in ceea ce priveste consumul de substante precum alcool, tutun, droguri; perceptia riscului si caracteristicile demografice si familiale pentru grupurile la risc; modelele de consum de droguri; motivul consumului si accesibilitatea la alcool, tutun, droguri; influenta, presiunea si complianta mediului social si familial; efectele secundare asupra starii de sanatate, asupra abilitatilor sociale, asupra performantei scolare pentru grade diferite de consum.

Studiul arata cum a evoluat fenomenul in timp, care sunt modificarile in ceea ce priveste modelele de practica la nivel individual, cat de raspandite sunt diferitele modele de practica.

Age Groups

16	16

Healthy Lifestyle in Europe by Nutrition in Adolescence

HELENA

Project Leader

Project Leader	Luis A. Moreno Aznar
Address	Universidad de Zaragoza
	E.U. Ciencias de la Salud,
	Domingo Miral s/n,
	50009 Zaragoza
	Spain
Executing Institution	Universidad de Zaragoza
Funding Agency	European Community (FP6-2003-Food-2-A, FOOD-CT-2005-007034)

Project Information

Start of Project	01/10/2006
End of Project	
Start of Data Collection	01/10/2006
End of Data Collection	
URL	http://www.helenastudy.com
Scope	European

Keywords

Abstract (English) The key to health promotion and disease prevention in the twenty-first century is to establish an environment that supports positive health behavior and healthy lifestyle. Most diseases have their origin during childhood and adolescence, but the relationship between the development of noncommunicable diseases and the adolescence process is poorly understood.

Adolescence is a crucial period in life and implies multiple physiological and psychological changes that affect nutritional needs and habits. The HELENA proposal includes cross-sectional, crossover, and pilot community intervention multi-center study, as an integrated approach to the above-mentioned problem. The following aspects will provide the full information about the nutritional status of the European adolescents:

- Dietary intake, nutrition knowledge, and eating attitudes
- Food choices and preferences
- Body composition
- Plasma lipids and metabolic profile
- Vitamin status
- Immune function related to nutritional status
- Physical activity and fitness
- Genotype (to analyse gene-nutrient and gene-environment interactions)

The requirements for health promoting foods will also be identified, and three sensory acceptable products for adolescents will be developed. Both scientific and technological objectives should result in reliable and comparable data of a representative sample of European adolescents, concerning: foods and nutrients intake, food choices and preferences, obesity prevalence, dislipidemia, insulin resistance, vitamin and minerals status, immunological markers for subclinical malnutrition, physical activity and fitness patterns, and variations of the nucleotide sequence in selected genes.

This will contribute to understand why health-related messages are not being as effective as expected in the adolescent population. A realistic intervention strategy will be proposed to achieve the goals of understanding and effectively enhancing nutritional and lifestyle habits of adolescents in Europe.

Abstract (Original Language)

Age Groups

13–16 old adolescents

Europe Alimentation

EURALIM

Project Leader

Project Leader	Alfredo Morabia
Address	Division d'Epidémiologie Clinique
	Hôpitaux Universitaires de Genève
	24 rue Micheli-du-Crest
	1211 Genève 14 - Suisse
Executing Institution	
Funding Agency	European Community

Project Information

Start of Project	07/09/1990
End of Project	07/09/1996
Start of Data Collection	07/09/2006
End of Data Collection	07/09/2006
URL	http://www.epidemiology.ch/euralim/index.htm
Scope	European

Keywords

Abstract (English)   The EURALIM (EURope ALIMentation) project is a European collaborative study, aimed to determine and describe the extent to which European data on risk factor distributions from different populations could be pooled and harmonised in a common database for international comparisons.

Abstract (Original Language)

Age Groups

40	59

Health Behavior in School-Aged

Svenska skolbarns hälsovanor

Project Leader

Project Leader	Ulla Marklund
Address	Statens folkhälsoinstitut, Swedish National Institute of Public Health
	Olof Palmes gata 17
	SE-103 52 Stockholm
	Sweden
Executing Institution	Swedish National Institute of Public Health
Funding Agency	

Project Information

Start of Project	01/11/2005
End of Project	31/12/2005
Start of Data Collection	01/11/2005
End of Data Collection	31/12/2005
URL	http://www.fhi.se/templates/page____9577.aspx
Scope	European

Keywords

Abstract (English) This report is primarily based on the data collected from 11, 13, and 15-year-olds in November to December 2005, within the framework of the cross-sectional study "Health Behavior in School-Aged Children". Since 1985/1986, this study has taken place every fourth year around the world, most recently in over 40 different countries, within the framework of a WHO collaborative project. As a result, this report also contains some data from previous years. International comparisons are, however, published in a separate report from WHO. Here is a brief summary of some of the results presented in this report along with the sex, age, and trend differences discovered.

It is not that easy to summarize in just a few words how children of these ages feel as things look very different depending on the subject areas studied. In general, the report ascertains that children's health, lifestyles, social relations, and opinions about the school environment change depending on their age and that there are often differences between boys and girls. At the age of 11, children on the whole feel better, live more healthily, and have a more positive attitude toward school than when they are older (13–15 years). Self-rated health, somatic and mental problems, and general well-being all worsen as children get older, and the difference between boys and girls increases. The majority feel that they are in good health and seen over time, the proportion of those who feel they are in very good health has remained unchanged.

Historically, somatic and mental problems have increased among both boys and girls, with the exception of 11-year-old girls. According to the most recent study, however, this generally negative trend was broken. It is still the case, however, that girls of all the ages are less happy with life than boys of the same age. This difference has become more marked between 1985 and 2005, and the contentment of 13- and 15-year-old girls in particular has diminished. Boys feel that they are too thin and girls feel that they are too fat, the older they become, and this also influences the extent to which they want to alter their weight.

Both tobacco and alcohol habits are established during the later compulsory school years (13- to 16-years old). More girls than boys smoke but the proportion of those who smoke at least once a week has fallen both among girls and boys between 2001 and 2005. More boys use oral smokeless tobacco than girls; however, and if we look at total tobacco consumption, there are more regular tobacco users among 15-year-old boys than among girls.

As regards alcohol use, about 15% of 15-year-olds say that they have drunk enough alcohol to make them drunk on at least four occasions. Seen over time, binge drinking (drinking until one becomes drunk) increased between 1985 and 2001, but since then has decreased both among girls and boys.

The proportion of those eating breakfast decreases with age and mostly among girls. The fact that children's eating habits change and deteriorate with age can also be noticed when they are asked questions whether they eat fruit, vegetables, sweets, and soft drinks. Boys generally eat less healthy food than girls. The proportion of physically active individuals diminishes with age, while the proportion of those who watch TV and use the computer for more than four hours a day increases with age. Seen over time, the proportion of those who are physically active at least four times a week has varied, and it is difficult to see a clear trend in this respect.

Social relations: The majority of those asked have three or four close friends. The patterns of social intercourse change over time to the extent that the proportion of those who meet their friends after school decreases between 11 and 15 years old, while more meet their friends in the evenings as they get older. Common to both boys and girls is that they find it more difficult to talk to their parents as they get older, while they find it easier to talk to friends of the opposite sex. Contact with parents has not changed over time.

Children feel less content at school as they get older and in contrast to many of the other questions asked, there is a difference between the opinions of boys and girls mostly in the youngest age group, where more girls say that they are very happy at school. At the same time, as school contentment decreases with age, the feeling of stress in connection with schoolwork increases and 15-year-old girls feel more stress than boys of the same age.

Seen over time, the proportion of those who like school very much remained basically unchanged between 1985 and 2001. When asked more in-depth questions about the school environment, opinions differ between the ages, and boys and girls basically feel the same way. As they get older, more of them feel that the demands on them increase, while fewer feel that they are able to influence their situation at school that they are treated fairly by their teachers and that they obtain help from the teachers when they need it.

Abstract (Original Language) Denna rapport bygger i första hand på uppgifter insamlade från 11-, 13- och 15-åringar i november– december år 2005, inom ramen för tvärsnittsundersökningen Skolbarns hälsovanor. Undersökningen äger sedan 1985/1986 rum vart fjärde år och genomförs i ett flertal länder, senast i ett drygt 40-tal länder, inom ramen för ett WHO-samarbete. I denna rapport finns därför även vissa uppgifter från tidigare år. Internationella jämförelser publiceras dock i en separat rapport utgiven av WHO. Nedan följer en kort sammanfattning över några av resultaten som redovisas i denna rapport och de köns-, ålders- och trendskillnader som hittats.självskattad hälsa och allmänt välbefinnande Att kortfattat återge hur barn i dessa åldrar mår är inte helt enkelt då det ser mycket olika ut beroende på vilka frågeområden som studeras. Generellt framkommer i denna rapport att hälsan, levnadsvanorna, de sociala relationerna samt uppfattningen om skolmiljön förändras över åldrarna och att det ofta skiljer sig mellan pojkar och flickor. Vid 11 års ålder mår man som regel bättre, lever sundare och upplever skolan mer positivt än då man kommer upp i högstadiet (13–15-årsåldern). Såväl självskattad hälsa, somatiska och psykiska besvär, som allmänt välbefinnande försämras med stigande ålder och skillnaden mellan pojkar och flickor ökar. Majoriteten skattar att de har en bra hälsa och sett över tid har andelen som skattar sig som mycket friska varit oförändrad. Sett över tid har de somatiska och psykiska besvären ökat bland både pojkar och flickor, med undantag av de 11-åriga flickorna. Ändå är det fortsatt så att flickorna trivs i mindre utsträckning med livet än pojkarna i alla åldrarna. Denna skillnad har blivit mer märkbar under åren 1985–2005, då framför allt de 13-åriga och 15- åriga flickornas trivsel minskat. Pojkar uppfattar att de är för smala och flickor att de är för tjocka med stigande ålder och detta påverkar också i vilken utsträckning de vill förändra sin vikt. tobak och alkohol Såväl tobaks- som alkoholvanor etableras under högstadietiden. Flickor röker i högre tsträckning än pojkar. Andelen som röker minst varje vecka har dock minskat både bland flickor och pojkar mellan åren 2001 och 2005. Pojkar snusar dock i högre utsträckning än flickor och ser man till den totala tobakskonsumtionen brukar 15-åriga pojkar i högre utsträckning tobak regelbundet än flickor. När det gäller alkoholbruk uppger cirka 15 procent av 15-åringarna att de druckit så mycket alkohol att de blivit fulla fyra gånger eller mer. Sett över tid ökade berusningsdrickandet mellan 1985 och 2001 bland flickorna, men har sedan dess minskat bland såväl flickor som pojkar. matvanor och fysisk aktivitet Andelen som äter frukost minskar med åldern och mest bland flickorna. Att matvanorna förändras och försämras med åldern märks även då frågor ställts om de dagligen äter frukt, grönsaker, godis och läsk. Generellt äter pojkarna i mindre utsträckning nyttigheter än flickorna.

Andelen som är fysiskt aktiva minskar med åldern, samtidigt som andelen som tittar på tv och använder datorn mer än fyra timmar om dagen ökar med åldern. Sett över tid har andelen som varit fysiskt aktiva minst fyra gånger i veckan varierat och det är svårt att se en tydlig trend avseende detta. sociala relationer Majoriteten har tre eller fler nära vänner. Umgängesmönstret förändras över åldrarna så till vida att andelen som träffar kompisar efter skolan minskar mellan 11 år och 15 år, samtidigt som fler träffar kompisar på kvällarna ju äldre de blir.

Gemensamt för pojkar och flickor är att de får svårare att tala med sina föräldrar ju äldre de blir, samtidigt som de får lättare att tala med vänner av motsatt kön. Kontakten med föräldrarna har inte förändrats över tid. skolan Skoltrivseln minskar med åldern och till skillnad från många andra frågor skiljer sig pojkars och flickors uppfattning i denna fråga mest i den yngsta åldersgruppen, då flickorna uppger att de trivs mycket bra i skolan i högre utsträckning. Samtidigt som skoltrivseln minskar med åldern ökar känslan av att vara stressad av sitt skolarbete och i 15-års ålder känner sig flickorna mer stressade än pojkarna. Sett över tid har andelen som tycker mycket bra om skolan till stora delar varit oförändrad åren 1985–2001. Vid fördjupade frågor kring skolmiljön framkommer att uppfattningarna skiljer sig mellan åldrarna, medan pojkar och flickor i stort har samma uppfattning. Med stigande ålder är det fler som tycker att kraven ökar, samtidigt som det är färre som tycker att de har möjlighet att påverka sin skolsituation, att de blir rättvist behandlade av sina lärare och att de får hjälp från lärare då de behöver det.

Age Groups

Subjects are 11, 13, and 15-year-old young adolescents

Dietary Quality, Lifestyle Factors, and Healthy Ageing in Europe: the SENECA Study

SENECA

Project Leader

Project Leader	Annemien Haveman-Nies
Address	Department of Human Nutrition and Epidemiology, Wageningen University, Bomer weg 4, 6703 HD Wageningen, The Netherlands.
Executing Institution	Department of Human Nutrition and Epidemiology, Wageningen University, Wageningen
	The Netherlands
Funding Agency	European Union

Project Information

Start of Project	01/01/1988
End of Project	30/04/1999
Start of Data Collection	
End of Data Collection	
URL	http://ageing.oxfordjournals.org/cgi/reprint/32/4/427
Scope	European

Keywords Diet; Lifestyle; Mortality; Healthy ageing; SENECA

Abstract (English) *Objective:* To identify dietary and lifestyle factors that contribute to healthy ageing.

Subjects: For the analyses, data of the longitudinal SENECA study were used. The study population consisted of 1,091 men and 1,109 women aged 70–75 years from Belgium, France, Denmark, Italy, The Netherlands, Portugal, Spain, Switzerland, and Poland.

Methods: This European study started with baseline measurements in 1988–1989 and lasted until 30 April 1999. The study includes data on diet, lifestyle, and health. The study population is followed for 10 years, and measurements were performed in 1988/1989 (baseline), 1993, and 1999. The relationships of the three lifestyle factors diet, physical activity, and smoking habits to survival and maintenance of health at old age were investigated. Finally, it is discussed whether the relationships of healthy lifestyle habits to survival and health contribute to healthy ageing.

Results: The unhealthy lifestyle habits, smoking, having a low-quality diet, and being physically inactive were singly related to an increased mortality risk (hazard ratios ranged from 1.2 to 2.1). In addition, inactive and smoking persons had an increased risk for a decline in health status when compared with active and non-smoking people. The net effect of a healthy lifestyle on the process of healthy ageing is likely to go together with a compressed cumulative morbidity.

Conclusions: A healthy lifestyle at older ages is positively related to a reduced mortality risk and to a delay in the deterioration in health status. This postponement of the onset of major morbidity is likely to go together with a compressed cumulative morbidity. Therefore, health promotion at older ages can contribute to healthy ageing.

Abstract (Original Language)

Age Groups

70	75

Estrategy on European Community Health Indicators

ECHI

Project Leader

Project Leader	Pieter Kramers
Address	P.O. Box 1
	3720 BA Bilthoven
	A. van Leeuwenhoeklaan 9
	NL – Bilthoven
Executing Institution	National Institute of Public Health and the Environment
Funding Agency	EU

Project Information

Start of Project	14/09/1999
End of Project	14/09/2005
Start of Data Collection	14/09/2006
End of Data Collection	14/09/2006
URL	
Scope	European

Keywords European Community; Monitoring programme; Health indicators

Abstract (English) The EU Health Monitoring Programme (HMP) wants to establish data collection, exchange, and reporting in the field of Public Health, to facilitate the monitoring of trends, differences, and policy impact throughout the EU. During 1999 and 2000, the ECHI project has been funded to define the areas of data and indicators to be included in the system; to define generic indicators in this areas, and to imply a high degree of flexibility in the indicator set, by defining subsets of indicators, or "user-windows" tuned to specific users.

Abstract (Original Language)

Age Groups

The project involves definitions of indicators

European Food Consumption Survey Method

EFCOSUM

Project Leader

Project Leader	Michiel R.H. Löwik
Address	P.O Box 360
	NL-3700 AJ Zeist
Executing Institution	Tno Nutrition and Food Research Institute
Funding Agency	DG SANCO F/3

Project Information

Start of Project	01/10/1999
End of Project	30/03/2000
Start of Data Collection	
End of Data Collection	
URL	
Scope	European

Keywords

Abstract (English) The project "European Food Consumption Survey Method" (EFCOSUM) was undertaken within the framework of the EU Programme on Health Monitoring. The purpose of this EU programme is to contribute to the establishment of a Community health monitoring system, which allows for measurement of health status, trends, and determinants throughout the Community, facilitating, planning, monitoring and evaluation of Community programmes and actions, and providing Member States with appropriate health information to make comparisons and support their national health policies. The aim of EFCOSUM was to define a method for monitoring food consumption in nationally representative samples of all age-sex categories in Europe in a comparable way. Additionally, the project aimed to indicate how to make existing food consumption data comparable and available to the health monitoring system (HIEMS).

Abstract (Original Language)

Age Groups

Survey in Europe on Nutrition and the Elderly, a Concerted Action

EURONUT-SENECA

Project Leader

Project Leader	Wija van Staveren
Address	P.O. Box 9101
	6700 HB Wageningen
	The Netherlands
Executing Institution	Wageningen University, Department of Agrotechnology and Food
	Sciences, Division of Human Nutrition and Epidemiology
Funding Agency	EU

Project Information

Start of Project	07/09/1986
End of Project	07/09/1999
Start of Data Collection	07/09/1988
End of Data Collection	07/09/1989
URL	
Scope	European

Keywords

Abstract (English) In 1988, EURONUT, the umbrella European Community (EC) Concerted Action on Nutrition and Health initiated a major European multicenter study, named SENECA to study cross-cultural differences in nutritional issues and life-style factors affecting health and performance of elderly people in Europe.

Abstract (Original Language)

Age Groups

70	75

European Health Promotion Indicators Development

EUHPID

Project Leader

Project Leader	John Davies
Address	Mithras House
	Lewes RoadUK-BN2 4AT
	Brighton
Executing Institution	University of Brighton
Funding Agency	EU

Project Information

Start of Project	01/11/2001
End of Project	01/11/2003
Start of Data Collection	15/09/2006
End of Data Collection	15/09/2006
URL	http://www.brighton.ac.uk/euhpid/
Scope	European

Keywords European Community; Health promotion indicators

Abstract (English) The general aims to the EUHPID project are to establish a European Health Promotion Monitoring System, including a common set of health promotion indicators, to recommend suitable methodology and systems to collect the above data on health promotion indicators and activate the monitoring system and to recommend appropriate user-friendly dissemination strategies that provide practical relevance and value to the work of both policy makers and practitioners concerned with promotion policy and practice at Community level and within the Member States.

Abstract (Original Language)

Age Groups

The project involves definition of health promotion indicators

Health Behaviors and Health Awareness Among European College Students

Project Leader

Project Leader	Prof. Dr. Andrew Steptoe
Address	University College of London
Executing Institution	University College of London
Funding Agency	

Project Information

Start of Project	01/09/1999
End of Project	30/06/2000
Start of Data Collection	01/10/1999
End of Data Collection	30/11/1999
URL	
Scope	European

Keywords

Abstract (English)

Abstract (Original Language)

Age Groups

18	25

Scottish Health Survey 2003

SHS

Project Leader

Project Leader	Catherine Bromley
Address	
Executing Institution	Scottish Center for Social Research
Funding Agency	Scottish Executive Health Department

Project Information

Start of Project	01/06/2003
End of Project	31/12/2004
Start of Data Collection	01/06/2003
End of Data Collection	31/12/2004
URL	http://www.scotland.gov.uk/Publications/2005/11/25145024/50251
Scope	European

Keywords

Abstract (English) The 2003 Scottish Health Survey was the third in a series of surveys, the previous two having been conducted in 1995 and 1998. All surveys have provided data about the health of the population living in private households in Scotland. The 2003 survey covered the adult population aged 16 and over, and children aged 0–15. The 2003 Scottish Health Survey was the third in a series of surveys, the previous two having been conducted in 1995 and 1998. All surveys have provided data about the health of the population living in private households in Scotland. The 2003 survey covered the adult population aged 16 and over, and children aged 0–15.

Abstract (Original Language)

Age Groups

Some questions related to children under 2; under 4; under 12; under16
Some questions related to adults 17–74

Young Person's Behavior and Attitudes Survey 2003

Project Leader

Project Leader	Central Survey Unit
Address	Central Survey Unit,
	McAulay House,
	2–14 Castle Street
	Belfast
	BT1 1SY
Executing Institution	Northern Ireland Statistics and Research Agency
Funding Agency	Northern Ireland consortium of government departments and public bodies

Project Information

Start of Project	01/10/2003
End of Project	30/11/2003
Start of Data Collection	01/10/2003
End of Data Collection	30/11/2003
URL	http://www.csu.nisra.gov.uk/archive/Surveys/YPBAS/ RESULTS/YPBAS%202003%20Technical%20Report.pdf
Scope	European

Keywords

Abstract (English) A school-based survey of a representative sample of 11- to 16-year-old son a wide range of topics relevant to young people today.

Abstract (Original Language)

Age Groups

11	12
12	13
13	14
14	15
15	16
11.4.	Project Identity Cards: National Projects

10.4. Project Identity Cards: National Projects

Austria

1. Österreichischer Männergesundheitsbericht

Project Leader

Project Leader	Claudia Habl; Andreas Birner; Anton Hlava; Petra Winkler
Address	Stubenring 6
	A-1010 Wien
Executing Institution	Österreichisches Bundesinstitut für Gesundheitswesen (ÖBiG)
Funding Agency	Bundesministerium für soziale Sicherheit, Generationen und
	Konsumentenschutz (BMSG); Männerpolitische
	Grundsatzabteilung (Sektion V, Abteilung 6)

Project Information

Start of Project	
End of Project	31/03./2004
Start of Data Collection	01/01/1991
End of Data Collection	01/01/1991
URL	http://www.oebig.at/upload/files/CMSEditor/PUBLIKATION_
	Maennergesundheitsbericht_2004.pdf
Scope	National

Keywords

Abstract (English)   The first nationwide report on Men's Health was commissioned by the Federal Ministry of Social Security, Generations and Consumer Protection and published by the "Österreichisches Bundesinstitut für Gesundheitswesen" (Austrian Federal Insitute of Health).

The report outlines the influence of health determinants (e.g., lifestyle and working conditions) and epidemiological data as well as data collection and analyses of health behavior of Austrian men. The study aimed at identifying models of best practice in men's health and at proposing target group oriented prevention measures.

Abstract (Original Language)   Im vorliegenden ersten bundesweiten Männergesundheitsbericht, den das ÖBIG (Österreichisches Bundesinstitut für Gesundheitswesen) im Auftrag der männerpolitischen Grundsatzabteilung des Bundesministeriums für soziale Sicherheit, Generationen und Konsumentenschutz (BMSG) erstellt hat, wurden oben stehende Erkenntnisse mit Daten belegt und - zumindest in Ansätzen - Erklärungen dafür gefunden.

Weitere Berichtsinhalte sind die Darstellung von gesundheitlichen Einflussgrößen (z. B. Lebensstil, Arbeitsbedingungen, Belastungssituationen) und von epidemiologischen

Daten sowie eine Erhebung und Analyse des Gesundheitsverhaltens bzw. -handelns der österreichischen Männer. Aufgabe der Studie war ergänzend die Identifizierung von Best-Practice Modellen der Männergesundheit verbunden mit Vorschlägen für zielgruppengerechte Vorsorgemaßnahmen.

Age Groups

16	24
25	29
30	34
35	39
40	44
45	49
50	54
55	59
60	64
65	69
70	and older

1. Wiener Ernährungsbericht

Project Leader

Project Leader	I. Elmadfa
Address	Althanstraße 14
	A - 1090 Wien
Executing Institution	Institut für Ernährungswissenschaften der Universität Wien
Funding Agency	Gemeinde Wien

Project Information

Start of Project	
End of Project	31/12/1994
Start of Data Collection	
End of Data Collection	
URL	https://www.wien.gv.at/who/downloads.htm
Scope	National

Keywords

Abstract (English) With the compilation of the first Vienna Nutrition Report an important foundation was laid. The following topics were dealt with in the first Report:

Group specific data on food availability are important to characterise the general situation. Efficient planning of target group oriented measures requires details on the originalities of the nutrition situation of the respective population group. The characteristics of the individual population groups were specified and attempts were made to define obvious risk areas.

Communal feeding offers the chance to start measures in nutrition policy as individual nutritional responsibility has been passed on to others. An optimised nutrition situation can be reached with the help of improved offers and structured information.

The communication of nutrition information is of central importance to the realisation of many measures in nutrition policy. As there are no such data available for the Vienna region, the report attempted to provide a short description.

Abstract (Original Language) Mit der Erstellung des ersten Wiener Ernährungsberichtes wurden wichtige grundlegende Schritte gesetzt. Folgende Schwerpunkte wurden in diesem ersten Bericht behandelt:

Gruppenspezifische Grunddaten zur Lebensmittelversorgung sind für die Charakteristika der allgemeinen Ausgangssituation wichtig.

Die effiziente Planung der zielgruppenspezifischen Maßnahmen benötigt Information zu den Eigenarten der Ernährungssituation der entsprechenden

Bevölkerungsgruppen. Die Charakteristika der einzelnen Bevölkerungsgruppen wurden spezifiziert und es wurde dabei auch versucht, deutliche Risikobereiche festzulegen.

Eine Möglichkeit, ernährungspolitische Maßnahmen zu setzen, stellt das Gebiet der Gemeinschaftsverpflegung dar, wo die individuelle Verantwortung für die Verpflegung an Dritte weitergegeben wird. Über ein verbessertes Angebot verbunden mit einer strukturierten Information ist es sehr gut möglich, zur Optimierung der Ernährungssituation beizutragen.

Von zentraler Bedeutung bei der Realisation vieler Maßnahmen der Ernährungspolitik ist die Vermittlung von Ernährungsinformation. Da für den Raum Wien diesbezüglich ebenfalls noch keine Daten vorliegen, wurde versucht eine kurze Charakteristik vorzunehmen.

Age Groups

2. Wiener Ernährungsbericht 2004

Project Leader

Project Leader	I. Elmadfa
Address	Althanstraße 14
	A - 1090 Wien
Executing Institution	Institute of Nutritional Sciences, University of Vienna, Austria
Funding Agency	Bereichsleitung für Sozial- und Gesundheitsplanung sowie Finanzmanagement (BGF) der Stadt Wien

Project Information

Start of Project	
End of Project	31/05/2005
Start of Data Collection	
End of Data Collection	
URL	https://www.wien.gv.at/who/downloads.htm
Scope	National

Keywords

Abstract (English) The second Vienna Nutrition Report provides a good overview on the nutrition situation in the population of Vienna. It lists what measures have been taken in recent years and also what aims shall be targeted in nutrition policy. This concerns the measures for the elimination of the mentioned forms of malnutrition, further implementation of health reporting, dissemination of nutrition information as well as extended health promoting strategies.

Abstract (Original Language) Der 2. Wiener Ernährungsbericht gibt einen guten Überblick über die Ernährungssituation in der Wiener Bevölkerung. Er zeigt auf, welche Maßnahmen in den letzten Jahren gesetzt wurden, aber auch welche ernährungspolitischen Ziele für die Zukunft anvisiert werden sollten. Darunter fallen die Fortsetzung der Maßnahmen zur Beseitigung der aufgezeigten Formen der Fehlernährung, die Weiterführung der Ernährungsberichterstattung, die Verbreitung von Ernährungsinformationen sowie die Ausweitung gesundheitsfördernder Strategien.

Age Groups

Survey Chapter 6.1:

- schoolchildren (7–14 years)
- AHS-pupil (14–19 years)
- Trainees (14–36 years)
- Undergraduates (18–35 years)
- Adults (19–65 years)
- Elderly (>55 years)
- Expectant mother (25–45 years)

Survey Chapter 6.2:

- Schoolchildren
- 7–9 years
- 10–12 years
- 13–14 years

Survey Chapter 6.5:

- <24 years
- 25–50 years
- 54–64 years

>65 years

- <24 years
- 25–50 years
- 54–64 years
- >65 years

Burgenländischer Gesundheitsbericht 2002

Project Leader

Project Leader	Dr. Sebastian Kux
Address	Stubenring 6
	A-1010 Wien
Executing Institution	ÖBIG (Österreichisches Bundesinstitut für Gesundheitswesen)
Funding Agency	Amt der Burgenländischen Landesregierung, Abt. 6 Gesundheit

Project Information

Start of Project	
End of Project	
Start of Data Collection	01/01/1991
End of Data Collection	31/12/2000
URL	http://neu.burgenland.at/gesundheit_soziales/Images/BGLD-Gesundheitsbericht_2002_KF_tcm30-42245.pdf#search=%22 burgenl%C3%A4ndischer%20gesundheitsbericht%22
Scope	National

Keywords

Abstract (English) The Burgenland Health Report 2002 describes the health situation of the Burgenland population as well as important features of the health care system. The report covers the period between 1991 and 2000. Provided that regional data are available the report also includes regional analyses. The report addresses several target groups:

- Health policy makers in the Burgenland
- Interested stakeholders
- Broad public

The report is not only to draw attention to health problems and trends but also provide a sound basis for intervention measures in the area of health care and health promotion as well as for the further development of the Burgenland health care system.

Abstract (Original Language) Der burgenländische Gesundheitsbericht 2002 beschreibt die gesundheitliche Lage der burgenländischen Landesbürger sowie die wichtigsten Merkmale des Gesundheitsversorgungssystems im Land. Die Inhalte des Berichts beziehen sich grundsätzlich auf den Zeitraum 1991 bis 2000. Sofern es die Datenlage zulässt, erfolgen Analysen auf der regionalen Ebene. Der Bericht wendet sich an mehrere Zielgruppen, und zwar:

- an die (gesundheits-) politischen Entscheidungsträger im Land
- an die interessierte Fachöffentlichkeit und nicht zuletzt auch
- an die breite Öffentlichkeit.

Der Bericht soll nicht nur das Erkennen von gesundheitlichen Problemfeldern und Trends ermöglichen, sondern auch eine fundierte Grundlage für gesundheitspolitische Interventionen im Bereich der Gesundheitsvorsorge und -förderung sowie zur Weiterentwicklung des burgenländischen Gesundheitsversorgungssystems bilden.

Age Groups

Ernährung älterer Menschen in Wien

Project Leader

Project Leader	Prof. Dr. Ibrahim Elmadfa
Address	
Executing Institution	Institut für Ernährungswissenschaften der Universität Wien
Funding Agency	Stadt Wien

Project Information

Start of Project	
End of Project	31/12/1996
Start of Data Collection	
End of Data Collection	
URL	https://www.wien.gv.at/who/forms/
Scope	European

Keywords

Abstract (English) The report focuses on characterising the nutrition situation of the elderly in Vienna. The introductory chapter points out that the elderly in Vienna, 350,000 inhabitants aged over 60, make up a considerable part of the population. There have been no representative data on the nutrition situation of the elderly available. The nutrition situation of this group could be estimated by evaluating the nutrition status of Viennese living in homes for the aged and by evaluating food provision in private homes.

On the basis of the results lined out in Chaps. 2 and 3, the report attempts to develop concrete and target group oriented proposals for the improvement of the nutrition situation of elderly Viennese.

Abstract (Original Language) Der vorliegende Bericht hat die Charakteristik der Ernährungssituation älterer Menschen in Wien zum Gegenstand. Im einleitenden Kapitel wird dargestellt, dass ältere Menschen in Wien mit etwa 350.000 Menschen über 60 Jahren einen beträchtlichen Anteil der Bevölkerung stellen. Repräsentative Angaben zur Ernährungssituation dieser Gruppe lagen bis dato nicht vor. Über die Evaluation des Ernährungsstatus von Bewohnern Wiener Pensionistenheime und die ernährungswissenschaftliche Bewertung der Angebote der mobilen Mahlzeitdienste konnte eine Abschätzung der Ernährungssituation dieser Gruppe durchgeführt werden.

Auf der Grundlage der im Kapitel 2 und 3 vorgelegten Ergebnisse soll zusammenfassend versucht werden, konkrete zielgruppenspezifische Vorschläge für die Verbesserung der aktuellen Ernährungssituation älterer Menschen in Wien zu entwerfen.

Age Groups

Frauengesundheitsbericht 2003 für die Steiermark

Project Leader

Project Leader	Dr. Thomas Amegah
Address	
Executing Institution	
Funding Agency	Amt der Steiermärkischen Landesregierung, Fachabteilung 8B – Gesundheitswesen

Project Information

Start of Project	
End of Project	
Start of Data Collection	
End of Data Collection	
URL	http://www.verwaltung.steiermark.at/cms/ziel/3763997/DE/
Scope	National

Keywords

Abstract (English) It is the high ranking aim of Styria health reporting to compile health reports that use a holistic health term. Valid and representative health data (in contrast to routine data on disease) have not been available for Styria. The collection and evaluation of data are not only of basic importance for goal-oriented health planning but also cause costs, which are momentarily not sufficiently covered in the Styria budget. The report focuses on those areas that show a high cost-benefit ratio (i.e., high benefit due to data quality for costs adequate to the health budget of the country). For that reason, the report was limited to demographic, social, and political developments, main causes of death, most important diseases, utilisation of preventive medical check-up, and gender-specific differences in diabetes. On top of that the report is characterised by the optimum use of available data and good quality of used data as well as good evaluation of statistics.

Abstract (Original Language) Das übergeordnete Ziel der steirischen Gesundheitsberichterstattung ist es Gesundheitsberichte zu erstellen, die einen umfassenden ganzheitlichen Gesundheitsbegriff verwenden. Valide und repräsentative Gesundheitsdaten (in Abgrenzung von Routinedaten aus dem Krankheitsbereich) sind nach wie vor für die Steiermark nicht erhältlich. Die Erhebung und Auswertung dieser Daten ist nicht nur von unumgänglicher Wichtigkeit für die zielorientierte Gesundheitsplanung, sondern verursacht auch Kosten, die zum aktuellen Zeitpunkt im Landesbudget nicht ausreichend bedeckt sind. Der Bericht konzentriert sich daher auf jene Bereiche, die einen hohen Kosten-Nutzen-Effekt (im Sinne von hohem Nutzen durch gute Datenqualität für Kosten, die dem Gesundheitsbudget des Landes angemessen sind) zeigen. Somit wurde der Bericht auf die Bereiche der demographischen, sozialen und politischen Entwicklung, der Haupttodesursachen, der wichtigsten Erkrankungen, der Inanspruchnahme von Vorsorgeuntersuchungen und der geschlechtsspezifischen Unterschiede im Bereich Diabetes eingeschränkt. Darüber hinaus zeichnet sich der Bericht durch die optimale Nutzung vorhandener und die gute Qualität verwendeter Daten aus, sowie durch die gute statistische Auswertung.

Age Groups

Gesundheit in Wien

Project Leader

Project Leader	Mag. Monika Csitkovics
Address	
Executing Institution	
Funding Agency	Stadt Wien, Bereichsleitung für Gesundheitsplanung und Finanzmanagement

Project Information

Start of Project	
End of Project	31/03/2003
Start of Data Collection	
End of Data Collection	
URL	https://www.wien.gv.at/who/downloads.htm
Scope	National

Keywords

Abstract (English) This brochure aims at providing an overview on basic aspects of the Vienna health care system. The headline "What We Know" summarises current data and facts on the health status and health-related behavior of the Viennese in the first part of the brochure. The part "What We Want" contains policy guidelines and approaches. The third part "What We Do" describes important parts of the health care system from the hospitals to health promotion.

Abstract (Original Language) Die vorliegende Broschüre soll einen Überblick über wesentliche Aspekte des Wiener Gesundheitswesens geben. Im ersten Teil der Broschüre werden unter dem Titel "Was wir wissen" aktuelle Daten und Fakten zum Gesundheitszustand sowie zum Gesundheitsverhalten der Wienerinnen und Wiener wiedergegeben. Im Abschnitt "Was wir wollen" befinden sich Leitbilder und programmatische Ansätze. Im dritten Teil, "Was wir tun", werden wichtige Bereiche des Gesundheitssystems beschrieben - vom Spitalswesen bis hin zur Gesundheitsförderung.

Age Groups

Gesundheitsbericht 2003

Project Leader

Project Leader	Anton Hlava
Address	Stubenring 6
	A - 1010 Wien
Executing Institution	Österreichisches Bundesinstitut für Gesundheitswesen
Funding Agency	Bundesministerium für Gesundheit und Frauen

Project Information

Start of Project	
End of Project	31/12/2004
Start of Data Collection	
End of Data Collection	
URL	http://www.bmgf.gv.at/cms/site/attachments/4/1/7/CH0083/
	CMS1087997708602/gesundheitsbericht-2003-komplett.pdf
Scope	National

Keywords

Abstract (English) The Health Report 2003 is a reply to the request of the Parliament from 16 December 1988 to provide a description of the development in the Austrian health care system every three years. The Austrian Ministry of Health was commissioned to compile the health report. In contrast to the "Gesundheits-statistischen Jahrbuch", which is published every year, the following criteria are to be met by the health report:

- Analyse of the current state of development of the Austrian health care system considering historical development and international comparison
- Provide reference to the health policy aims of the government, European Union, and the WHO (especially referring to the concept "Health for All", which was set up for the European region)
- Describe perspectives of Austrian health policy

Abstract (Original Language) Mit dem vorliegenden "Gesundheitsbericht 2003" wird nunmehr zum vierten Mal dem Ersuchen des Nationalrats vom 16. Dezember 1988 entsprochen, alle drei Jahre eine Darstellung der Weiterentwicklung des österreichischen Gesundheitswesens vorzulegen. Mit der Erstellung des vorliegenden Gesundheitsberichts war das ÖBIG (Österreichisches Bundesinstitut für Gesundheitswesen) betraut, das eng mit Mitarbeiterinnen und Mitarbeitern des Gesundheitsressorts zusammenarbeitete. In Abgrenzung zum jährlich vom Gesundheitsressort in Zusammenarbeit mit der Bundesanstalt "Statistik Österreich" herausgegebenen "Gesundheitsstatistischen Jahrbuch" sind für die Erstellung des Gesundheitsberichts an den Nationalrat folgende Gesichtspunkte maßgebend:

- Standortbestimmung des österreichischen Gesundheitswesens unter Berücksichtigung der historischen Entwicklung und im internationalen Vergleich
- Bezugsetzung der Aktivitäten des Gesundheitsressorts im Berichtszeitraum zu den gesundheitspolitischen Zielsetzungen der Bundesregierung, der Europäischen Union und der Weltgesundheitsorganisation (insbesondere zu den für die europäische Region formulierten Zielen zum Rahmenkonzept "Gesundheit für alle")
- Darstellung der Perspektiven der österreichischen Gesundheitspolitik

Age Groups

Gesundheitsbericht Österreich 2004

Health Report Austria 2004

Project Leader

Project Leader	Gerhard Fülöp
Address	Stubenring 6
	A - 1010 Wien
Executing Institution	Österreichisches Bundesinstitut für Gesundheitswesen
Funding Agency	Österreichisches Bundesinstitut für Gesundheitswesen

Project Information

Start of Project	
End of Project	31/05/2004
Start of Data Collection	01/01/1992
End of Data Collection	01/01/1992
URL	http://www.bmgf.gv.at/cms/site/attachments/9/0/1/CH0083/
	CMS1091709051535/gboe_2004_internet_korrigiert.pdf
Scope	National

Keywords

Abstract (English) "Gesundheit und Krankheit in Österreich" was primarily designed as an epidemiological health report. It addresses health policy decision makers as well as the interested experts and offers comprehensive analyses of the different aspects of the health system. Special attention is paid to health status of the population, important factors influencing health, health prevention, and health promotion as well as to health care facilities.

Abstract (Original Language) "Gesundheit und Krankheit in Österreich" ist primär als epidemiologischer Basisgesundheitsbericht konzipiert. Er richtet sich an die gesundheitspolitischen Entscheidungsträger sowie an die interessierte Fachöffentlichkeit und bietet umfangreiche Analysen zu den unterschiedlichsten Aspekten des Gesundheitswesens, insbesondere zum Gesundheitszustand der Bevölkerung, zu wesentlichen Einflussfaktoren auf die Gesundheit, zu Gesundheitsvorsorge und -förderung sowie zu den Einrichtungen des Gesundheitswesens.

Age Groups

Gesundheitsbericht Wien 1996

Vienna Health Report 1996

Project Leader

Project Leader	Dr. Eleonore Bachinger
Address	
Executing Institution	
Funding Agency	MA 15 - Gesundheitswesen der Stadt Wien

Project Information

Start of Project	
End of Project	31/10/1997
Start of Data Collection	
End of Data Collection	
URL	https://www.wien.gv.at/who/downloads.htm
Scope	National

Keywords

Abstract (English) The Vienna Health report is part of health planning activities in Vienna. It is a particular concern and task of the Vienna Health Report to provide a comprehensive overview on the health of the Vienna population and the health care system in Vienna. The reports are structured this way that they meet the expectations of the different target groups. Among these there is an audience of specialists from the field of medicine, health and social science, health politicians and other decision makers in health care, experts from the field of health management and social security, journalists, teachers and students of public health, nursing and interested laymen.

Abstract (Original Language) Die Wiener Gesundheitsberichterstattung ist Teil der Wiener Gesundheitsplanung. Es ist insbesondere Anliegen und Aufgabe der Wiener Gesundheitsberichterstattung, einen umfassenden Überblick über die Gesundheit der Wiener Bevölkerung und das Wiener Gesundheitswesen zu geben. Die Berichte sind so aufgebaut, dass sie den Erwartungen und Anforderungen der verschiedenen und sehr unterschiedlichen Zielgruppen gerecht werden. Diese umfassen das Fachpublikum aus den Bereichen Medizin, Gesundheits- und Sozialwissenschaften, Gesundheits-politikerInnen und andere EntscheidungsträgerInnen im Gesundheitswesen, ExpertInnen aus dem Bereich Gesundheitsverwaltung und Sozialversicherung, JournalistInnen, Unterrichtende und Studierende in den Bereichen Public Health, Kranken- und Altenpflege, sowie interessierte Laien.

Age Groups

Gesundheitsbericht Wien 1997

Vienna Health Report 1997

Project Leader

Project Leader	Dr. Eleonore Bachinger
Address	
Executing Institution	
Funding Agency	MA 15 - Gesundheitswesen der Stadt Wien, Dezernat III - Gesundheitsplanung

Project Information

Start of Project	
End of Project	
Start of Data Collection	
End of Data Collection	
URL	https://www.wien.gv.at/who/downloads.htm
Scope	National

Keywords

Abstract (English) The Vienna Health report is part of health planning activities in Vienna. It is a particular concern and task of the Vienna Health Report to provide a comprehensive overview on the health of the Vienna population and the health care system in Vienna. The reports are structured this way that they meet the expectations of the different target groups. Among these there is an audience of specialists from the field of medicine, health and social science, health politicians and other decision makers in health care, experts from the field of health management and social security, journalists, teachers and students of public health, nursing and interested laymen.

Abstract (Original Language) Die Wiener Gesundheitsberichterstattung ist Teil der Wiener Gesundheitsplanung. Es ist insbesondere Anliegen und Aufgabe der Wiener Gesundheitsberichterstattung, einen umfassenden Überblick über die Gesundheit der Wiener Bevölkerung und das Wiener Gesundheitswesen zu geben. Die Berichte sind so aufgebaut, dass sie den Erwartungen und Anforderungen der verschiedenen und sehr unterschiedlichen Zielgruppen gerecht werden. Diese umfassen das Fachpublikum aus den Bereichen Medizin, Gesundheits- und Sozialwissenschaften, GesundheitspolitikerInnen und andere EntscheidungsträgerInnen im Gesundheitswesen, ExpertInnen aus dem Bereich Gesundheitsverwaltung und Sozialversicherung, JournalistInnen, Unterrichtende und Studierende in den Bereichen Public Health, Kranken- und Altenpflege, sowie interessierte Laien.

Age Groups

Gesundheitsbericht Wien 1998

Vienna Health Report 1998

Project Leader

Project Leader	Dr. Eleonore Bachinger
Address	
Executing Institution	
Funding Agency	Magistratsabteilung für Angelegenheiten der
	Landessanitätsdirektion, Dezernat II – Gesundheitsplanung

Project Information

Start of Project	
End of Project	
Start of Data Collection	
End of Data Collection	
URL	https://www.wien.gv.at/who/downloads.htm
Scope	National

Keywords

Abstract (English) The Vienna Health report is part of health planning activities in Vienna. It is a particular concern and task of the Vienna Health Report to provide a comprehensive overview on the health of the Vienna population and the health care system in Vienna. The reports are structured this way that they meet the expectations of the different target groups. Among these there is an audience of specialists from the field of medicine, health and social science, health politicians and other decision makers in health care, experts from the field of health management and social security, journalists, teachers and students of public health, nursing and interested laymen.

Abstract (Original Language) Die Wiener Gesundheitsberichterstattung ist Teil der Wiener Gesundheitsplanung. Es ist insbesondere Anliegen und Aufgabe der Wiener Gesundheitsberichterstattung, einen umfassenden Überblick über die Gesundheit der Wiener Bevölkerung und das Wiener Gesundheitswesen zu geben. Die Berichte sind so aufgebaut, dass sie den Erwartungen und Anforderungen der verschiedenen und sehr unterschiedlichen Zielgruppen gerecht werden. Diese umfassen das Fachpublikum aus den Bereichen Medizin, Gesundheits- und Sozialwissenschaften, GesundheitspolitikerInnen und andere EntscheidungsträgerInnen im Gesundheitswesen, ExpertInnen aus dem Bereich Gesundheitsverwaltung und Sozialversicherung, JournalistInnen, Unterrichtende und Studierende in den Bereichen Public Health, Kranken- und Altenpflege, sowie interessierte Laien.

Age Groups

Gesundheitsbericht Wien 2000

Vienna Heatlh Report 2000

Project Leader

Project Leader	Dr. Eleonore Bachinger, Mag. Monika Csitkovics, Mag. Klaudia Wais
Address	
Executing Institution	
Funding Agency	Magistratsabteilung für Angelegenheiten der Landessanitätsdirektion, Dezernat II – Gesundheitsplanung

Project Information

Start of Project	
End of Project	30/11/2000
Start of Data Collection	
End of Data Collection	
URL	https://www.wien.gv.at/who/downloads.htm
Scope	National

Keywords

Abstract (English) The Vienna Health report is part of health planning activities in Vienna. It is a particular concern and task of the Vienna Health Report to provide a comprehensive overview on the health of the Vienna population and the health care system in Vienna. The reports are structured this way that they meet the expectations of the different target groups. Among these there is an audience of specialists from the field of medicine, health and social science, health politicians and other decision makers in health care, experts from the field of health management and social security, journalists, teachers and students of public health, nursing and interested laymen.

Abstract (Original Language) Die Wiener Gesundheitsberichterstattung ist Teil der Wiener Gesundheitsplanung. Es ist insbesondere Anliegen und Aufgabe der Wiener Gesundheitsberichterstattung, einen umfassenden Überblick über die Gesundheit der Wiener Bevölkerung und das Wiener Gesundheitswesen zu geben. Die Berichte sind so aufgebaut, dass sie den Erwartungen und Anforderungen der verschiedenen und sehr unterschiedlichen Zielgruppen gerecht werden. Diese umfassen das Fachpublikum aus den Bereichen Medizin, Gesundheits- und Sozialwissenschaften, GesundheitspolitikerInnen und andere EntscheidungsträgerInnen im Gesundheitswesen, ExpertInnen aus dem Bereich Gesundheitsverwaltung und Sozialversicherung, JournalistInnen, Unterrichtende und Studierende in den Bereichen Public Health, Kranken- und Altenpflege, sowie interessierte Laien.

Age Groups

Gesundheitsbericht Wien 2001

Vienna Health Report 2001

Project Leader

Project Leader	Dr. Eleonore Bachinger, Mag. Monika Csitkovics
Address	
Executing Institution	
Funding Agency	Magistrat der Stadt Wien, Bereichsleitung für Gesundheitsplanung und Finanzmanagement, Gesundheitsberichterstattung

Project Information

Start of Project	
End of Project	30/11/2001
Start of Data Collection	
End of Data Collection	
URL	https://www.wien.gv.at/who/downloads.htm
Scope	National

Keywords

Abstract (English) The Vienna Health report is part of health planning activities in Vienna. It is a particular concern and task of the Vienna Health Report to provide a comprehensive overview on the health of the Vienna population and the health care system in Vienna. The reports are structured this way that they meet the expectations of the different target groups. Among these there is an audience of specialists from the field of medicine, health and social science, health politicians and other decision makers in health care, experts from the field of health management and social security, journalists, teachers and students of public health, nursing and interested laymen.

Abstract (Original Language) Die Wiener Gesundheitsberichterstattung ist Teil der Wiener Gesundheitsplanung. Es ist insbesondere Anliegen und Aufgabe der Wiener Gesundheitsberichterstattung, einen umfassenden Überblick über die Gesundheit der Wiener Bevölkerung und das Wiener Gesundheitswesen zu geben. Die Berichte sind so aufgebaut, dass sie den Erwartungen und Anforderungen der verschiedenen und sehr unterschiedlichen Zielgruppen gerecht werden. Diese umfassen das Fachpublikum aus den Bereichen Medizin, Gesundheits- und Sozialwissenschaften, Gesundheits- politikerInnen und andere EntscheidungsträgerInnen im Gesundheitswesen, ExpertInnen aus dem Bereich Gesundheitsverwaltung und Sozialversicherung, JournalistInnen, Unterrichtende und Studierende in den Bereichen Public Health, Kranken- und Altenpflege, sowie interessierte Laien.

Age Groups

Gesundheitsbericht Wien 2002

Vienna Health Report 2002

Project Leader

Project Leader	Dr. Eleonore Bachinger, MSc
Address	
Executing Institution	
Funding Agency	Magistrat der Stadt Wien, Bereichsleitung für Gesundheitsplanung
	und Finanzmanagement, Gesundheitsberichterstattung

Project Information

Start of Project	
End of Project	30/11/2002
Start of Data Collection	
End of Data Collection	
URL	https://www.wien.gv.at/who/downloads.htm
Scope	National

Keywords

Abstract (English) The Vienna Health report is part of health planning activities in Vienna. It is a particular concern and task of the Vienna Health Report to provide a comprehensive overview on the health of the Vienna population and the health care system in Vienna. The reports are structured this way that they meet the expectations of the different target groups. Among these there is an audience of specialists from the field of medicine, health and social science, health politicians and other decision makers in health care, experts from the field of health management and social security, journalists, teachers and students of public health, nursing and interested laymen.

Abstract (Original Language) Die Wiener Gesundheitsberichterstattung ist Teil der Wiener Gesundheitsplanung. Es ist insbesondere Anliegen und Aufgabe der Wiener Gesundheitsberichterstattung, einen umfassenden Überblick über die Gesundheit der Wiener Bevölkerung und das Wiener Gesundheitswesen zu geben. Die Berichte sind so aufgebaut, dass sie den Erwartungen und Anforderungen der verschiedenen und sehr unterschiedlichen Zielgruppen gerecht werden. Diese umfassen das Fachpublikum aus den Bereichen Medizin, Gesundheits- und Sozialwissenschaften, Gesundheits-politikerInnen und andere EntscheidungsträgerInnen im Gesundheitswesen, ExpertInnen aus dem Bereich Gesundheitsverwaltung und Sozialversicherung, JournalistInnen, Unterrichtende und Studierende in den Bereichen Public Health, Kranken- und Altenpflege, sowie interessierte Laien.

Age Groups

Gesundheitsbericht Wien 2004

Vienna Health Report 2004

Project Leader

Project Leader	Dr. Eleonore Bachinger, MSc(EPH)
Address	
Executing Institution	
Funding Agency	Magistrat der Stadt Wien, Bereichsleitung für Soziales- und Gesundheitsplanung sowie Finanzmanagement, Gesundheitsberichterstattung

Project Information

Start of Project	
End of Project	30/10/2005
Start of Data Collection	
End of Data Collection	
URL	https://www.wien.gv.at/who/downloads.htm
Scope	National

Keywords

Abstract (English) The Vienna Health report is part of health planning activities in Vienna. It is a particular concern and task of the Vienna Health Report to provide a comprehensive overview on the health of the Vienna population and the health care system in Vienna. The reports are structured this way that they meet the expectations of the different target groups. Among these there is an audience of specialists from the field of medicine, health and social science, health politicians and other decision makers in health care, experts from the field of health management and social security, journalists, teachers and students of public health, nursing and interested laymen.

Abstract (Original Language) Die Wiener Gesundheitsberichterstattung ist Teil der Wiener Gesundheitsplanung. Es ist insbesondere Anliegen und Aufgabe der Wiener Gesundheitsberichterstattung, einen umfassenden Überblick über die Gesundheit der Wiener Bevölkerung und das Wiener Gesundheitswesen zu geben. Die Berichte sind so aufgebaut, dass sie den Erwartungen und Anforderungen der verschiedenen und sehr unterschiedlichen Zielgruppen gerecht werden. Diese umfassen das Fachpublikum aus den Bereichen Medizin, Gesundheits- und Sozialwissenschaften, Gesundheits-politikerInnen und andere EntscheidungsträgerInnen im Gesundheitswesen, ExpertInnen aus dem Bereich Gesundheitsverwaltung und Sozialversicherung, JournalistInnen, Unterrichtende und Studierende in den Bereichen Public Health, Kranken- und Altenpflege, sowie interessierte Laien.

Age Groups

Lebensstile in Wien

Lifestyle in Vienna

Project Leader

Project Leader	Univ.-Prof. Dr. Wolfgang Freidl, Univ.-Prof. Dr. Willibald-Julius Stronegger, Dr. Christine Neuhold
Address	
Executing Institution	
Funding Agency	Magistrat der Stadt Wien, Bereichsleitung für Gesundheitsplanung und Finanzmanagement, Gesundheitsberichterstattung

Project Information

Start of Project	
End of Project	30/06/2003
Start of Data Collection	
End of Data Collection	
URL	https://www.wien.gv.at/who/downloads.htm
Scope	National

Keywords

Abstract (English) Health is not only influenced by biological, psychological, and socio-economic factors but also by health-related behavior. Health behavior includes health promoting and health preserving behavior such as physical activity, healthy diet, or vaccination as well as risk behaviour such as smoking or excessive consumption of alcohol. To gain an in depth description of the health-related behavior of the Vienna population, the city of Vienna instructed the Institute of Social Medicine of the University of Graz to carry out a study in this regard. This report "Lifestyles in Vienna" is based on data of the Vienna Health and Social Survey and describes health-related behaviour, consumption of food and drugs, physical activity and body mass index, utilization of medical care as well as activity and regenerative behavior. The mentioned patterns of behavior are analysed according to age and gender, and where relevant also according to social and internal resources as well as state of health.

The results of the study show that health-related behavior is influenced by gender and age as well as the financial situation, level of education, quality of social networks, and additionally by work satisfaction and work load. Despite the fact that some indicators deviate the study concludes that positive health-related behaviour can be predominantly found in women, the elderly, persons with a higher income and education and a low workload.

Abstract (Original Language) Die Gesundheit wird nicht nur von biologischen, psychologischen und sozioökonomischen Faktoren, sondern auch von gesundheitsrelevanten Verhaltensweisen beeinflusst. Der Begriff Gesundheitsverhalten schließt sowohl gesundheitsfördernde und -erhaltende Verhaltensweisen wie körperliche Aktivität, gesunde Ernährung oder Impfungen als auch Risikoverhaltensweisen wie Rauchen oder exzessiven Alkoholkonsum ein.

Um erstmals eine vertiefende Darstellung der gesundheitsrelevanten Verhaltensweisen der Wienerinnen und Wiener zu erhalten, beauftragte die Stadt Wien das Institut für Sozialmedizin der Universität Graz mit der Erstellung einer diesbezüglichen Studie. Der nun vorliegende Bericht "Lebensstile in Wien" beschreibt – basierend auf den Daten des Wiener Gesundheits- und Sozialsurveys – die gesundheitsrelevanten Verhaltensweisen, Suchtmittel- und Nahrungsmittelkonsum, körperliche Bewegung und body mass index, die Inanspruchnahme der medizinischen Versorgung sowie Aktivität und regeneratives Verhalten. Die genannten Verhaltensweisen werden durchgehend nach Alter und Geschlecht und – wo sinnvoll – auch nach sozialen und internen Ressourcen sowie nach dem Gesundheitszustand analysiert.

Aus den Ergebnissen der Studie lässt sich ersehen, dass gesundheitsrelevante Verhaltensweisen sowohl vom Geschlecht und Alter als auch von der finanziellen Situation, der Bildungshöhe, der Qualität der sozialen Netzwerke sowie der Arbeitszufriedenheit und Arbeitsbelastungen beeinflusst werden. Trotz Abweichungen bei einzelnen Indikatoren kann aus der Studie der Schluss gezogen werden, dass ein positives Gesundheitsverhalten bei Frauen, älteren Menschen, Personen mit höherem Einkommen und Bildung sowie geringerer Arbeitsbelastung vermehrt zum Tragen kommt.

Age Groups

Linzer Gesundheitsbericht 2001

Project Leader

Project Leader	Dr. Claudia Pass
Address	
Executing Institution	
Funding Agency	Stadt Linz

Project Information

Start of Project	
End of Project	
Start of Data Collection	
End of Data Collection	
URL	http://www.linz.at/images/GBVorwort.pdf#search=%22gesundh eitsbericht%20ober%C3%B6sterreich%22
Scope	National

Keywords

Abstract (English) This descriptive overview report summarises a variety of data, research results, and statistical evaluations with the aim to develop a basis for health policy and for the development of health aims. Following this the focus will be on analysing emerging problem areas in more detail and to start necessary counteractive measures.

Abstract (Original Language) In diesem deskriptiven Überblicksbericht werden eine Vielzahl von Daten, Untersuchungsergebnissen und statistischen Auswertungen zusammengefasst, mit dem Ziel, eine Grundlage für die Gesundheitspolitik und die Entwicklung von Gesundheitszielen zu erarbeiten. In der Folge wird es vor allem darum gehen, Problembereiche, die sich hier herauskristallisieren, eingehender zu analysieren und notwendige Gegenmaßnahmen zu setzen.

Age Groups

Mikrozensus 1999: Ergebnisse zur Gesundheit in Wien

Microcensus 1999: Results on Health in Vienna

Project Leader

Project Leader	Dr. Richard Költringer, Dr. Elfriede Urbas
Address	
Executing Institution	
Funding Agency	Magistrat der Stadt Wien, Bereichsleitung für Gesundheitsplanung und Finanzmanagement, Gesundheitsberichterstattung

Project Information

Start of Project	
End of Project	31/12/2002
Start of Data Collection	
End of Data Collection	
URL	https://www.wien.gv.at/who/downloads.htm
Scope	National

Keywords

Abstract (English) The Microcensus is a survey that is carried out by Statistics Austria on a quarterly basis. For the Microcensus about 60,000 Austrians, about 6,000 of whom are Viennese, are questioned. The permanent basic set of questions on the structure of the population, household, and apartment as well as jobs and unemployment is complemented by a set of extra questions. The extra set of questions on health were last included in the survey in 1991 and 1999. The set of questions in 1999 was basically adapted to the questions of the previous year so that results could be compared. The questions on health cover aspects such as lifestyle and workload, utilization of preventive health care services, health status as well as utilization medical services. The Microcensus dataset on population health was evaluated and analysed by the Institute for Panel research on request of the city of Vienna. The report "Microcensus 1999 – Findings on Health in Vienna" provides an overview on the most important results. This report distinguishes between gender and age, partly considers differences in income and education, nationality, and regional location. Comparisons with previous surveys and between Vienna and Austria make the complete.

Abstract (Original Language) Der Mikrozensus ist eine Stichprobenerhebung, die von der Statistik Austria vierteljährlich in Privathaushalten durchgeführt wird. Dabei werden in Österreich fast 60.000 Personen, davon rund 6.000 in Wien, befragt. Das gleich bleibende Grundprogramm mit Fragen zur Bevölkerungs-, Haushalts- und Wohnungsstruktur sowie zur Erwerbstätigkeit und Arbeitslosigkeit wird durch

Sonderprogramme ergänzt. Das Sonderprogramm "Gesundheit" wurde zuletzt in den Jahren 1991 und 1999 erhoben. Dabei wurde der Fragenkatalog des Jahres 1999 in seinen Grundzügen den vorangegangenen Erhebungen angepasst, sodass ein zeitlicher Vergleich der Ergebnisse möglich ist. Das Sonderprogramm zur Gesundheit erfasst die Merkmale Lebensstil und Belastungen, Teilnahme an Vorsorgemaßnahmen, Gesundheitsstatus sowie die Beanspruchung medizinischer Leistungen. Der Mikrozensusdatensatz zur Gesundheit der Bevölkerung wurde im Auftrag der Stadt Wien vom Institut für Panel Research ausgewertet und analysiert. Der nun vorliegende Bericht "Mikrozensus 1999 – Ergebnisse zur Gesundheit in Wien" gibt einen Überblick über die wichtigsten Ergebnisse, wobei Differenzierungen nach Geschlecht und Alter, zum Teil auch nach Erwerbsstatus, Bildung, Nationalität und regionaler Lage vorgenommen wurden. Zeitliche Vergleiche und der Vergleich Wiens mit Österreich runden diesen Bericht ab.

Age Groups

0	14
15	29
30	44
45	59
60	74
75	and older

Niederösterreichischer Gesundheitsbericht 2002

Project Leader

Project Leader	Andreas Birner
Address	Stubenring 6
	A-1010 Wien
Executing Institution	Österreichisches Bundesinstitut für Gesundheitswesen (ÖBiG)
Funding Agency	Niederösterreichische Landesregierung, Gruppe "Gesundheit und Soziales", Abteilung "Gesundheitswesen/ Sanitätsdirektion"

Project Information

Start of Project	
End of Project	31/12/2002
Start of Data Collection	01/01/1991
End of Data Collection	31/12/2000
URL	http://www.noel.gv.at/service/gs/gs1/Downloads/ Gesundheitsbericht_NOE.pdf
Scope	National

Keywords

Abstract (English)

The Health Report for Lower Austria 2002 describes the health situation of the population in Lower Austria as well as most important features of the health care system in the country. The report addresses several target groups:

- Health policy makers in the Burgenland
- Interested stakeholders
- Broad public

The report is not only to draw attention to health problems and trends but also provide a sound basis for intervention measures in the area of health care and health promotion as well as for the further development of health care system in Lower Austria.

Abstract (Original Language)

Der Niederösterreicherische Gesundheitsbericht 2002 beschreibt die gesundheitliche Lage der niederösterreichischen Landesbürger sowie die wichtigsten Merkamale des Gesundheitsversorgungssystems im Land. Der Bericht wendet sich damit an mehrere Zielgruppen, und zwar:

- an die (gesundheits-)politischen Entscheidungsträger im Land,
- an die interessierte Fachöffentlichkeit,
- an die breite Öffentlichkeit.

Der Bericht soll nicht nur die Indentifikation von gesundheitlichen Problemfeldern und Trends ermöglichen, sondern auch eine fundierte Grundlage für gesundheitspolitische Interventionen im Bereich der Prävention und Gesundheitsförderung bzw. zur Weiterentwicklung des niederösterreichischen Gesundheitsversorgungssystem bilden.

Age Groups

Österreichischer Ernährungsbericht 1998

Project Leader

Project Leader	Prof. D. I. Elmadfa
Address	Althanstraße 14
	A - 1090 Wien
Executing Institution	Institut für Ernährungswissenschaften der Universität Wien
Funding Agency	Bundesministerium für Frauenangelegenheiten und
	Verbraucherschutz, Bundesministerium für Arbeit,
	Gesundes und Soziales

Project Information

Start of Project	
End of Project	31/12/1998
Start of Data Collection	
End of Data Collection	
URL	http://www.univie.ac.at/nutrition/oeeb/OEEB.PDF
Scope	National

Keywords

Abstract (English) This report provides a description of food consumption in Austria between 1947 and 1997. The report focuses on the nutrition status of the Austrian population, different aspects of food quality, and communal feeding. It furthermore contains information on mortality of nutrition-related diseases from 1950 to 1995 and on some areas of health care and prevention. The report furthermore focuses on recommendation and guidelines for an optimum nutrition situation.

Abstract (Original Language) Der vorliegende Bericht enthält eine vergleichende Darstellung des Lebensmittelverbrauchs hierzulande in der Zeit von 1947 bis 1997. Seine Schwerpunkte bilden Kapitel über den Ernährungszustand der österreichischen Bevölkerung und über verschiedene Aspekte der Lebensmittelqualität und Gemeinschaftsverpflegung. Ferner enthält er Informationen über die Mortalität an ernährungsabhängigen Erkrankungen von 1950 bis 1995 und einige Bereiche der Gesundheitsförderung/Prävention. Ein weiterer Schwerpunkt sind die Empfehlungen bzw. Richtlinien zur Optimierung der Ernährungssituation.

Age Groups

Österreichischer Ernährungsbericht 2003

Austrian Nutrition Report 2003

Project Leader

Project Leader	
Address	
Executing Institution	Institut für Ernährungswissenschaften der Universität Wien
Funding Agency	Bundesministwerium für Gesundheit und Frauen

Project Information

Start of Project	
End of Project	
Start of Data Collection	
End of Data Collection	
URL	http://www.univie.ac.at/Ernaehrungswissenschaften/oeeb/ OEB2003.htm
Scope	European

Keywords

Abstract (English) The heterogeneity and complexity of data collection, documentation, and interpretation in the area of food quality, health promotion, and prevention of nutrition-related diseases give rise to the necessity to regularly take stock and analyse available and relevant information. Such descriptions shall help health politicians and decision makers to recognise problems and to develop and implement short term and medium term measures and strategies. Many countries/states followed the necessity of fundamental consideration and the aim of continuity documentation in the food and health policy sector by regularly publishing official nutrition reports every four or five years.

After the Austrian nutrition report 1998 now the next Austrian nutrition report 2003 is available. This report is based predominantly on study data and projects which the Institute of Food Sciences conducted either in cooperation or on request of the Federal Ministry for Teaching and Arts, the Federal Chancellery, Section VI and Section VIII, the municipality of Vienna (WHO project) and institutes of the university in Vienna. The Austrian Nutrition Report was initiated by the Institute for Nutrition Science and on request of the Ministry for Health and Women.

Abstract (Original Language) Die Vielfalt und Komplexität der Datenerhebung, Dokumentation und Interpretation auf dem Gebiet der Lebensmittelqualität, Gesundheitsförderung und der Prävention ernährungsabhängiger Erkrankungen machen eine regelmäßige Bestandsaufnahme und Analyse relevanter vorhandener Informationen erforderlich. Solche Darstellung soll dem Gesundheitspolitiker und Entscheidungsträger helfen, Probleme zu erkennen und kurz- und mittelfristige

Maßnahmen und Strategien zur Abhilfe zu entwickeln und einzuleiten. Von der Notwendigkeit dieser grundsätzlichen Betrachtung und Zielsetzung der Kontinuität der Dokumentation auf dem ernährungs- und gesundheitspolitischen Sektor gingen viele Länder/Staaten aus, indem sie offizielle und regelmäßige, in vier- bis fünfjährigen Zeitabständen erscheinende "Ernährungsberichte" veröffentlichen.

Nach dem Österreichischen Ernährungsbericht 1998 liegt nun auch der neue Östereichische Ernährungsbericht 2003 vor. Dieser Ernährungsbericht fußt hauptsächlich auf Daten von Studien und Projekten, die das Institut für Ernährungswissenschaften in Zusammenarbeit oder im Auftrag vom Bundesministerium für Unterricht und Kunst, dem Bundeskanzleramt, Sektion VI und Sektion VIII, der Gemeinde Wien (WHO-Projekt) und Instituten der Universität Wien durchgeführt hat. Er ist als Initiative des Instituts für Ernährungswissenschaften und im Auftrag vom Bundesministerium für Gesundheit und Frauen zustande gekommen.

Age Groups

Österreichischer Frauengesundheitsbericht 2005/2006

Project Leader

Project Leader	Prof. Dr. Beate Wimmer-Puchinger
Address	
Executing Institution	Ludwig Boltzmann Institut für Frauengesundheitsforschung
Funding Agency	Bundesministerium für Gesundheit und Frauen

Project Information

Start of Project	
End of Project	30/04/2006
Start of Data Collection	
End of Data Collection	
URL	http://www.bmgf.gv.at/cms/site/attachments/2/7/3/CH0330/ CMS1114154451979/frauengesundheitsbericht_2005-2006_ 11_4_2006.pdf
Scope	National

Keywords

Abstract (English) The report shows the wide range of multidisciplinary topics in women's health and follows the criteria recommended by the WHO in 1995. The working fields in women's health are defined and now need to be analysed in more detail by implementing more concrete measures. The existing data on the health situation of women in Austria are a starting point for further strategy development to reach a gender specific health system.

Abstract (Original Language) Der vorliegende Bericht gibt die große Bandbreite und die multidisziplinäre Themenstellung der Frauengesundheit wieder, er orientiert sich dabei an den von der WHO 1995 empfohlenen Kriterien. Die Handlungsfelder der Frauengesundheit sind somit abgesteckt und bedürfen einer Vertiefung durch die Entwicklung konkreter Maßnahmen für die Umsetzung. Die vorliegenden Daten zur gesundheitlichen Lage von Frauen in Österreich sind als Ausgangspunkt für die weitere Strategieentwicklung zur Erlangung eines geschlechtsgerechten Gesundheitssystem zu sehen.

Age Groups

Sport und Gesundheit

Die Auswirkungen des Sports auf die Gesundheit - eine sozio-ökonomische Analyse

Project Leader

Project Leader	Otmar Weiß, Christian Halbwachs
Address	
Executing Institution	
Funding Agency	Bundesministerium für soziale Sicherheit und Generationen

Project Infomation

Start of Project	
End of Project	
Start of Data Collection	
End of Data Collection	
URL	http://www.bmgf.gv.at/cms/site/attachments/7/8/9/CH0083/ CMS1051889989527/studie_sport_und_gesundheit.pdf
Scope	National

Keywords

Abstract (English) Health economists, sports physicians, and social scientists have developed together cost-benefit-model for recreational exercise in Austria. With the help of a model, the economic costs of sport injuries and accidents and the economic benefit from physical activity were calculated for Austria in 1998. The report aimed at providing an objective view on positive and negative effects of exercise on health.

Abstract (Original Language) Gesundheitsökonomen, Sportmediziner und Sozialwissenschafter haben interdisziplinär ein wohlfahrtsökonomisches Cost-Benefit-Modell des Breiten- und Freizeitsports in Österreich entwickelt. Mit Hilfe dieses Modells wurden einerseits die volkswirtschaftlichen Kosten von Sportverletzungen und -unfällen, andererseits der gesundheitsökonomische Nutzen sportlicher Aktivitäten für das Jahr 1998 in Österreich berechnet. Ziel war, die Frage der positiven und negativen Wirkungen des Sports auf die Gesundheit zu objektivieren.

Age Groups

Statistische Mitteilungen zur Gesundheit in Wien 1999/2

Gesundheit der Wiener Bevölkerung im regionalen Vergleich

Project Leader

Project Leader	Dr. Gerhard Fülöp, Mag. Petra Ofner
Address	
Executing Institution	Österreichisches Bundesinstitut für Gesundheitswesen (ÖBIG)
Funding Agency	MA-L, Gesundheitsplanung

Project Information

Start of Project	
End of Project	30/11/1999
Start of Data Collection	
End of Data Collection	
URL	https://www.wien.gv.at/who/downloads.htm
Scope	National

Keywords

Abstract (English) This edition of the "Statistischen Mitteilungen zur Gesundheit in Wien" from 1999/2000 covers the topic of health of the Vienna population and is a regional comparison. For that reason boroughs of Vienna, the surrounding of Vienna, and the remaining Austrian states are compared with regard to central health data on life expectancy, mortality, carcinoma incidence, etc. Following that the report compares the above-mentioned health indicators of the Vienna population on a regional level with the general health conditions.

Abstract (Original Language) Die vorliegende Ausgabe der Statistischen Mitteilungen zur Gesundheit in Wien 1999/2 befasst sich mit dem Thema "Gesundheit der Wiener Bevölkerung im regionalen Vergleich". Dabei werden für zentrale Gesundheitsdaten wie Lebenserwartung, Mortalität, Krebsinzidenz etc. sowohl Vergleiche auf Bezirksebene innerhalb Wiens angestellt, als auch Wiener Bezirke mit dem gesamten Bundesgebiet und den Bezirken der anderen österreichischen Bundesländer verglichen. Daran anschließend werden die angesprochenen Indikatoren zur Gesundheit der Wiener Bevölkerung auf regionaler Ebene den gesundheitlichen Rahmenbedingungen gegenübergestellt.

Age Groups

Statistische Mitteilungen zur Gesundheit in Wien 2001/1

Gesundheit von Lehrlingen in Wien

Project Leader

Project Leader	Univ.-Prof. Dr. Brigitte Rollett, Mag. Martin Busch, Angelika Drabek, Tina Holzer, Mag. Karin Waldherr
Address	
Executing Institution	
Funding Agency	Magistratsabteilung für Angelegenheiten der Landessanitätsdirektion, Dezernat II – Gesundheitsplanung

Project Information

Start of Project	
End of Project	30/04/2001
Start of Data Collection	
End of Data Collection	
URL	https://www.wien.gv.at/who/downloads.htm
Scope	National

Keywords

Abstract (English) Prof Brigitte Rollet describes in the first part of the "Statistischen Mitteilungen zur Gesundheit in Wien 2001/1" available survey results on the health situation of trainees and the influencing factors. The second part presents results of the "Wiener Jugendlichenuntersuchung" (Vienna Adolescence Study), carried out by Mrs. Waldherr on request of the city of Vienna. In Austria, all compulsory insured adolescent employees aged 15–19 are invited to take part in a trainee survey, which shall contribute to health prevention. Every year these surveys focus on a particular health aspect. The result of the 1981 survey of the Vienna trainees were statistically evaluated and interpreted. The analysis is about the survey of the first training year, which covered the self-reported health state and aspects of health behavior of the adolescents.

Abstract (Original Language) Im ersten Teil der vorliegenden Ausgabe der "Statistischen Mitteilungen zur Gesundheit in Wien 2001/1" mit dem Titel "Gesundheit von Lehrlingen in Wien" werden von Frau Univ.-Prof. Dr. Brigitte Rollett die bereits vorhandenen Untersuchungsergebnisse über die gesundheitliche Situation von Lehrlingen und deren Einflussfaktoren dargestellt.

Im zweiten Teil werden die Ergebnisse der Wiener Jugendlichenuntersuchung, die von Frau Mag. Waldherr im Auftrag der Stadt Wien durchgeführt wurde, wiedergegeben. In Österreich werden alle pflichtversicherten jugendlichen ArbeitnehmerInnen zwischen 15 und 19 Jahren zu einer Lehrlingsuntersuchung eingeladen, die der Gesundheitsvorsorge dienen soll und für jedes Lehrjahr auf einen speziellen Schwerpunkt ausgerichtet ist. Die Resultate dieser Untersuchung wurden für die Wiener Lehrlinge des Jahrgang 1981 statistisch ausgewertet und interpretiert. Die Analyse bezieht sich auf die Untersuchung im ersten Lehrjahr, die den selbstberichteten Gesundheitszustand und Aspekte des Gesundheitsverhaltens der Jugendlichen erfasst.

Age Groups

Statistische Mitteilungen zur Gesundheit in Wien 2001/2002

Einfluss von Ernährung und Training auf Leistungsparameter bei alten Menschen

Project Leader

Project Leader	Univ.-Prof. Dr. Ibrahim Elmadfa
Address	
Executing Institution	
Funding Agency	Magistratsabteilung für Angelegenheiten der Landessanitätsdirektion, Dezernat II – Gesundheitsplanung

Project Information

Start of Project	
End of Project	30/06/2001
Start of Data Collection	
End of Data Collection	
URL	https://www.wien.gv.at/who/downloads.htm
Scope	National

Keywords

Abstract (English)   The following is a study of nutrition and physical activity and how they effect performance parameters of elderly people. To begin with, nutrient status ($n = 53$), nutrient intake ($n = 20$), metabolism parameters ($n = 37$), and physical efficiency of seniors in their eighth and ninth decade of life were determined. Thirty-seven seniors were then subjected to the following test situations for a total of 12 weeks: physical activity combined with nutrient optimisation, physical activity only, nutrient optimisation only, check-up (without physical activity or nutrient optimisation). Follow-up measurements of nutrient status and physical efficiency were taken to complete the intervention. Ergospirometry was applied to test people's physical efficiency. Their nutrient status and metabolism parameters were measured biochemically.

Abstract (Original Language)   In der vorliegenden Studie wurde der Einfluss von Ernährung und Training auf Leistungsparameter bei alten Menschen untersucht. Zu Beginn der Studie wurden der Nährstoffstatus (n = 53), die Nährstoffaufnahme (n = 20), Stoffwechselparameter (n = 37) und die Leistungsfähigkeit (n = 37) von SeniorInnen der achten und neunten Lebensdekade bestimmt. Danach erfolgte bei 37 SeniorInnen eine Intervention über die Dauer von 12 Wochen in vier Versuchsbedingungen: Training und Nährstoffoptimierung, nur Training, nur Nährstoffoptimierung, Kontrolle (ohne Training und ohne Nährstoffoptimierung). Nach der Intervention wurde nochmals eine Messung des Nährstoffstatus und der Leistungsfähigkeit vorgenommen. Die Bestimmung der Leistungsfähigkeit erfolgte dabei mittels Spiroergometrie, der Nährstoffstatus und die Stoffwechselparameter wurden biochemisch untersucht.

Age Groups

The DAFNE IV Project: Trends in food availability in Austria

Project Leader

Project Leader	I. Elmadfa
Address	Althanstraße 14
	A - 1090 Wien
Executing Institution	Institute of Nutritional Sciences, University of Vienna, Austria
Funding Agency	European Commission

Project Information

Start of Project	01/10/2002
End of Project	30/09/2004
Start of Data Collection	01/11/1999
End of Data Collection	31/10/2000
URL	http://ec.europa.eu/health/ph_projects/2002/monitoring/ monitoring_2002_04_en.htm
Scope	National

Keywords

Abstract (English) The Austrian Household Budget Survey (HBS) is a national survey, collecting data about expenses and income of private households. Additionally, the HBS records data on the quantity of food and beverages acquired at household level. The Austrian HBS records all purchases, own production, and payment in kind.

The Austrian data provided to the DAFNE IV project are based on the HBS carried out in 1999/2000. The DAFNE food classification system and socio-economic categories were applied to Austrian HBS data, to provide data comparable between countries. Valid estimations of food availability concerning food habits of the entire Austrian population and of population subgroups defined on the basis of their socio-economic characteristics were reproduced. The DAFNE databank allows international comparisons and monitoring of daily food availability.

The present report presents data on the availability of the main DAFNE food groups among the Austrian population in 1999/2000. Food availability values are further monitored in relation to four socio-demographic factors affecting food choices (namely, education and occupation of the household head, and household's locality and composition).

Abstract (Original Language) Die Österreichische Haushaltsbudgeterhebung ist eine nationale Erhebung, bei der Daten zum Einkommen und den Ausgaben von privaten Haushalten erhoben werden. Zudem erhebt diese Studie Daten zu der Menge an Lebensmitteln und Getränken, die auf Haushaltsebene erworben werden. Die Österreichische Haushaltsbudgeterhebung erfasst alle Einkäufe und Eigenproduktion. Die Daten zu Österreich, die in das DAFNE IV Projekt einflossen, basierten auf einer Haushaltbudgeterhebung von 1999/2000. Die

DAFNE Lebensmittelklassifizierung und sozioökonomischen Kategorien wurden auch für die Österreichische Haushaltsbudgeterhebung genutzt, um die international Vergleichbarkeit der Daten zu gewährleisten. Die DAFNE Datenbank ermöglicht den internationalen Vergleich und die Überwachung der täglichen Verfügbarkeit von Lebensmitteln.

Der aktuelle Bericht beinhaltet Daten über die Verfügbarkeit der hauptsächlichen DAFNE Lebensmittelgruppen in der Österreichischen Bevölkerung in 1999/2000. Die Verfügbarkeit von Lebensmitteln wird weiter in Bezug auf vier sozio-demographische Faktoren überwacht, die Einfluss auf die Wahl der Lebensmittel haben (Bildung und Beruf des Familienoberhauptes, Lage des Haushaltes und die Haushaltszusammensetzung).

Age Groups

Food availability was estimated for eight types of household composition:
- Households of a single adult
- Households of two adult members
- Households of one adult resident and children (lone parents)
- Households of two adult members and children
- Households of adult and elderly residents
- Households of children, adult and elderly residents
- Households of single elderly
- Households of two elderly residents

Children were defined as up to 18 years of age, adults from 19–65 years of age and elderly as more than 65-years old.

Tiroler Gesundheitsbericht 2002

Project Leader

Project Leader	Mag. Josef Danner, Dr. Gerhard Fülöp
Address	Stubenring 6
	A-1010 Wien
Executing Institution	Österreichisches Bundesinstitut für Gesundheitswesen (ÖBIG)
Funding Agency	Amt der Tiroler Landesregierung

Project Information

Start of Project	
End of Project	30/06/2003
Start of Data Collection	01/01/1991
End of Data Collection	31/12/2000
URL	http://www.tirol.gv.at/themen/gesundheit/gruppe-gesundheit und-soziales/gesundheitsbericht/
Scope	National

Keywords

Abstract (English) The Tyrolean Health Report 2002 was laid out as a basis health report and describes the health situation of the Tyrolean population as well as the most important features of the Tyrolean health care system. The report considered the time between 1991 and 2000, and the regional level provided that regional data are available. The report is not only supposed to identify health problems and trends but to provide a sound basis for health interventions in the area of prevention and health promotion and respectively contribute to the further development of the Tyrolean health care system. It is furthermore to reveal information and data gaps to tackle concerted improvement of data availability.

Abstract (Original Language) Der vorliegende Tiroler Gesundheitsbericht 2002 ist als Basisgesundheitsbericht konzipiert und beschreibt die gesundheitliche Lage der Tiroler Landesbürger sowie die wichtigsten Merkmale der Gesundheitsversorgung im Land. Die Inhalte des Berichts beziehen sich grundsätzlich auf den Zeitraum 1991 bis 2000 bzw. auf die Ebene der politischen Bezirke (Zuordnung nach dem Wohnortprinzip), so weit entsprechende Daten vorliegen (vgl. dazu Abschnitt "Bemerkungen zu Daten und Datenqualität" im Anhang).

Der Bericht soll nicht nur die Identifikation von gesundheitlichen Problemfeldern und Trends ermöglichen, sondern auch eine fundierte Grundlage für gesundheitspolitische Interventionen im Bereich der Prävention und Gesundheitsförderung bzw. bei der Weiterentwicklung des Tiroler Gesundheitsversorgungssystems bilden. Des Weiteren soll er auch Informations- und Datenlücken aufzeigen, um gezielt an einer Verbesserung der Datenlage ansetzen zu können.

Age Groups

Voralberger Gesundheitsbericht 2002

Project Leader

Project Leader	
Address	Stubenring 6
	A-1010 Wien
Executing Institution	Österreichischen Bundesinstitut für Gesundheitswesen (ÖBiG)
Funding Agency	Vorarlberger Landesregierung Abteilung "Sanitätsangelegenheiten"

Project Information

Start of Project	
End of Project	31/12/2002
Start of Data Collection	01/01/1991
End of Data Collection	31/12/2000
URL	http://www.vorarlberg.at/pdf/gesundheitsbericht2002.pdf
Scope	National

Keywords

Abstract (English) The Voralberger Health Report 2002 is geared to the WHO recommendations for the evaluation of regional health situations. The 21 WHO goals for the twenty-first century were divided into chapters and analysed with respect to the grade of completion in the state of Voralberg. The health report shall thus allow identification of problem areas and trends in health and provide a basis for health intervention measures.

Abstract (Original Language) Der Vorarlberger Gesundheitsbericht 2002 orientiert sich an den Empfehlungen der WHO für die Beurteilung der gesundheitlichen Lage in einer Region. Dazu wurden die 21 WHO Ziele für das 21. Jahrhundert nach Kapiteln gegliedert und im Hinblick auf ihre Erfüllung im Bundesland Vorarlberg untersucht. Damit soll der Gesundheitsbericht die Identifikation von gesundheitlichen Problemfeldern und Trends ermöglichen und eine Grundlage für gesundheitspolitische Interventionen bilden.

Age Groups

Wiener Gesundheits- und Sozialsurvey

Vienna Health and Social Survey

Project Leader

Project Leader	Univ.-Prof. Dr. Wolfgang Freidl, Univ.-Prof. Dr. Willibald-Julius Stronegger, Dr. Christine Neuhold
Address	
Executing Institution	
Funding Agency	Magistrat der Stadt Wien, Bereichsleitung für Gesundheitsplanung und Finanzmanagement, Gesundheitsberichterstattung

Project Information

Start of Project	
End of Project	30/11/2001
Start of Data Collection	01/11/1999
End of Data Collection	31/03/2001
URL	https://www.wien.gv.at/who/downloads.htm
Scope	National

Keywords

Abstract (English) To survey the health state of the Vienna population comprehensively for the first time, the city of Vienna commissioned the Institute of Higher Studies to plan and put the Vienna Health and Social Survey 1999/2001 into practice. In two survey periods 4,000 Viennese were interviewed about their state of health during the winter months in 1999/2000 and 2000/2001. The questions focused on subjective health, chronic and acute diseases, intake of medicine and utilization of medial centers. At the same time, health-related behaviour such as lifestyle, socioeconomic situation, work environment, workload, living situation, social networks, individual coping strategies, and critical life situations were covered.

Abstract (Original Language) Um den Gesundheitszustand der Wiener Bevölkerung erstmals umfassend zu erheben, beauftragte die Stadt Wien das Institut für Höhere Studien mit der Planung und Durchführung des Wiener Gesundheits- und Sozialsurveys 2000/2001. In zwei Befragungswellen wurden in den Wintermonaten der Jahre 1999/2000 und 2000/2001 insgesamt 4.000 Wienerinnen und Wiener in Form von mündlichen Interviews zu ihrer gesundheitlichen Lage befragt. Die Fragen bezogen sich dabei auf die Bereiche subjektive Gesundheit, chronische und akute Erkrankungen, Medikamenteneinnahme und Inanspruchnahme medizinischer Einrichtungen. Gleichzeitig wurden auch gesundheitsrelevante Lebensbereiche wie Lebensstil, sozioökonomische Situation, Arbeitswelt, Belastungen, Wohnsituation, soziale Netzwerke, subjektive Bewältigungsstrategien und kritische Lebensereignisse erfasst.

Age Groups

16	and older

Wiener Jugendgesundheitsbericht 2002

Vienna Youth Health Report 2002

Project Leader

Project Leader	Mag. Ingrid Kromer, Mag. Monika Csitkovics
Address	
Executing Institution	
Funding Agency	Magistrat der Stadt Wien, Bereichsleitung für Gesundheitsplanung und Finanzmanagement, Gesundheitsberichterstattung

Project Information

Start of Project	
End of Project	30/09/2002
Start of Data Collection	
End of Data Collection	
URL	https://www.wien.gv.at/who/downloads.htm
Scope	National

Keywords

Abstract (English) The Vienna Youth Health Report shows that health problems in adolescents are heterogeneous. Especially gender, social standing and nationality have a considerable influence. There is deficient dentition in migrants and their movement behavior, especially in girls, is alarming. Female students more often report about stress than male students. After starting a professional career, there is increased alcohol consumption in adolescents and young adults. There is a need for more information on sexuality of students at secondary schools and in polytechnic vocational training.

Abstract (Original Language) Der Wiener Jugendgesundheitsbericht zeigt auf, dass gesundheitliche Probleme bei Jugendlichen heterogen verteilt auftreten. Vor allem nach Geschlecht, sozialer Lage und Nationalität kommt es zu unterschiedlichen Betroffenheiten: So weisen MigrantInnen einen mangelhaften Zahnstatus auf; auch ist ihr Bewegungsverhalten – vor allem bei Mädchen – besorgniserregend. Schülerinnen wiederum berichten häufiger von Stress als Schüler. Einen erhöhten Alkoholkonsum jedoch weisen Jugendliche und junge Erwachsene nach dem Einstieg ins Berufsleben auf. Eine Verbesserung des Wissensstandes bezüglich Sexualität ist bei HauptschülerInnen und SchülerInnen des Polytechnischen Lehrganges anzustreben.

Age Groups

Wiener Kindergesundheitsbericht 2000

Project Leader

Project Leader	Univ.-Prof. Dr. Brigitte Kwizda-Gredler
Address	
Executing Institution	
Funding Agency	Magistratsabteilung für Angelegenheiten der Landessanitätsdirektion, Dezernat II – Gesundheitsplanung

Project Information

Start of Project	
End of Project	30/09/2000
Start of Data Collection	
End of Data Collection	
URL	https://www.wien.gv.at/who/downloads.htm
Scope	National

Keywords

Abstract (English) The Vienna Child Health Report 2000 describes in detail the physical and psychological situation of children in Vienna and furthermore provides an overview on the demographic situation, risks and dangers, sexuality, health care, health prevention, as well as framework requirements for children. The report considers in this context the legal position of children, social circumstances as well as family and school environment of children.

This comprehensive description of the health situation in children allows identifying relevant health problems, so that suitable measures of health promotion and health prevention can be taken. Additionally, there is a need for preventive health policy in this area to counteract the growing trend of chronic diseases as early as possible.

Abstract (Original Language) Der Wiener Kindergesundheitsbericht 2000 beschreibt ausführlich die physische und psychische Situation der Wiener Kinder und gibt darüber hinaus einen Überblick über die demographische Situation, Risiken und Gefährdungen, Sexualität, Gesundheitsvorsorge, Gesundheitsversorgung sowie über weitere Rahmenbedingungen für die Gesundheit von Kindern. Dabei wird etwa auf die rechtliche Position, die sozialen Umstände und das familiäre und schulische Umfeld der Kinder eingegangen.

Diese umfassende Darstellung der gesundheitlichen Situation von Kindern ermöglicht die Identifizierung von relevanten Gesundheitsproblemen, um in der Folge geeignete gesundheitsfördernde und präventive Maßnahmen setzen zu können. Eine vorsorgende Gesundheitspolitik in diesem Bereich ist zudem notwendig, um dem steigenden Trend zu chronischen Krankheiten so früh wie möglich entgegenzuwirken.

Age Groups

Wiener Männergesundheitsbericht 1999

Project Leader

Project Leader	ao. Univ.-Prof. Dr. Anita Schmeiser-Rieder, o. Univ.- Prof. Dr. Michael Kunze
Address	
Executing Institution	
Funding Agency	Magistratsabteilung für Angelegenheiten der Landessanitätsdirektion, Dezernat II,

Project Information

Start of Project	
End of Project	31/07/1999
Start of Data Collection	
End of Data Collection	
URL	https://www.wien.gv.at/who/downloads.htm
Scope	National

Keywords

Abstract (English) Men are affected worldwide by premature morbidity and mortality. Despite that there is little research on men's health. To counteract the deficit, the city of Vienna commissioned Prof Anita Schmeiser-Rieder and Prof Michael Kunze to compile the Vienna report on men's health. This report analyses men's health in Austria for the first time explicitely. The report provides findings on the health status and special health risks for male Viennese. It furthermore deals with demographic conditions and trends as well as the social situation and effects on health of Viennese men.

Special attention is paid to those health areas that are of central importance to the health status and life expectancy of male inhabitants, such as cardio-vascular disease, lifestyle, gender-specific, and age-specific diseases as well as education and social behavior.

The essential result of the report is that male Viennese show that there is considerable need for prevention in men. Promoting prevention by relevant health promoting and preventive measures can contribute to increased life expectancy and general improvement of the health status of the population.

Abstract (Original Language) Männer sind weltweit von vorzeitiger Morbidität und Mortalität betroffen. Trotzdem stellt das Thema Männergesundheit ein bisher kaum erforschtes Gebiet dar. Um diesem Defizit entgegenzuwirken, beauftragte die Stadt Wien Univ.-Prof. Dr. Anita Schmeiser-Rieder und Univ.-Prof. Dr. Michael Kunze mit der Erstellung eines Wiener Männergesundheitsberichtes. Mit diesem Bericht wird in Österreich das Thema Männergesundheit erstmals explizit einer genauen Analyse unterzogen. Der Bericht gibt Auskunft über den Gesundheitszustand und spezielle gesundheitliche Risiken der männlichen Wiener

Bevölkerung. Zudem beschäftigt er sich mit demographischen Gegebenheiten und Trends sowie der sozialen Situation und deren Auswirkungen auf die Gesundheit der Wiener Männer.

Ein besonderes Augenmerk gilt jenen Gesundheitsbereichen, die für den Gesundheitszustand und die Lebenserwartung der männlichen Bevölkerung von zentraler Bedeutung sind – wie Herz-Kreislauf-Erkrankungen, Lebensstil, geschlechts- und altersspezifische Erkrankungen sowie Bildung und Sozialverhalten.

Das wesentliche Ergebnis des Berichtes ist die Erkenntnis, dass die männliche Bevölkerung über ein besonders großes präventives Potential verfügt. Die Förderung dieses Potentials – durch entsprechende gesundheitsfördernde und präventive Maßnahmen – kann eine weitere Steigerung der Lebenserwartung und eine allgemeine Verbesserung des Gesundheitszustandes für die gesamte Bevölkerung bewirken.

Age Groups

Belgium

Food Consumption Survey Belgium

VCP Belgium

Project Leader

Project Leader	Herman van Oyen
Address	Wetenschappelijk Instituut Volksgezondheid
	J. Wytsmanstraat 4
	1050 Brussel
Executing Institution	Scientific Institute of Public Health
Funding Agency	Federal authorities

Project Information

Start of Project	01/01/2004
End of Project	
Start of Data Collection	01/01/2004
End of Data Collection	
URL	http://www.iph.fgov.be/epidemio/epinl/foodnl/table04.htm
Scope	National

Keywords Survey; Food consumption; Diet assessment; 24-h recall

Abstract (English) Food-based dietary guidelines (FBDG) transcribe nutrient-based guidelines in a practical tool to promote balanced food consumption. Data of the Belgian Food Consumption Survey are used to evaluate the compliance to FBDG.

Using a multistage stratified sampling from the national register, subjects, aged 15 years and older, were selected. Two 24-h diet recalls (interval of 6 weeks) were obtained for 3,083 subjects, by trained dietitians using EPIC-SOFT. Interviews were done covering the whole year and spread over all days of the week. Data were analyzed, weighted for the Belgian population, season and interview day. The Nusser method (Nusser, J Am Soc, 1440, 1996) was used to estimate the distribution of usual dietary intake by repeated measurement. The abstract focuses on fruit consumption.

The FBDG for the population 15–18 years is three pieces of fruit or at least 375 grams/day (g/d). Over the age of 18 years, the FBDG recommend 250–375 g/d. The mean usual intake was 134.4 g/d (Standard deviation (SD) 76.6) in women and 99.4 g/d (SD 85.2) in men. The minimal recommended usual consumption was reached by 7.9% of the women and 6.0% of the men. Under the age of 18, none of the females or males passed the threshold. The proportion of females and males reaching the threshold increased to 24.8% and 18.1% when adding fruit juices to the fruit consumption. Next to seasonal variation, the fruit consumption was higher in households with no more than two persons (129.5 vs. 108.8 g/d). The consumption increased with increasing body mass index (138.8 in obese vs. 110.7 g/d in normal weight subjects). Physically inactive persons (109.9 g/d) had the lowest intake compared with minimally (129.5 g/d) and very active (119.5 g/d) subjects.

Abstract (Original Language) België is een van de weinige landen in Europa waar tot op heden geen systematische gegevensverzameling gebeurde die informatie verschaft over de voedselconsumptie in de algemene bevolking. Het laatste onderzoek in België waarin ook voedingsgewoonten werden onderzocht dateerde immers reeds van de jaren 1980. Informatie over de voedingsgewoonten is nochtans onontbeerlijk voor het plannen en het uitvoeren van een gezondheidsplan, een voedingsplan en een voedselveiligheidsbeleid gebaseerd op evidentie.

Voor de voedselconsumptiepeiling 2004 werd een representief staal van de bevolking 15 jaar en ouder gekozen uit het Rijksregister. Deze personen werden twee maal aan huis bezocht door getrainde diëtisten. Tijdens het eerste bezoek werden algemene vragen gesteld, o.a. over de gezondheid en de leefgewoonten van de respondent. Ook de lengte en het gewicht van de respondent werden mondeling door de persoon zelf gerapporteerd. Het belangrijkste onderdeel van de bevraging was de 24-uursvoedingsnavraag. Hierbij wordt alles in detail gerapporteerd wat door de bevraagde persoon sinds het opstaan de vorige dag tot het opstaan op de dag van de bevraging is gegeten en gedronken. Omdat dit niet eenvoudig is voor de respondenten werden zij daarbij geholpen door de diëtist-enquêteur. Om de bevraging te stroomlijnen en te standaardiseren gebeurde de 24-uursvoedingsnavraag via een draagbare computer en met een specifiek programma, nl. EPIC-SOFT. Tijdens het tweede bezoek, ongeveer 2 tot 8 weken later, werd een tweede 24-uursvoedingsnavraag afgenomen. Ondertussen diende de respondent zelf nog een schriftelijke vragenlijst te beantwoorden i.v.m. de frequentie waarbij zij/hij bepaalde voedingsmiddelen eet en waarin gepeild werd naar de kennis over en de houding t.o.v. richtlijnen rond voedingshygiëne. De persoon van het huishouden die het eten bereidt beantwoordde ook een schriftelijke vragenlijst over hoe hij/zij omgaat met voedingsmiddelen (o.a. het ontdooien, het bewaren van restjes, het toepassen van richtlijnen rond voedingshygiëne, …). Tijdens de huisbezoeken werd de lendenomtrek van de respondent gemeten, alsook de temperatuur in de koelkast en de diepvries. De voornaamste reden waarom twee huisbezoeken noodzakelijk zijn, is het feit dat een persoon van dag tot dag verschillend eet. Voor een correcte evaluatie van de verdeling van de inname van voedingsmiddelen binnen de bevolking in vergelijking met de voedingsaanbevelingen en voor het bepalen van normen voor voedselveiligheid is minimum informatie over twee dagen nodig. Door middel van statistische analyse kan dan een schatting gemaakt worden van de inname over een langere periode. Hierbij is dan enkel de spreiding tussen personen belangrijk en niet de intra-individuele dag-tot-dag verschillen. We spreken hier over de gebruikelijke inname. In het rapport ligt de nadruk op de gebruikelijke inname in de totale bevolking en niet deze van de gebruikers alleen.

De body mass index (BMI) werd berekend op basis van door de respondent zelf-gerapporteerde lengte en gewicht, wat mogelijks een vertekening is van de reële BMI. Zo tonen studies aan dat personen met overgewicht vaker hun lichaamsgewicht (en bijgevolg ook BMI) onderschatten dan personen met een normaal gewicht, terwijl personen met ondergewicht meer hun lichaamsgewicht overschatten. Hoewel de prevalenties van overgewicht en obesitas dus onderschat kunnen zijn, blijkt althans uit deze gevens dat een belangrijk deel van de bevolking overgewicht heeft of zelfs zwaarlijvig is. Dit is zo bij respectievelijk 23.5% en 11.6% van de vrouwen. Bij mannen is het percentage overgewicht en zwaarlijvigheid respectievelijk 37.6% en 9.9%. Het aandeel van de bevolking met overgewicht en zwaarlijvigheid neemt toe met de leeftijd. Personen met een lagere opleiding hebben vaker last van overgewicht en obesitas. Zwaarlijvigheid komt ook vaker voor bij personen die lichamelijke inactief zijn. De lendenomtrek wordt ingedeeld in 3 groepen (normaal, limiet en te groot) op basis van leeftijds- en geslachtsspecifieke grenswaarden. De verdeling bij vrouwen is respectievelijk 40.1%, 21.4% en 38.4%. De lendenomtrek ligt op de grens of is te groot bij respectievelijk 26% en 25% van de mannen. Een te grote lendenomtrek komt frequenter voor in de oudere leeftijdsgroepen. Mensen met een lagere opleiding of personen die inactief zijn hebben minder frequent een normale lendenomtrek, maar frequenter een te grote lendenomtrek. De lendenomtrek neemt ook toe in functie van het lichaamsgewicht. Het niveau van lichamelijke activiteit in de algemene bevolking is ondermaats. Zo zijn 45.1% en 33.1% van de vrouwen respectievelijk inactief of maar minimaal lichamelijk actief. Bij mannen is dit respectievelijk 36.8% en 29.2%. Bij vrouwen is het gebrek aan voldoende lichaamsbeweging al uitgesproken in de leeftijdsgroep 15–18 jaar.

Figuur 1 toont in welke mate de gebruikelijke inname van voedingsmiddelen afwijkend is van de aanbevelingen uit de voedingsmiddelendriehoek. Indien de voedingsmiddeleninname van onze bevolking zou voldoen aan de aanbevelingen van de voedingsdriehoek, dan zouden alle vakken van de reële voedingsdriehoek dezelfde oppervlakte moeten hebben als deze in de aanbevolen driehoek. Binnen elk vak van de reële voedingsdriehoek werden eventuele tekorten in gebruikelijke inname aangegeven door een deel van het totale oppervlak wit te maken. Wanneer de helft van het vak wit is, betekent dit dat de reële inname ongeveer de helft van de aanbeveling bedraagt. Is de inname van een voedingsmiddelengroep groter dan de aanbeveling, dan komt het gekleurde oppervlak buiten de grenzen van de driehoek.

Het witte oppervlak is dus een maat voor het procentuele verschil tussen de gebruikelijke inname van een voedingsmiddelengroep en de aanbeveling. In Tabel

1 worden deze cijfers van gebruikelijke inname, samen met het percentage van de bevolking dat voldoet aan de aanbeveling, gegeven volgens geslacht.

De basisrij van de driehoek verwijst naar het belang van lichamelijke beweging. Slechts 27% van de bevolking heeft een voldoende lichamelijke beweging. De gebruikelijke inname van dranken (water, koffie, thee en bouillon) in de algemene bevolking is 1.2 liter en bedraagt 80% van de aanbeveling van 1.5 liter per dag. Brood, beschuiten of ontbijtgranen worden te weinig gegeten (133 g/dag), gezien maar 76% van de aanbeveling (175–420 g/dag of 5 tot 12 sneden brood) wordt bereikt. De inname van 306.6 g aardappelen en/of deegwaarden per dag ligt binnen de grenzen van de aanbeveling (210–350 g/dag of 3 tot 5 aardappelen). Van groenten wordt verwacht dat men er dagelijks 350 g eet (100 g rauw en 200 g gekookt (= 250 g rauw product)). De gebruikelijke groente-inname van 138.3 g/d is dus ondermaats en net geen 40% van de aanbeveling. Hetzelfde geldt voor de fruitconsumptie. De gebruikelijke fruitinname is amper 118.2 g/dag, terwijl de ondergrens van de aanbeveling 250 g of 2 stukken fruit is. Melkproducten met exclusie van kazen worden ook te weinig ingenomen gezien de gebruikelijke inname van 158.6 g/dag maar ongeveer 35% van de ondergrens van de aanbeveling (450–600 g/ dag of 3 à 4 glazen) bedraagt. De gebruikelijke inname van kaasproducten is 30.2 g/ dag, wat binnen de aanbeveling valt van 20–40 g/dag (1 à 2 sneden kaas). Voor vlees en/of vleesvervangers is de inname 1.6-maal te groot in vergelijking met de bovengrens van de aanbeveling (75–100 g/d). Voor vetten kan enkel een vergelijking gemaakt worden met de aanbeveling voor smeervetten (maximaal 5 g/snede brood). De gebruikelijke inname is 21.2 g/dag, wat overeenkomstig is met de geobserveerde gebruikelijke broodinname. Voedingsmiddelen uit de restgroep (gesuikerde en alcoholische dranken, koek en gebak, …) zijn niet nodig in een evenwichtige voeding. De gebruikelijke inname toont duidelijk dat de realiteit heel ver staat van deze verwachting gezien de inname gemiddeld 481.2 g/dag is wanneer alcoholische dranken ook bij de restgroep worden gerekend en nog 266.3 g/dag indien alcoholische dranken niet in rekening worden gebracht. Met uitzondering van smeervetten worden de aanbevelingen voor geen enkele voedingsmiddelengroep bereikt door de helft van de bevolking. Voor groenten, fruit, melkproducten en de restgroep (inclusief alcohol) is het percentage van de bevolking dat aan de aanbeveling voldoet minder dan 10% (Tabel 1).

De gebruikelijke totale energie-inname in de bevolking 15 jaar en ouder is gemiddeld 2046 kcal. Bij vrouwen is dit 1651 kcal in vergelijking met 2472 kcal bij mannen. De gebruikelijke energie-inname neemt in beide geslachten af met toenemende leeftijd. Wanneer de individuele energie-inname vergeleken wordt met het minimale energieverbruik of het basaal metabolisme, wat berekend wordt op basis van het lichaamsgewicht, het geslacht en de leeftijd, dan is bij 20% van de personen de gerapporteerde energie-inname extreem laag. Er zijn meerdere oorzaken van een te lage rapportering, o.a. enkele methodologische problemen zoals het foutief rapporteren, een onderschatting van de energiewaarde in de voedingsmiddelentabellen maar ook het feit dat mensen een dieet volgen of ziek waren op de dag die bevraagd werd. Bij het uitsluiten van deze personen is de gebruikelijke energie-inname gemiddeld 2268 kcal: 1855 kcal bij vrouwen en 2648 kcal bij mannen. De gebruikelijke energie-inname bij personen met overgewicht en obesitas is lager dan bij personen met een gezond gewicht of ondergewicht. De energie-inname is ook lager bij inactieve personen en personen die minimaal lichamelijk actief zijn. De voornaamste energiebronnen in onze Belgische voeding zijn graan en graanproducten, vnl. brood. Daarna volgen vers vlees, aardappelen, cake en gebak, kaas, margarines en sauzen.

Er zijn vier verschillende soorten energieleverende macronutriënten die elk een verschillende hoeveelheid energie aanleveren: nl. vetten die 9 kcal per gram leveren, koolhydraten en eiwitten die beide 4 kcal per gram vrijstellen en uiteindelijk alcohol dat 7 kcal per gram kan vrijstellen. De aanbevelingen die de procentuele bijdrage van de nutriënten vet, eiwit en koolhydraten aan de totale energie-inname bepalen gaan ervan uit dat de energie afkomstig van alcohol gelijk is aan nul. Daarom wordt de energiebijdrage door alcohol (3.6 energiepercent (en%) bij vrouwen en 6.2 en% bij mannen) van de totale energie-inname afgetrokken om de vergelijking te maken met de aanbevelingen van de Hoge Gezondheidsraad.

De gebruikelijke dagelijkse procentuele bijdrage van het macronutriënt vet aan de totale energie-inname in de bevolking, 15 jaar en ouder, bedraagt gemiddeld 37.0 en% bij vrouwen en 38.9 en% bij mannen (Tabel 2). De gebruikelijke procentuele bijdrage van vet neemt in beide geslachten toe met de leeftijd tot 39.6 en% bij vrouwen en 40.2 en% bij mannen in de leeftijdsgroep 75 jaar en ouder. De aanbeveling om een dagelijkse procentuele bijdrage van vet niet hoger dan 30 en% te hebben, wordt maar bereikt door ongeveer 14% van de vrouwen en 7% van de mannen. Volgens de aanbeveling mag de aanvoer van verzadigde vetten niet meer zijn dan 10 % van de ingenomen energie. Minder dan 5% van zowel vrouwen als mannen voldoet aan deze aanbeveling. De aanvoer van mono-onverzadigde vetten moet liggen tussen 10 en% en 14.7 en%; de bijdrage van en polyonverzadigde vetten moet liggen tussen 5.3% en 10% van de ingenomen energie. Deze aanbevelingen worden respectievelijk gehaald door 62.3% en 59.1% van de vrouwen en door 56.7% en 65.5% van de mannen. Vetten, vnl. margarines en boter, zijn de voornaamste energiebron van vet in onze voeding. Daarnaast volgen vlees en vleesproducten, melkproducten, cake, koek, gebak en puddingen en sauzen.

De gebruikelijke bijdrage door koolhydraten is gemiddeld 46.4 en% bij vrouwen en 45.0 en% bij mannen. De proportie van de bevolking, die de aanbeveling van minstens 55 en% koolhydraten haalt, is respectievelijk 9.0 en% en 5.7 en% bij vrouwen en mannen. De gebruikelijke inname van koolhydraten neemt in beide geslachten licht af met toenemende leeftijd. De inname van suikers (mono- en disacchariden) is te hoog in vergelijking met de aanbeveling, terwijl de inname van polysacchariden veel te laag is. Brood is de voornaamste bron van koolhydraten in onze voeding, gevolgd door aardappelen, limonades, fruit, zoete toespijs, cake en gebak, deegwaren en rijst.

De gebruikelijke procentuele bijdrage van eiwit aan de totale energie-inname in de algemene populatie, 15 jaar en ouder, bedraagt gemiddeld 16.6 en% bij vrouwen en 16.0 en% bij mannen. In totaal voldoet 99%, zowel bij vrouwen als bij mannen aan de minimum aanbeveling van 10 en% eiwit. Algemeen kan hieruit besloten worden dat er binnen de bevolking, 15 jaar en ouder, nauwelijks problemen zijn betreffende een te lage eiwitinname. Er zijn weinig verschillen volgens leeftijd voor de procentuele eiwitinname. Vlees en vleesproducten zijn de voornaamste bronnen van eiwitten in onze voeding. Daarnaast komt de energiebijdrage van eiwitten vooral uit granen en graanproducten, melkproducten en vis en schaaldieren.

De inname van drie micronutriënten werd geëvalueerd. De gemiddelde gebruikelijke inname van vitamine C in de algemene bevolking ligt voor alle leeftijdsgroepen en voor zowel vrouwen als mannen boven de aanbeveling. De gemiddelde calciuminname ligt voor zowel vrouwen als mannen voor alle leeftijdsgroepen onder de leeftijdspecifieke dagelijkse aanbeveling. In tegenstelling tot volwassen mannen, voor wie de gemiddelde dagelijkse ijzerinname hoger is dan de leeftijdspecifieke aanbevelingen, ligt de gebruikelijke dagelijkse ijzerinname bij vrouwen voor alle leeftijdsgroepen onder de aanbeveling.

Age Groups

15	18
19	59
60	74
74	and older

Gezondheidsenquete Door Middel van Interview (Health Survey Through Interview)

Project Leader

Project Leader	Dr. Jean Tafforeau
Address	J. Wytsmanstraat 14
	1050 Brussel
Executing Institution	Scientific Institute of Public Health
Funding Agency	Ministry of Health

Project Information

Start of Project	01/01/1997
End of Project	
Start of Data Collection	01/01/1997
End of Data Collection	
URL	
Scope	National

Keywords

Abstract (English) *Objectives:*

Identification of health problems
Description of the health status and health needs of the population
Estimation of prevalence and distribution of health indicators
Analysis of social (in)equality in health and access to the health services
Study of health consumption and its determinants
Study of possible trends in the health status of the population
Methods

General principles:

- Performing fieldwork during one year (1997, 2001, 2004)
- Task of the IPH: choice of themes, sample design, supervision of the data collection, analyse of the results, reporting
- Sample of all inhabitants of Belgium, stratified per region, province and community, and constructed on the basis of the National Register using the household as sample unit
- Sample of more than 10,000 respondents (with the possibility of an oversampling of provinces and/or specific groups)

Instruments : Three sorts of questionnaires:

- Oral questionnaire to be filled out by the household
- Face to face questionnaire to be filled out by each selected person (with a maximum of 4 persons per household), this could also be filled out by a proxy)
- Written questionnaire to be filled out by each selected person over 15 years (this could not be filled out by a proxy)

Choices concerning the content:
Fields considered:
Health status
Lifestyle
Prevention
Consumption of care
Health and society
Arguments for the choice of the domains
Domains depending on the conceived objectives
Comparison the results with other countries is possible
Possibility of comparing the results in time

Abstract (Original Language)

Age Groups

All ages are included

Investigation of the Current Quantitative and Qualitative Pattern of Physical Activity, Sport Participation, Physical Fitness, and General Health of the Flemish Population

Project Leader

Project Leader	Prof. J. Lefevre, Prof. R. Philippaerts en Prof. W. Duquet
Address	Steunpunt Sport, Beweging en Gezondheid, Studentenwijk Arenberg
	13001 Heverlee Belgium
Executing Institution	Steunpunt Sport, Beweging en Gezondheid Policy Research Centre Sport, Physical Activity and Health
Funding Agency	Flemish Government

Project Information

Start of Project	01/03/2002
End of Project	31/12/2006
Start of Data Collection	01/10/2002
End of Data Collection	01/02/2004
URL	http://www.steunpuntsbg.be
Scope	National

Keywords Physical activity; Physical fitness; Health

Abstract (English) The objective of the study was to get insight in the physical activity, sport participation, physical fitness, and general health of the Flemish population. A representative sample of the Flemish population was assessed in a fitobiel, which drove from city to city. The results give an overview of the physical activity, health and fitness of this population. Advises are given for policy.

Abstract (Original Language)

Age Groups

18	24
25	29
30	34
35	39
40	44
45	49
50	54
55	59
60	64
65	69
70	74

Research on the Fiber-Intake and Determinants of Fiber-Intake

VEKA project

Project Leader

Project Leader	Lea Maes
Address	G. Schildknechtstraat 9
	1020 Brussel
	Belgium
Executing Institution	University of Gent and The Scientific Institute of Public Health
Funding Agency	Flemish government

Project Information

Start of Project	01/07/1995
End of Project	01/06/1998
Start of Data Collection	01/01/1996
End of Data Collection	01/04/1998
URL	http://www.vig.be > gezonde voeding (for documents and information)
Scope	National

Keywords Dietary fiber; Food education; Poverty; Determinants

Abstract (English)

Abstract (Original Language)

Age Groups

16	74

Voedingsbeleid in Bedrijven (Onderzoek);

Food Policy in Companies (Research)

Project Leader

Project Leader	Linda de Boeck
Address	G. Schildknechtstraat 9
	1020 Brussel
	Belgium
Executing Institution	Vlaams Instituut voor Gezondheidspromotie (The Scientific Institute of Public Health)
Funding Agency	Flemish government

Project Information

Start of Project	01/01/2003
End of Project	
Start of Data Collection	01/01/2003
End of Data Collection	
URL	http://www.vig.be
Scope	National

Keywords Food policy; Healthy workplace; Nutrition education

Abstract (English) The Flemish institute for health promotion investigated in 2003 in collaboration with Local Health networks (LOGO's) the food policy in companies with over 50 employees. In total, questionnaires were send to 4,297 companies of which 2,191 questionnaires were returned. It appeared that efforts of food education and interventions are very limited at work.

Abstract (Original Language)

Age Groups

Voedingsbeleid in Scholen (Onderzoek);

Food Policy in Schools (Research)

Project Leader

Project Leader	Linda de Boeck
Address	G. Schildknechtstraat 9
	1020 Brussel
	Belgium
Executing Institution	Flemish institute of health policy
Funding Agency	Flemish government

Project Information

Start of Project	01/01/2003
End of Project	
Start of Data Collection	01/01/2003
End of Data Collection	
URL	http://www.vig.be
Scope	National

Keywords Food policy; Healthy school; Nutrition education

Abstract (English) The Flemish institute for health promotion investigated in 2003 in collaboration with Local Health networks (LOGO's) the food policy in schools in the school year 2003–2004. In total, questionnaires were send to 3,917 primary schools and 1,433 secondary schools of which 1,854 and 804 questionnaires were returned, respectively. It appeared that the attention for food education becomes less in secondary school. The supply of drinks and snacks can become healthier.

Abstract (Original Language)

Age Groups

Bulgaria

National Dietary and Nutritional Status Survey of the Population in Bulgaria, 1997

Project Leader

Project Leader	Prof. Stefka Petrova
Address	
Executing Institution	National Center of Hygiene, Medical Ecology and Nutrition and GALLUP – BBSS
Funding Agency	United Nations Developmenet Program (UNDP)

Project Information

Start of Project	01/05/1997
End of Project	30/05/1997
Start of Data Collection	01/05/1997
End of Data Collection	30/05/1997
URL	
Scope	National

Keywords

Abstract (English) A national survey of dietary and nutritional status of the population of Bulgaria has been conducted in May 1997 by the National Center of Hygiene, Medical Ecology, and Nutrition and GALLUP – BBSS. The survey was supported by United Nations Development Program (UNDP).

The primary objectives of the survey include: to identify the current nutrition problems of the population in Bulgaria, to define their severity and prevalence, to identify the risk population groups in order to determine priorities for humanitarian assistance and intervention measures, to provide base line data for monitoring the nutrition situation.

The survey design was a complex, multistage, stratified, probability cluster sample throughout the country. The survey was carried out in field on the basis of the consumer panel sample of 1,000 households, which were nationally representative with respect to age, sex urban/rural distribution, main social strata, and ethnicity maintained by BBSS. The effective sample size was 2,833 individuals aged 1 years and over. Data were collected in May 1997.

Dietary data were obtained by personal in-house face-to-face interviews using 24-h recall. These data were translated into energy and nutrient intake values using specially designed computer programme for calculating the chemical composition of Bulgarian foods, dishes, and beverages, including nutrient losses during preparation of foods and cooking.

Nutritional status was assessed on the basis of self-reported data for height and weight (for children up to 10 years reported by parents) applying the recommended by WHO anthropometric indices height and weight, indicators and criteria for underweight, normal weight, and overweight.

Validation study on anthropometric parameters was carried on subsample of 402 subjects including urban and rural population of the same age groups, and the nutritional status was assessed on the basis of reported and measured values.

Average energy daily intakes of children, adolescents, and elderly people were higher or close to the recommended values for the corresponding ages and sex groups. A prevalence of deficient daily energy intake (40.2%) amongst the children 3–6 years of age was observed, which corresponded to the high frequency of wasting in this age group. The mean energy intake values for adults' 30–60 years of age were relevant to the recommended energy intakes for low level of physical activity. A proportion of 28.6% amongst the female's 18–30 years of age had deficient energy intake under 1,500 kcal per day and this corresponded to the observed high frequency of low body mass index (14.5–16%) in this age group. The rural population from each age/sex group had higher energy intake than the urban subsamples.

Mean protein intake of the total studied sample, as well as of urban and rural population subgroups, adjusted by age and sex, was over the reference nutrient intakes (RNI) for Bulgaria population. There was a significant percentage of individuals in some population groups, however, at a risk of inadequate protein intakes assessed on the basis of the accepted cut-off of 67% RNI. The percentage of subjects at risk of protein deficient intake was over 10% in the age groups over 18 years. The highest prevalence was observed in the urban subgroup of females aged 18–30 years (25.5%).

Average carbohydrate intake by most of the age and sex subgroups was under the recommended proportion of the total daily energy intake (E%) – 53 E% for children 1–10 years and under 55 E% for the other age/sex groups.

The high fat intake is a serious problem for the whole studied population. The energy derived from fat was 33 E% – 44 E% of the total daily food energy intake. All age and sex groups from rural regions had lower total daily fat energy intake but higher intake of animal fat.

The average vitamin and mineral intakes by most population groups were below RNI for the corresponding age/sex subgroups. The prevalence of the subjects at risk of inadequate intake of the micronutrients estimated on the basis of the cut-off 67% RNI is in the range 15–61% for calcium, 9.4–62.5% for iron, 17.2–69.8% for riboflavin, 35–65.6% for vitamin B6, 10.3–59.5% for folate, and 10%–53%–33.7% for vitamin C). Children aged 1–6 years were defined as at highest risk concerning some vitamin and mineral deficiencies. Children and adolescents aged 6–18 years were at highest risk for deficient intake of calcium and vitamin B2. Females over 10 years of age are at highest risk for inadequate intake of iron, calcium, vitamin C, and folale.

The analysis of regional distribution in relation to food and nutrient intake of groups aged 18–60 years revealed that the most serious problems concern Montana and Lovech districts.

The observed data from the national survey indicate that the dietary pattern of the population of Bulgaria is unbalanced with high fat and insufficient carbohydrates intake. Significant proportion of the population is at risk for deficient intakes of micronutrients as well as some population groups are also at risk for protein inadequate intake. The identified groups at highest risk for deficient nutrient intakes are children, adolescents, young women, and elderly people. Children aged 3–6 years and young women 18- to 30-years old are defined also as the most risk group for undernutrition. These problems concern all of the country regions.

The unfavorable characteristics of the nutrient intake are related to the food consumption pattern. The median value of the levels of consumption of fish, milk, fruit, potatoes, and legumes is low for all studied population groups, defined by age, sex, urban/rural distribution. The added fat consumption is traditionally high.

Parallel to the estimated problem of wasting and underweight for some population groups, overweight and obesity remain a common and serious problem for adults over 30 years of age, with prevalence of overweight grade I reaches 58.2% and overweight grade II/III – 28.9% for some population subgroups. It is a serious problem that the prevalence of overweight is high for the children aged 1–10 years (30.4%).

The identified problems for the dietary and nutritional status of the population of Bulgaria, their magnitude and distribution, require urgent measures to improve the nutritional situation, adequate humanitarian aid for defined risk groups, investigations for estimation of risk factors, monitoring and control of the nutritional situation in Bulgaria.

Abstract (Original Language) Осъществено е национално проучване на хранителния прием и хранипелния статус на населението в България през 1997 г. от Националния център по хигиена, медицинска екология и хранене и Галъп-ввSS. Проучването е по поръчка на Програмата за развитие към ООН (United Nations Development Program).

Основните задачи на проучването включват: идентифициране на настоящите проблеми на храненето на населението в България, определяне на тяхната тежест и разпространение, и дефиниране на рисковите популационни групи с оглед очертаване на приоритетите за хуманитарна помощ и други интервенционни мерки, създаване на база данни за мониторинг на хранителната ситуация.

Проучването е извършено на базата на извадка на домакински панел от 1000 домакинства, поддържана от ГАЛЪП-ввSS, която е национално представителна по отношение на възраст, пол, градско/селско местоживеене, основни социални и етнически групи. Ефективният размер на извадката включва 2833 лица на възраст над 1 година, от които: градско население – 72.9%, селско население – 27.1%; лица от мъжки пол – 46.7%, лица от женски пол – 53.3%.

Данните за хранителния прием са получени чрез персонални инитервюта, като е използван методът "възстановяване по памет на хранителната консумация за 24 часа". Използвана е компютърна програма за изчисляване на химичния състав на наличните на пазара български и вносни храни и напитки, както и на базата на общоприетите рецептури на българските ястия. Отчитани са загубите на хранителни вещества при кулинарната обработка на храните.

Хранителният статус е оценен на базата на препоръчаните антропометрични индекси ръст и телесна маса, индикатори и критерии за оценка на поднормено, нормално и свръхтегло и тяхното разпространение (СЗО, 1995). Данните за ръст и телесна маса на лицата са събирани на базата на лична информация. За децата до 10 години всички данни са съобщавани от родителите или друг взрастен член на семйството. За оценка на точността на съобщените от изследваните лица данни за ръстта и теглото е направено валидизационно проучване върху 402 лица от двата пола от всички дефинирани възрастови групи в основното проучване върху градска и селска популация, като хранителният статус е оценен на базата на съобщени и измерени стойности.

Средният прием на енергия при децата, юноиште и старите хора е по-висок или близък до определените средни потребности за съответниите групи. При 40.2% от децата на възраст 3–6 години обаче се открива енергиен прием по-нисък от средните потребности за тази възрастова група, като тези данни съответстват на установения значителен дял деца с поднормено тегло (15.6%). Средните стойнос¬ти на енергийния прием при изследваните групи .мъже и жени на възраст 30–60 години съответстват на средните енергийни потребност ¬и за тази възраст и при двата пола за ниска физическа активност. Жените на възраст 18–30 години имат среден прием на енергия по-нисък от средните енергийни потребности, като при 28.6% той е под 1500 ккал/ден. Това съответства на установената голяма често¬та на поднормено тегло (14.5–16%) в тази възрастова група. Обобщено селската популалация има по-висок енергиен прием в сравнение с тази с градско местоживеене.

Средният прием на белтък при цялата изследвана група, както при селските и градските подгрупи, диференцирани по възраст и пол, покриват референтните стойности за хранителен прием на белтък. В групите над 18 години обаче се установява риск за дефицитен белтъчен прием (под 67% от референтните стойности) при над 10% от индивидите. Най-висока честота на лица с риск за дефицитен прием на белтък се открива при жените на 18–30 години с градско местоживеене (25.5%).

Средният прием на въглехидрати е под препоръчаните 53 Е% при децата от 10 години и под 55 Е% при останалите възрастови групи.

Високият прием на мазнини е сериозен проблем за цялото население. Енергията, получена от мазнини, е в интервала 33–44% от общия приелм на енергия с храната, включително и при децата. Групите със селско местоживеене имат по-нисък енергиен прием от общите мазнини, но относителният дял на животинските мазнини е по-висок.

Средният прием на витамини и минерални вещества при повечето популационни групи е под референтните стойности за хранителен прием за съответната възраст и пол. Относителният дял на лицата с риск за дефицитен прием на микронутриенти (<67% от съответните референтни стойности) при различните групи е в интервала 15% – 61% за калция, 9.4% – 62.5% за желязото, 17.2% – 69.8% за рибофлавина, 35% – 65.6% за витамин B6, 10.3% – 59.5% за фолата и за витамин С – от 10% до 53%. Децата във възрастовия период 1–6 години са дефинирани като група с най-висок риск по отношение на дефицитен прием на витамини и минерали. Децата и юношите на възраст 6 – 18 години са с най-висок риск за дефицитен прием на калций и витамин B1. Лицата от женски пол над 10-годишна възраст са най-рискови по отношение на хранителния прием/ на желязо. калций. витамин С и фолат.

Направеният анализ на данните за хранителния прием на възрастовите групи от 18до 60 години показва, че най-сериозни са проблемите в област Монтана и Ловешка област.

Получените данни показват, че храненето на населението в България е небалансирано, с висок прием на мазнини и недостатъчно съ¬държание на въглехидрати, като значителен процент от цялото българско население е с риск за дефицтен прием на витамини и мине¬рални вещества, а при някои популационни групи – и с риск за дефицитен прием на белтък. При децата и младите жени също се устано¬вява енергиен дефицит и голяма честота на поднормено тегло. Обобщено групите с най-висок риск за дефицитен прием на хранителни вещества са децата и юношите, младите жени и старите хора.

Неблагоприятните характеристики на хранителния прием са свързани с модела на хранене. При всички популационни групи, дефинирани по възраст, пол и градско/селско местоживеене е иедостатьчен приемът на мляко и млечни продукти, пресни плодове и зеленчуци много ниска е консумацията на риба. Приемът на добавените мазнини е традиционно висок.

Наред с установения проблем с недохранването при някои популационни групи, свръхтеглото и затлъстяването остават общ и сериозен проблем и за възрастните хора над 30 години, като относителната честота на свръхтегло I-ва степен достига 58.2%, а свръхтегло 2-ра и 3-та степен – до 28.9% при някои популационни подгрупи. Тревожно е, че и при децата на възраст 1–10 години се установява висок относителен дял със свръхтегло (30.4%).

Дефинираните проблеми в хранителния прием и хранителния статус на населението в България, тяхната степен и разпространение изискват прилагането на ефективни мерки за подобряване на храненето, адекватно насочена хуманитарна помощ към идентифицираните рискови групи, извършване на проучвания за установяване на рисковите фактори, наблюдение и контрол на хранителната ситуация в страната.

Age Groups

1	3
3	6
6	10
10	14
14	18
18	30
30	60
60	75
75	999

National Dietary and Nutritional Status Survey of the Population in Bulgaria, 1998

Project Leader

Project Leader	Prof. Stefka Petrova
Address	
Executing Institution	National Center of Hygiene, Medical Ecology and Nutrition and GALLUP - BBSS
Funding Agency	

Project Information

Start of Project	23/03/1998
End of Project	31/03/1998
Start of Data Collection	23/03/1998
End of Data Collection	31/03/1998
URL	
Scope	National

Keywords

Abstract (English) A national survey of dietary and nutritional status of the population in Bulgaria has been conducted in 1998 by the National Center of Hygiene, Medical Ecology and Nutrition and GALLUP – BBSS. The primary objectives of the survey include the following: to assess the current nutrition and nutritional status of the population, to identify the risk population groups for inadequate dietary intake, to monitor changes in dietary and nutritional status of the Bulgarian population in order to provide a basis for development of a National Nutrition Policy.

The survey was carried out on the basis of quota sample that was multistage stratified and defined by random route method. It was achieved an effective nationally representative sample size of 2,757 individuals aged 1 year and over, including 69.1% respondents with urban residence and 30.9% with rural residence, males were 68% and females were 51.6%. Information to outline main socio-economic characteristics of respondents was collected. Dietary data were collected using 24-h recall. To assess possible underreporting of dietary intake the ratio of energy intake to basal metabolic rate was calculated. Nutritional status was assessed on the basis of self-reported data for weight and height using anthropometric indices, indicators and criteria, recommended by WHO. To assess the accuracy of reported data for weight and height, a validation study was conducted on 612 individuals both sexes from all age groups.

Mean values of daily energy intakes for all age groups were higher or close to the recommended average energy levels, with the exception of female adults aged 18–60 years, whose mean energy intakes were lower than the respective recommendations. The medians of energy intakes were lower than the corresponding mean levels, implying higher relative frequency of lower energy intakes. Risk for inadequate energy intakes was determined for the population groups of children under 10 years of age with rural residence as well as for women aged 18–60 years, both with urban and rural residence. Corresponding to these data, higher prevalence of underweight and low height-for-age was apparent among children of age under 10 years, and low body mass index among the women of age 18–30 years. In the similar study conducted in 1997, children and young women were identified as most risk population groups for undernutrition, assessed on the basis of anthropometric indices. Overweight prevalence was high and was determined as serious problem for the most of population groups in the both surveys.

Mean protein intakes, expressed as g/day and g/kg body weight were over the corresponding Reference Nutrient Intakes (RNI). The animal protein was 55.6% of total protein intake for young children, as it was declined with the increasing of age up to 40.3%. It was determined prevalence of 10–22% among women of age over 30 years and men aged over 75 with risk for inadequate protein intake, the group of women 30- to 60-years old with urban residence was identified as the most risk group.

Mean values of fat intakes of all population groups were higher than the recommendations. It was observed great prevalence (50–80%) of subjects of all age groups with fat intakes over the recommended upper limits. Mean intakes of saturated fatty acids of all defined groups were over the recommended upper levels of 10 E%. Mean cholesterol intakes over 300 mg per day were observed only for population groups of males aged 10–60 years.

Average daily intakes of carbohydrates were lower than the recommendations. Mean intakes of total dietary fibers were adequate for defined groups of adult males but for adult women they were lower than the recommended values.

Values of mean daily intakes of thiamin, riboflavin, and folate were below the corresponding RNI for the most population groups being in the range 56–94% RNI for the different vitamins. Mean intakes of vitamin A. E, C, B6, and niacin for all defined groups were adequate. Great prevalence (10–51%) of individuals with risk for deficient intakes of the most vitamins was observed despite of the adequate average intakes on population level. The most serious problem was identified concerning folate, especially for females aged over 10 years. Twenty to thirty-five percent individuals among this population were with almost certainly inadequate folate intake (below Lower Reference Nutrient Intakes).

Mean daily intakes of macro and microelements for the most of the population groups were below the corresponding RNI. Medians of mineral intakes for all defined groups were lower than the mean values, implying higher relative frequency of lower intakes. Prevalence of individuals with risk for inadequate calcium intake is the most higher for the groups of females of age 10–14, 18–60 years. The prevalence of subjects with risk for inadequate magnesium intakes was lower than those for Ca, it was the most high among male adolescents aged 14–18 years, both genders of subjects aged 18–30 years and those over 75 years. Iron intakes were especially low among children aged 1–6 years (both genders) and for the girls 10- to 18-years old. The relative frequency of individuals with risk for inadequate zinc intakes is high among children of age 1–3 years with rural residence and for all ages over 18 years.

Differences in the intakes of energy and some nutrients in connection with the socio-economic status of the household were observed.

Unbalanced dietary intakes and inadequate intakes of micronutrient corresponded to the observed unhealthy characteristics of the dietary pattern: high consumption of added fats, great proportion of red meats within the meat and meat products food group, low fish and milk consumption, intakes of vegetables and fruits under recommendations. High alcohol intakes were determined among adult men. An increase in consumption of meat and meat products, better distribution of intakes of potatoes, fruits and milk products, but lower milk consumption, great season differences in raw vegetable and fruit intakes were observed in this study compared with the data obtained in the survey in 1997.

Abstract (Original Language) През 1998 гоуина е осъществено национално репрезентативно проучване на храненето и хранителния статус на население ¬то в България от Националния център по хигиена, медицинска екология и хранене и GALLUP-ввSS. Основни цели на проучването са: оценка на храненето и хранителния статус, идентифициране на популационните групи с най-висок риск за неадекватен храни¬телен прием, мониторинг на промен—ите в хранителната консумация и хранителния статус на населението в България с оглед създаването на база за разработване на национална хранителна политика.

Извадката е квотна, многостепенна и рандомизирана, включваща 2757 лица, представшпелни за населението в България над 1¬годишна възраст, от които с градско местоживееене – 69.1%, със селско местоживееене – 30.9%; лица от мъжки пол – 49.5%, лица от женски пол – 51.5%. Събирана е информация за основни социално-икономически характеристики на изследваните лица. Данните за хранителния прием са получени чрез метода "24-часова хранителна консумация". Приемът на енергия е валидизиран чрез изчис¬ляване на отношението на енергийния прием към основната обмяна. Хранителният статус е оценен чрез антропометрични индекси, индикатори и критерии на СЗО на базата на телесното тегло и ръста, съобщени от изследваните лица. Акуратността на съобщените данни за теглото и ръста е оценена чрез валидизационно проучване върху 612 лица от двата пола от всички възрастови групи.

Средните стойности на дневен енергиен прием при всички възрастови групи са по-високи или близки до препоръчаните нива, с изключение на популацията на жените на възраст 18–60 години, при която са по-ниски. Медианите на прием са с по-ниски стойнос¬ти от съответните средни нива. показващи по-висока относителна честота на по-нисък енергиен прием. Риск за неадекватен енерговнос се открива по отношение на децата до 1О-годишна възраст от селата, както и при жените на възраст 18–60 години, независимо от местоживееенето. Съответно при децата до 10 години се установява по-висок относителен дял с поднормено тегло и нисък ръст за съответната възраст. При жените от 18 до 30 години също се наблюдава по-голяма честота на лица с нисък индекс на телесна маса в сравнение с другите популационни групи. В аналогичното национално проучване, извършено през 1997 г. също се наблюдава, че децата и младите жени са най-рискови по отношение на недохранването, оценено на базата на антропометрични индекси. И в двете проучвания се установява, че свръхтеглото е сериозен проблем за голяма част от популационните групи.

Средният прием на белтък, изразен като g/ден и g/kg телесно тегло при всички дефинирани групи, е над съответните референ¬ни стойности за хранителен прием (РСХП). Животинският белтък е 55.6% от тоталния белтъчен прием при малките деца, като неговият дял намалява с увеличаването на възрастта до 40.3%. При 10–22% от жените над 30 години и мъжете над 75 години се установява риск за неадекватен приелм на белтък, като с най-висок риск са жените на 30–60 години с градско местоживеене.

Всички популационни групи имат средни нива на прием на мазнини по-висок от препоръчаните, като се наблюдава висок относителен дял лица (50–80%) от всички възрастови групи с консумация на мазнини над горната препоръчвана граница. Средният прием на наситени мастни киселини за всички дефинирани групи е над горните препоръчани нива от 10 Е%. Само при групите от мъжки пол от 10 до 60-годишна възраст средният дневен прием на холестерол е над препоръчаната горна граница 300 mg дневно.

При всички популационни групи средният прием на въглхидрати е по-нисък от препоръчания. Средният прием на хранителни влакнини е адекватен за дефинираните групи при мъжете, но при жените е по-нисък от препоръчаната долна граница за прием.

Стойностите на средния дневен прием на тиамин, рибофлавин и фолат при почти всички дефинирани групи са по-ниски от съответните РСХП, като при различните витамини са в интервала 56–94% от РСХП. Средният прием на витамин А, Е, С, В6 и ниацин при всички групи е адекватен. За повечето витамини се намира висок относителен дял (10–51%) на лица с риск за дефицитен внос, независимо от адекватния среден прием на популалационно ниво. Най-сериозен е проблемът по отношение на фолата, особено при групите от женски пол над 10 години, при които 20–35% са с почти сигурен дефицитен прием (под долните референтни стойности за хранителен прием).

Средният дневен прием на макро- и микроелементи в повечето популационни групи е нисък. Медианите на прием при всички дефининираи грутпи са по-ниски от съответните средни стойности – показател за дистрибуция на приема към ниски стойности. Относителният дял на лица с риск от неадекватен внос на Са е най-висок при групите от женски пол на възраст 10–14, 18–60 години. С риск за дефицитен прием на магнезий са относително по-малък брой лица, като най-голяма честота се наблюдава сред юношите на 14–18 години, лицата от двата пола на 18–30 години и над 75 години. Средният прием на желязо е особено нисък при децата до 6-годишна възраст от двата пола, момичетата на 10–18 години и при старите хора. Честотата на индивидите с риск за неадекватен внос на цинк е висока при децата на 1–3 години от селата и при всички възрасти над 18 гоуини. Групите на жените на 10–14 години и хората над 75 години се идентифицират като най-високо рискови за дефицити от микроелементи.

Установяват се различия в приема на енергия и някои хранителни вещества във връзка със социално-икономическия статус на домакинството.

Небалансираният характер на хранителния прием и неадекватният внос на голяма част от микронутриентите са свързани с установените в проучването неблагоприятни характеристики на хранителния модел: висока консумация на добавени мазнини, висок относителен дял на червени меса, ниска консумация на риба и мляко, недостатъчен прием на зеленчуци и плодове. Открива се и висок прием на алкохол сред мъжете в зряла възраст. В сравнение с данните от проучването през 1997г. се установява увеличаване на консумацията на месо и месни продукти за по-голяма част от населението, подобряване в в разпределението на приема на картофи, плодове и млечни продукти, но по-ниска консумация на мляко, изразени сезонни различия в консумацията на сурови зеленчуци и плодове.

Age Groups

1	3
3	6
6	10
10	14
14	18
18	30
30	60
60	75
75	999

National Dietary and Nutritional Status Survey of the Schoolchildren in Bulgaria, 1998

Project Leader

Project Leader	Prof. Stefka Petrova
Address	Sofia 1431
	boul D. Nestorov 15
Executing Institution	National Center of Hygiene, Medical Ecology and Nutrition
Funding Agency	

Project Information

Start of Project	10/03/1998
End of Project	31/03/1998
Start of Data Collection	23/03/1998
End of Data Collection	30/03/1998
URL	
Scope	National

Keywords Nutrition of schoolchildren; Nutritional problems

Abstract (English) In 1998, the National center of hygiene, medical ecology, and nutrition along with all 28 regional inspectorates for protection and control of the public health carried out a national representative transversal survey on nutrition and nutritional status of schoolchildren in Bulgaria. The survey included 7,100 schoolchildren aged 7–19. The sample size is representative not only on national level but also on regional levels. Dietary data were collected using 24-h recall and frequency of food consumption. To assess possible underreporting of dietary intake the ratio of energy intake to metabolic rate was calculated. To assess the anthropologic nutritional status, weight and height were measured. Using active questioning data about physical activity, incidence of acute respiratory diseases as well as data about the socio-economic status of the families of the schoolchildren were gathered.

Abstract (Original Language) През 1998 Националният център по хигиена съвместно с всички ХЕИ в страната проведе национално представително трансверзално проучване на храненето и хранителния статус на учениците в България върху общо 7100 ученици на възраст 7-19 години. Извадката, дефиринцирана по възраст и пол е представителна не само за страната, но и за всяка от 9-те области в страната. Храненето е изследвано чрез методите "24 часова хранителна консумация" и "Честота на консумация на храни". За оценка на антропометричния хранителен статус са измервани теглата и ръста. Чрез активно анкетиране са събирани данни за физическата активност, зболеваемостта от остри респираторни заболявания, информация зза някои основни социално-икономически характеристики на семейството на учениците.

Age Groups

7	9
10	13
14	17
18	19

National Nutrition Survey of Institutionalized Children Aged 7 – 16 Years

Project Leader

Project Leader	Prof. Blagoy Jordanov
Address	Sofia 1431
	boul D. Nestorov 15
Executing Institution	National Center of Hygiene, Medical Ecology and Nutrition
Funding Agency	

Project Information

Start of Project	01/10/1997
End of Project	30/11/1997
Start of Data Collection	01/10/1997
End of Data Collection	11/10/1997
URL	
Scope	National

Keywords National survey; Institutionalized children aged 7–16 years; Dietary and nutritional status

Abstract (English) National representative cross-sectional survey for assessment of dietary and nutritional status of a high risk population group of institutionalized children aged 7–16 years has been conducted in 1997. The study group comprised 362 children, both sexes, from 16 randomly selected Social Institutions (country total number 89). The main identified nutritional problems are the large variability of energy supply, macronutrients and micronutrients, reaching critical low levels in some institutions during different seasons of the year, low proportion of animal protein, and risk for micronutrient deficiencies – minerals and vitamins.

Abstract (Original Language) Проведено е Национално репрезентативно трансверсално епидемиологично проучване през 1997 година за оценка на храненето и хранителния статус на институционализирани деца на възраст 7 – 16 години, група с висок социално-здравен риск. Изследвани са 362 деца от двата пола в 16 случайно подбрани Домове за деца, лишени от родителски грижи (от общо 89 Домове за страната). Основни проблеми в храненето на децата представляват широката вариабилност в обезпечеността от енергия, макронутриенти и микронутриенти, достигащи критично ниски нива в някои домове през отделни периоди на годината, ниският относителен дял на животински белтък и риск за дефицити от микронутриенти (минерални вещества и витамини) в предлаганата храна.

Age Groups

7	10
10	14
14	16

Cyprus

National Study for Obestity and Nutrional Habits

National Study of Nutrition

Project Leader

Project Leader	Eliza Markidou
Address	Ministry of Health
	Markou Drakou 10 Pallouriotissa
	Nicosia Cyprus
Executing Institution	Ministry of Health
Funding Agency	Cyprus Government

Project Information

Start of Project	01/06/2006
End of Project	01/06/2007
Start of Data Collection	01/06/2006
End of Data Collection	31/12/2006
URL	
Scope	National

Keywords

Abstract (English) Obesity is a big problem in Cyprus. The most recent data of the prevalence of obesity is from a study done in the year 1989/1990 that has shown that 19% of men and 24% of women age 36- to 64-years old are obese. With this study, the percentage of obesity will be estimated as well as the BMI and the fat percentage. With the study, we will identify the nutrional habits of Cypriots and the healthy lifestyle components of everyday life.

Abstract (Original Language)

Age Groups

The Epidemiological Study to Define the Percentage of Obesity and Overweight as Well as the Nutritional Habits of Cypriots

Research Done by the Cyprus Dietetics Association

Project Leader

Project Leader	Photos Hatzigeorgiou
Address	
Executing Institution	
Funding Agency	Research Institue

Project Information

Start of Project	01/05/2006
End of Project	01/05/2009
Start of Data Collection	01/05/2006
End of Data Collection	
URL	
Scope	National

Keywords

Abstract (English)

Obesity is a big problem in Cyprus. The most recent data of the prevalence of obesity is from a study done in the year 1989/1990 that has shown that 19% of men and 24% of women age 36- to 64-years old are obese. With this study, the percentage of obesity will be estimated as well as the BMI and the fat percentage. Special attention to analysis of the nutritional habits of Cypriots.

Abstract (Original Language)

Age Groups

Denmark

Arctic Public Health Research

Project Leader

Project Leader	Peter Bjerregaard
Address	National Institute of Public Health
	Øster Farimagsgade 5 A, 2nd floor
	DK- 1399 Copenhagen
	Denmark
Executing Institution	National Institute of Public Health
Funding Agency	

Project Information

Start of Project	
End of Project	
Start of Data Collection	
End of Data Collection	
URL	http://www.si-folkesundhed.dk/Forskning/Befolkningens%20sund
	hedstilstand/Gr%C3%B8nland.aspx
Scope	National

Keywords

Abstract (English) In 1995, a professorship in Arctic public health was established at the NIPH. The main aim of the department for health research in Greenland including the professorship is to contribute to an improvement of public health in Greenland. Transferring of knowledge and experience to Greenland has top priority. The department has a close working relationship with the Directorate of Health of the Greenland Home Rule, with other institutions in Greenland, and arctic health research environments in Denmark, Canada, Alaska, and the Nordic countries.

The programme is covering a wide range of research themes: from mortality analyses, descriptions of the disease pattern in Greenland, analyses of psychosocial health, environmental medicine, diet, cardio-vascular diseases, and diabetes to evaluation of the Greenland health care system.

Activities in 2004 comprise the following:

– Preparation of a public health report for Greenland and contributions to the establishment of a public health programme for Greenland
– Inuit Health in Transition. A longitudinal study of the influence of diet, physical activity, life style, and living conditions on cardio-vascular disease and diabetes among Inuit in Greenland, Canada, and Alaska
– Follow-up of the Greenland health profile – an interview survey from 1993–1994
– A study of the health condition of infants in Greenland in relation to environmental pollution and other living conditions

- Analyses of diet, cardio-vascular disease, and diabetes, on the basis of population surveys
- The effect of population surveys on the services of the health care system
- Analyses of social inequality in health
- Analyses of health conditions in the elderly population
- A survey among children and adolescents regarding well-being and with a specific view to sexual abuse
- Development of common Greenlandic-Canadian methods in social epidemiology
- Survey and analysis of health promotion projects in Greenland and Arctic Canada
- Finalisation of the local community project in Qasigiannguit, where the population is involved in the planning and implementation of activities to promote quality of life and health

Abstract (Original Language)

Age Groups

Children, Food, and Excercise

Børn, Mad og Bevægelse

Project Leader

Project Leader	Anne-Marie Nybo Andersen
Address	Statens Institut for Folkesundhed
	Øster Farimagsgade 5
	1399 København K
	Denmark
Executing Institution	Statens Institut for Folkesundhed, National Institute of Public Health
Funding Agency	

Project Information

Start of Project	01/01/2002
End of Project	
Start of Data Collection	01/01/2002
End of Data Collection	31/12/2006
URL	http://www.boernmadogbevaegelse.dk/wm113505
Scope	National

Keywords

Abstract (English)

Abstract (Original Language) Modelprojektet var et samarbejde mellem Fyns Amt og 10 fynske kommuner. Formålet med projektet var at øge trivslen og sundheden blandt børn i alderen 3–10 år. Dette søges specifikt gjort gennem:

At formulere, implementere og gøre erfaringer med at efterleve mad-, måltids- og bevægelsespolitikker i daginstitutioner, skoler og fritidsordninger samt opsamle erfaringer om, hvordan institutioner kan integrere og støtte udviklingen af sunde mad- og bevægelsesvaner i børns hverdag.

At udvikle viden og kompetencer hos de professionelle, som børn møder i deres hverdag (f.eks. lærere, pædagoger, sundhedsplejersker og tandlæger), så de bliver i stand til at formidle viden om sammenhæng mellem sundhed og sygdom og mad og bevægelse samt igangsætte og støtte en udvikling af lokale aktiviteter.

At udvikle børns kompetencer, så de kan handle for at fremme egne og andres sunde mad- og bevægelsesvaner, samt at involvere forældre og familier i projektet sådan at det bliver et fælles anliggende.

At skabe fysiske og sociale miljøer for mad, måltider og bevægelse, f.eks. attraktive og udviklende spisestuer og legearealer.

De deltagende kommuner i projektet var: Assens, Fåborg, Glamsbjerg, Kerteminde, Odense, Rudkøbing, Svendborg, Sydlangeland, Tommerup,

Vissenbjerg. Herudover medvirker Sundhedsministeriet, Arkitektskolen i Århus og Idrætshistorisk Værksted i Gerlev.

Statens Institut for Folkesundhed stod for evalueringen af projektet (de første 5 projektmål). Det overordnede formål med evalueringen var at belyse, i hvilket omfang det lykkedes at opfylde de målsætninger, der var formuleret for projektet. For at sikre at projektets erfaringer blev samlet op løbende, tog evalueringen afsæt i en kortlægningsfase, der satte fokus på børn, mad og bevægelse og dermed samtidig fungerede som udgangspunkt for den endelige udformning af projektet.

Formålet med modelprojektet er at fremme børns sundhed og trivsel. Modelprojektet begyndte i 2002 og første fase blev afsluttet i januar 2005. I fase 2 er modelprojektet udvidet til at omfatte nye kommuner i regionen. I Modelprojektets anden fase (2005 og 2006) deltager følgende kommuner: Odense, Svendborg, Munkebo, Ringe, Egebjerg, Haarby og Ejby.

Formålet med modelprojektet er:

At bistå de udvalgte lokalområder i de deltagende kommuner med at udvikle mad- og bevægelsespolitikker gældende for børn i alderen 3–16 år og med de lokale politikker skabe sundhedsfremmende rammer i institutionerne, der kan styrke børn og voksnes muligheder for at fremme egen og andres sundhed i forhold til mad og bevægelse.

At bistå kommunale forvaltningers praktiske arbejde med sundhedsfremme og forebyggelse over for børn og unge i den nye kommunale struktur samt skabe grundlag for det kommunale arbejde med sundhedspolitikker

At dokumentere indsatsens betydning for børns mad- og bevægelsesvaner.

I Modelprojektet uddannes lærere og pædagoger og sundhedsplejersker fra en række fynske kommuner til lokal erfaringsskabelse og udvikling af sundhedsfremmende rammer i børnehaver, skoler og skolefritidsordninger. Målgruppen er børn i alderen 3–16 år.

Statens Institut for Folkesundhed evaluerer Fyns Amts modelprojekt Børn, Mad og Bevægelse – fase 2.

Formålet med evalueringen er at undersøge, om modelprojektets effekt på børnenes mad og bevægelsesvaner, således at en højere andel af børnene lever op til de officielle anbefalinger vedr. mad og bevægelse efter modelprojektets gennemførelse. Det vil sige, at evalueringen, efter aftale med Fyns Amt, fokuserer på projektmål 3.

Ved evalueringen benyttes CAPI (Computer Assisted Personal Interviews) som den primære dataindsamlingsmetode til skolebørn med deltagelse af elever fra 10 interventionsskoler og 5 kontrolskoler. Det internetbaserede spørgeskema suppleres af et mindre spørgeskema, der udfyldes af lærerne samt måling fysisk aktivitet på en mindre stikprøve.

Age Groups

3	16

Frame and Presumption for Diet and Physical Activity in 3- to 10-Year-Old Children

Rammer Og Vilkår for Kost og Fysisk Aktivitet for Børn i 3– 10 Års Alderen

Project Leader

Project Leader	Inge Lissau
Address	National Institute of Public Health
	Øster Farimagsgade 5 A, 2nd floor
	1399 Copenhagen K
	Denmark
Executing Institution	National Institute of Public Health
Funding Agency	

Project Information

Start of Project	01/01/1999
End of Project	31/12/2004
Start of Data Collection	01/01/1999
End of Data Collection	31/12/2004
URL	http://www.si-folkesundhed.dk/Forskning/Befolkningens%20sun
	dhedstilstand/B%C3%B8rnesundhed/Sundhedsv%C3%A6senets
	%20indsats/Kost%20og%20fysisk%20aktivitet.aspx
Scope	National

Keywords

Abstract (English)

Abstract (Original Language) Børns sundhed og velbefindende er blandt andet betinget af deres kost og af graden af fysisk aktivitet. En sund livsstil grundlægges i barndommen og skabes i et samspil mellem barnet og dets omgivelser. I de første år er forældrenes og hjemmets påvirkning den afgørende faktor, men senere øges indflydelsen fra andre arenaer, hvor barnet færdes, først og fremmest i daginstitutioner og skoler.

Denne rapport beskriver rammer og vilkår for mad og bevægelse i danske børnehaver, skoler og fritidshjem/skolefritidsordninger i 2004. Herunder en gennemgang af udviklingen på kostområdet på skoler og fritidshjem/skolefritidsordninger i perioden 1999–2004. Fritidshjem og kolefritidsordninger benævnes i rapporten samlet som skolefritidsordninger. Undersøgelsen er udført af Statens Institut for Folkesundhed og er delvist finansieret af Sundhedsstyrelsen.

Undersøgelsen omfatter en stikprøve på i alt 1875 institutioner eller 20% af alle landets børnehaver, skoler og skolefritidsordninger. På baggrund af besvarede spørgeskemaer fra 1323 institutioner fandt vi i hovedtræk følgende (oplysninger fra skolerne refererer hovedsageligt til 0.–3. klasse):

- Andelen af skoler og skolefritidsordninger med en skriftligt formuleret kostpolitik steg markant fra 1999 til 2004. For skoler steg andelen fra 3% til 17% og for skolefritidsordninger fra 4% til 18%

- Mere end dobbelt så mange børnehaver (38%) som både skoler (17%) og skolefritidsordninger (18%) havde i 2004 en skriftligt formuleret kostpolitik
- En nedskreven kostpolitik syntes at have en betydning i retning af et sundere udbud af mad- og drikkevarer i børnehaver og skoler samt i skolefritidsordninger i mere beskeden grad
- Der var i perioden 1999–2004 generelt sket en stigning i udbuddet af sunde mad- og drikkevarer og en nedgang i udbuddet af mindre sunde mad- og drikke-varer i skoler og skolefritidsordninger. For eksempel steg andelen af skoler med frugt- og grøntordning til næsten det dobbelte fra 18% til 33%
- Sodavandssalg, herunder sodavandsautomater, var stort set ikke-eksisterende på skolerne i 2004. I 1999 var der sodavandsautomat på 5% af skolerne, mens tallet i 2004 var 0,2%. I 1999 var der mulighed for at købe sodavand på 10% af skolerne, mens dette kun var muligt på 0,2% af skolerne i 2004. Andelen af skolefritidsordninger med sodavandssalg var i 1999 1% og i 2004 0,4%
- Flere skolebørn havde adgang til køleskab til opbevaring af medbragt mad i 2004 (78%) end i 1999 (53%)
- Mere end dobbelt så mange børnehaver (16%) og skolefritidsordninger (16%) som skoler (6%) havde i 2004 en skriftligt formuleret bevægelsespolitik
- Der sås ikke en entydig sammenhæng mellem en nedskreven bevægelsespolitik og omfanget af fysisk aktivitet. Flere børnehaver med bevægelsespolitik havde daglige voksenstyrede aktiviteter med aktiv leg og bevægelse end institutioner uden. For skoler fandt vi ingen tydelig mmenhæng mellem, om skolerne havde en bevægelsespolitik og omfanget af motorisk træning
- 40% af skolerne havde retningslinier for, hvor meget eleverne skulle opholde sig udendørs
- På godt halvdelen af skolerne blev mindst tre-fjerdedele af idrætsundervisningen varetaget af en idrætsuddannet lærer. 32% af børnehaverne havde en idrætsfaglig person ansat, og 37% af skolefritidsordningerne havde det. Børnehaver med idrætsfagligt personale var mere tilbøjelige til at tilbyde motorisk træning end børnehaver uden
- Ønsker om at øge omfanget af fysisk aktivitet var i flere børnehaver og skolefritidsordninger til stede blandt personalet end blandt forældre og forældrebestyrelser i. Der var dog fortsat 61–64% af institutionerne, hvor personalet ønskede at bevare status quo i aktivitetsniveau
- I 44% af skolefritidsordningerne havde børnene dagligt adgang til gymnastiksal/ idrætshal, mens eleverne kun på 7% af skolerne havde adgang hertil i frikvartererne
- I knapt hver tredje børnehave blev der dagligt arrangeret voksenstyrede aktiviteter med aktiv leg og bevægelse. Det samme var tilfældet i knapt halvde-len af skolefritidsordningerne. På 42% af skolerne medvirkede voksne aktivt til at sætte aktiviteter i gang i frikvartererne.

Age Groups

3	10

Sundheds- Og Sygelighedsundersøgelserne

SUSY

Project Leader

Project Leader	Morten Grønbæk
Address	National Institute of Public Health
	Øster Farimagsgade 5 A, 2nd floor
	1399 Copenhagen K
	Denmark
Executing Institution	National Institute of Public Health
Funding Agency	

Project Information

Start of Project	01/05/2005
End of Project	31/03/2006
Start of Data Collection	01/05/2005
End of Data Collection	31/03/2006
URL	http://www.si-folkesundhed.dk/Forskning/Befolkningens %20sundhed stilstand/SUSY.aspx
Scope	National

Keywords

Abstract (English)

Abstract (Original Language) SUSY-undersøgelserne indsamles der data til brug for statslig, amtskommunal og kommunal planlægning og sundhedsovervågning og til brug for forskning og analyser. Undersøgelserne indsamler data om befolkningens sundhed og sygdom og om forhold af betydning herfor – fx risikofaktorer i livsstil og levevilkår. Det er informationer, som ikke findes i de eksisterende administrative registre indenfor sundhedsvæsenet og det sociale område.

Det overordnede formål med sundheds- og sygelighedsundersøgelserne er:

At beskrive forekomsten og fordelingen af sundhed og sygelighed i befolkningen

At opstille tidsserier, der kan beskrive udviklingen

At tilvejebringe datamateriale til brug for de enkelte amtskommuners sundhedsplanlægning og til brug for analyser af geografiske variationer

At danne grundlag for forløbs- og tværsnitsanalyser af sundheds- og sygelighedsforhold

At være reference- og kontrolmateriale for specifikke forskningsprojekter

SUSY-undersøgelserne veksler mellem generelle, brede undersøgelser og undersøgelser rettet mod specifikke emner.

Generelle, brede undersøgelser

I de generelle undersøgelser fra 1987, 1994 og 2000 tegnes der brede billeder af den voksne befolknings sundheds- og sygelighedstilstand, af sundhedsvanerne, af helbredsressourcer og helbredsrisici, og af sygdomsadfærd og sygdomskonsekvenser. Se Publikationer.

Den næste generelle, brede undersøgelse gennemføres i 2005, og resultaterne forventes offentliggjort i 2007.

Specifikke undersøgelser

I 1991 gennemførtes en specifik undersøgelse om muskel- og skeletsygdom - dækkende dels forekomsten og fordelingen af muskel- og skeletsygdom, dels befolkningens viden om og holdning til sundhedsfremme og forebyggelse generelt og i relation til muskel- og skeletsygdom.

I 2003 gennemførtes endnu en specifik undersøgelse. Det oprindelige formål var at indsamle data til et amerikansk forskningscenter om hvor belastende forskellige sygdomme vurderes at være (burden of disease). Undersøgelsens tilrettelæggelse gav tillige mulighed for at gennemføre en række metodestudier.

Age Groups

>16 y danish people

The Danish Nurse Cohort

The Danish Nurse Cohort 1999

Project Leader

Project Leader	Yrsa Andersen Hundrup
Address	The Danish Nurse Cohort
	Statens Institut for Folkesundhed
	Øster Farimagsgade 5
	1399 København K
	Denmark
Executing Institution	Statens Institut for Folkesundhed
Funding Agency	

Project Information

Start of Project	01/01/1999
End of Project	31/12/1999
Start of Data Collection	01/01/1999
End of Data Collection	31/12/1999
URL	http://www.si-folkesundhed.dk/Forskning/Generelt%20om %20 forskning/Sygeplejerskekohorten.aspx
Scope	National

Keywords Smoking cessation; Nurses; Work environment; Lifestyle, Breast neoplasm; Malignancy grade; Receptor status; Epidemiology; Oestrogen; Progestin; Hormone replacement therapy; Low-energy fractures; Osteoporosis; Prospective cohort study

Abstract (English) The Danish Nurse Cohort was established in 1993 when all female Danish nurses members of the Danish Nurses Organization were mailed a questionnaire collecting information on their health and illness behavior and morbidity. The purpose was to evaluate the long-term effect of women's use of postmenopausal hormone replacement therapy (HRT) on cardiovascular diseases, osteoporosis, and cancer diseases. On the basis of the current evidence, some of which originated from studies based on data from the US cohort The Nurses Health Study, and it was anticipated that women using HRT would have a 40–50% lower risk of coronary heart disease and fractures related to osteoporosis.

Furthermore, the purpose was to evaluate the preventive effect of the hormone therapy widely in Denmark, i.e., a combination of oestradiol and progestogene.

Since 2000, the cohort has been located at the National Institute of Public Health (NIPH). A steering group is responsible for the data.

The cohort comprises all Danish female nurses above the age of 44 years, who are either active or passive members of The Danish Nurses Organization.

The first survey was carried out in 1993. Altogether 23,170 nurses were invited to participate and of these 86% (N = 19,953) returned the questionnaire.

In 1999, the second survey was carried out inviting all responders from the 1993-survey plus all nurses, who in the meantime had become 45 years or above, altogether 31,642 and of these 77% (N = 24, 155) returned the questionnaire.

Abstract (Original Language)

Age Groups

Nurses above 44 year old

Estonia

Estonian Health Behavior Survey of Adult Population

HBAP

Project Leader

Project Leader	Mare Tekkel
Address	National Institute for Health Development
	Hiiu 42
	11619 Tallinn
	Estonia
Executing Institution	National Institute for Health Development
Funding Agency	Coordinated by Finbalt Health Monitor Survey since 1990

Project Information

Start of Project	01/01/2003
End of Project	31/03/2005
Start of Data Collection	28/04/2004
End of Data Collection	01/06/2004
URL	
Scope	National

Keywords Health self-assessment; Health behavior; Physical activity; Smoking and alcohol use; Nutrition

Abstract (English) The study Health Behavior among Estonian Adult population is conducted every other year starting from 1990 and forms a part of the FinBalt Health monitor (FinBalt) cooperative study in which Lithuania, Latvia, and Finland participate as well. The coordinator of the FinBalt study is the Finnish National Public Health Institute. Conducting the study each time on the basis of common methodology and employing a questionnaire that in a large part contains identical questions enables the monitoring and analysis of alterations of specific indicators of health behavior over a long period. The main topics studied are health self-assessment and the usage of medical aid, diet, physical activity, smoking and alcohol use, traffic behavior, as well as the respondents' opinions and attitudes toward health.

Summary: The study Health Behavior among Estonian Adult Population is conducted each even year starting from 1990. This forms a part of the Finbalt Health monitor (Finbalt) cooperative study in which Lithuania, Latvia, and Finland participate as well. The coordinator of the Finbalt study is the Finnish National Health Institute. Conducting the study each time on the basis of common methodology and employing a questionnaire that in a large part contains identical questions enables the monitoring and analysis of alterations of specific indicators of health behavior over a long period. Being a part of the cooperative project adds to Estonian data the element of comparison and helps to highlight the causes of alterations.

The main topics studied are health self-assessment, the usage of medical aid, diet, physical activity, smoking and alcohol use, traffic behavior, as well as the respondents' opinions and attitudes toward health. The study in 2004 was subscribed and financed by the Estonian Ministry of Social Affairs and conducted by the Department of Epidemiology and Biostatistics in the National Institute for Health Development.

For the purposes of the health behavior study, a simple random sample from the Estonian population aged between 16 and 64 was ordered from the Estonian population register; to enhance accuracy, the sample was increased up to 5,000 individuals. Like previous years, the study was conducted as a postal questionnaire survey. The questionnaires were compiled and mailed in both, Estonian and Russian. In two weeks after the initial mailing, a reminder in either Estonian or Russian was sent to those who had not responded because of an unknown reason. If a person still failed to respond after that the questionnaire was mailed to them for the second time after 2 weeks from the reminder. The questionnaires were mailed 28/04/2004–1/06/2004. The crude and adjusted response rates were 61.5% and 63.4%, respectively. Response rate was higher for women, rural inhabitants, and the elderly. The percentage of different age groups, Estonians, and urban inhabitants among respondents was not significantly different from the corresponding indicator for the population of Estonia in 01/01/2003. Data processing was done with the help of Visual FoxPro and STATA packages. Maximum question-specific nonresponse was 7%.

Abstract (Original Language) Eesti täiskasvanud rahvastiku tervisekäitumise uuring toimub igal paarisaastal alates aastast 1990 ning on siiani moodustanud osa Finbalt Health Monitor (Finbalt) ühisuuringust, milles osalevad veel Leedu, Läti ja Soome. Ühisuuringu koordineerija on Soome Rahvatervishoiu Instituut. Uuringu toimumine kõigil aastatel ühtse metoodika alusel ja suures osas samu küsimusi sisaldanud küsimustikuga võimaldab jälgida ja analüüsida tervisekäitumist iseloomustavate näitajate muutumist pikema aja vältel. Ühisprojektis osalemine lisab Eesti andmetele võrdluse lähiriikidega ning aitab paremini esile tuua muutuste põhjusi. Peamised uuritavad valdkonnad on tervise enesehinnang, arstiabi kasutamine, toitumine, kehaline aktiivsus, suitsetamine ja alkoholi tarvitamine, liikluskäitumine, samuti küsitletava arvamused, hoiakud ja suhtumine tervisesse.

Age Groups

16	64

Estonian Health Interview Survey 1996

EHIS

Project Leader

Project Leader	Mall Leinsalu
Address	National Institute for Health Development
	Hiiu 42
	11619 Tallinn
	Estonia
Executing Institution	National Institute for Health Development
Funding Agency	Coordinated: Working Group, WHO

Project Information

Start of Project	01/01/1996
End of Project	31/12/1998
Start of Data Collection	01/10/1996
End of Data Collection	01/03/1997
URL	
Scope	National

Keywords Public health; Health determinants; Health behavior

Abstract (English) After the reestablishment of independence in 1991, the Health Interview Survey (EHIS) was the first large-scale survey about the health status of the population in Estonia. As the third national survey after the Estonian Family and Fertility Survey (EFFS 1994) and the Estonian Labor Force Survey (ELFS 1995), it was a follow-up to a process initiated earlier to develop a person-related data collection system. As in the other subject areas, information about the population's health status had heretofore been mainly collected through the registration of certain life events by administrative units. As a result of the EHIS, in addition to the data obtained from the registration of births, deaths, causes of death, certain diseases, traumas, and medical services, we now have a survey-based dataset. This provides more extensive and diverse information about the health status and health behavior of the Estonian population.

When preparing the EHIS, the principles and definitions approved by the World Health Organization (WHO) were taken into account. Because of its conceptual and methodological compatibility with internationally accepted standards, the results of this survey are comparable with other countries that carry out analogous surveys. The data analyses will create the basis for elaborating a national health policy that takes account of both the special character of the Estonian transition economy and international experience. Implementing the survey fulfilled the decision of the Governmental Commission for Population Statistics in 1993 to begin regular health interview surveys.

As the survey results were intended to serve the interests of different data-users, it was very important to engage the cooperation of appropriate institutions, researchers, and officials in preparation of the survey. To secure conceptual and definitional compatibility with other surveys as well as with routine statistics, the issues of shared concepts and data definitions was of special concern in this survey. Because of this approach, it is possible to compare the results of national surveys with each other and to analyze health problems from much wider perspective than could be done within the frame of one specific study. In addition, this will assure the continuation of data development processes, which is significant for Estonia in joining to the network of international cooperation.

Abstract (Original Language) 1991 aastal taasiseseisvunud Eestis on Terviseuuring esimene ulatuslik rahva tervist käsitlev küsitlusuuring. Olles Eesti Pere-ja Sündimusuuringu (EPSV 1994)1,2 ja Eesti Tööjõu-uuringu (ETV 1995)3,4 järel arvult kolmandaks loenduse baasil läbiviidud riigiuuringuks, jätkati varem alustatud isikukeskse andmekogumissüsteemi väljaarendamist. Analoogselt teiste ainevaldkondadega koguti rahvastiku terviseseisundit iseloomustavat teavet senini valdavalt vaid ametkondade poolt isikusündmuste registreerimise kaudu. Terviseuuringu tulemusena on kõiksele sündide, surmade, surmapõhjuste, teatud haiguste, traumade ja meditsiiniliste teenuste registreerimisele lisandunud küsitluse teel kogutud andmestik. Seetõttu on tekkinud võimalus omada senisest märksa ulatuslikumat ja mitmekülgsemat teavet Eesti rahvastiku tervislikust olukorrast ja tervisekäitumisest.

Terviseuuringu ettevalmistamisel kasutati Maailma Tervishoiuorganisatsiooni (MTO) poolt heakskiidetud põhimõtteid ja andmedefinitsioone. Tänu uuringu kontseptuaalsele ja metoodilisele ühildumisele rahvusvaheliselt aktsepteeritud lähtekohtadega, on tulemused võrreldavad teiste analoogseid uuringuid korraldanud riikidega. Andmeanalüüs loob head eeldused pädeva riikliku tervisepoliitika väljatöötamiseks, mis arvestaks Eesti siirdemajanduse eripära ning rahvusvahelisi kogemusi antud valdkonnas. Ühtlasi täideti uuringu läbiviimisega Vabariigi Isikuandmekomisjoni poolt 1993. aastal vastuvõetud otsus alustada perioodiliste tervisealaste küsitlusuuringute läbiviimist.

Kuivõrd uuringu tulemused peavad teenima eri andmetarbijate huve, siis oli olulisel kohal asjast huvitatud institutsioonide, teadlaste ja ametnike koostöö süvendamine. Arvestades varasemaid tervise vallas tehtud töid ja riigiuuringute andmete sidumise vajadust, pöörati suurt tähelepanu uuringu metodoloogiliste lähtekohtade ning andmedefinitsioonide ühtlustamisele ja hoidmisele. Tänu sellele osutub võimalikuks riigiuuringute andmeid omavahel võrrelda ning avada tervisetemaatikat märksa laiemalt kui ühe konkreetse uuringu raames tavapäraseit teha saab. Ühtlasi tähendab see andmekindlustatuse jätkuvust, mis on tähendusrikas Eesti taotlustes asuda rahvusvahelise koostöö võrgustikku.

Age Groups

15	79

Estonian Social Survey

ESS

Project Leader

Project Leader	Mari Toomse
Address (Project Leader)	Estonian Statistical Office,
	Endla 15
	15174 Tallinn
	tel +372 625 9300
Executing Institution	Estonian Statistical Office
Funding Agency	Coordinated by EUROSTAT in the frame of EU-SILC

Project Information

Start of Project	01/01/2004
End of Project	31/12/2004
Start of Data Collection	19/03/2004
End of Data Collection	31/08/2004
URL	
Scope	National

Keywords Income; Living conditions

Abstract (English) EU-SILC (European Union Statistics on Income and Living Conditions) is a sample survey designed to obtain comparative and reliable statistics on income distribution, living conditions, and social exclusion at European level. The survey results are used to study the social and economic development of the society and to plan and evaluate socio-political decisions.

All Member States and a few countries not belonging to the EU are involved in the survey. These survey data are based on nationally representative probability samples to permit detailed analysis by population subgroups.

Regulations to ensure the overall comparability of national surveys are declared by European Commission. Still the Member States have some flexibility in the design of EU-SILC. These data are required in both cross-sectional (pertaining to a given time in a certain time period) and longitudinal (pertaining to individual-level changes over time) dimensions. Therefore, households and their members are surveyed on an annual basis, maximally during four consecutive years.

The Statistical Office of Estonia runs the survey since the year 2004, pilot surveys were organized in the period 2002–2003. The present publication summarises the data collected by the survey in 2004.

All published estimates have been calculated for the total population (or for the population of a respective region). The sample sizes have been determined on the basis of the estimated total population provided by the Statistical Office. Because of rounding, the column sums are not always equal with the total, the difference may be up to some last decimal places. It is a panel survey, with one panel included in a survey for four years. Health module included three MEHM questions.

Abstract (Original Language) Saada teavet aastasissetuleku ja materiaalse heaolu kohta, mille abil saadakse ka püsiv vaesuse indikaator. Järgida Euroopa Parlamendi ja Euroopa Nõukogu määrust COM (2001) 754 final, mis puudutab Euroopa Liidu sissetulekute ja eluolu statistikat. Uuringu andmestik koosneb andmetest, mida kogutakse aasta kohta (läbilõikelised andmed), ning andmetest, mida kogutakse 3 aasta kohta (paneelandmed, st samadelt inimestelt küsitakse kolm aastat järjest). Tervisemoodul sisaldab 3 küsimust terviseseisundi minimoodulist.

Age Groups

14	and older

Finland

Health Behavior and Health Among the Finnish Adult Population, Spring 2005

Suomalaisen aikuisväestön terveyskäyttäytyminen ja terveys, kevät 2005

Project Leader

Project Leader	Antti Uutela
Address	National Public Health Institute
	Department of Health Promotion and Chronic Disease Prevention
	Mannerheimintie 166
	FI - 00300 Helsinki
	Finland
Executing Institution	Department of Epidemiology and Health Promotion, Health Promotion Research Unit
Funding Agency	Ministry of Social Affairs and Health in Finland

Project Information

Start of Project	04/04/2005
End of Project	
Start of Data Collection	04/04/2005
End of Data Collection	
URL	
Scope	National

Keywords Health behavior; Smoking; Food habits; Alcohol consumption; Physical activity

Abstract (English) Since 1978, the National Public Health Institute (KTL), with financial support from the Ministry of Social Affairs and Health, has carried out an annual postal survey entitled "Health Behaviour and Health among the Finnish Adult Population." This report presents the results of the spring 2005 survey. The primary purpose of the monitoring is to obtain information on smoking, food habits, consumption of alcohol and physical activities, and on changes in them in the long and short term.

For this survey, a random sample (n = 5,000) of Finnish adults between 15 and 64 years of age was drawn from the Population Register. A questionnaire was mailed in April 2005, and three reminders were sent. The number of respondents was 3,287 (response rate 66%).

Daily smoking remained at the same level as in the previous year. In 2005, 26% of men and 18% of women smoked daily. Smoking among men has decreased since the late 1970s, whereas smoking among women has remained at the same level since the mid-1980s. In 2005, 29% of men and 45% of women told that they eat fresh vegetables daily. Forty percent of men told that they drink skimmed or 1-milk (fat 1%), and the corresponding rate among women was 47%. In the longterm, food habits have moved in the direction of dietary recommendations. In 2005, the consumption of alcohol was at the same level as in the previous year when consumption increased compared with the previous years. In 2005, 60% of men and 68% of women told that they pursue leisure-time physical activities at least twice a week.

The differences between educational groups with respect to daily smoking are clear: the highest educated smoke the least and the differences between educational groups have widened. In contrast, the differences in healthy food habits between educational groups have diminished. The differences in men's alcohol consumption have almost disappeared, because weekly alcohol consumption among the lowest-educated men increased during the study period 2004–2005. Among women, the differences between educational groups have remained: weekly alcohol consumption was the highest among the highest-educated women.

Abstract (Original Language) Kansanterveyslaitos on toteuttanut vuodesta 1978 alkaen vuosittain "Suomalaisen aikuisväestön terveyskäyttäytyminen ja terveys" (AVTK) -postikyselytutkimuksen sosiaalija terveysministeriön tuella. Tässä raportissa esitetään tulokset keväältä 2005. Keskeisinä tavoitteina on kartoittaa terveyskäyttäytymisen pitkän ja lyhyen aikavälin muutoksia.

Tutkimuksen tärkeimmät terveyskäyttäytymisen osa-alueet ovat tupakointi, ruokatottumukset, alkoholinkäyttö ja liikunta. Vuoden 2005 tutkimusaineistoksi poimittiin väestörekisteristä valtakunnallisesti edustava 5 000 henkilön satunnaisotos 15–64-vuotiaista suomalaisista. Kyselylomake postitettiin huhtikuussa 2005. Vastaamatta jättäneille lähetettiin kolme uusintakyselyä. Kyselyyn vastasi 3 287 henkilöä (vastausaktiivisuus 66 %).

Päivittäistupakointi pysytteli edellisen vuoden tasolla. Vuonna 2005 miehistä tupakoi päivittäin 26 prosenttia ja naisista 18 prosenttia. Pitkällä aikavälillä miesten tupakointi on vähentynyt ja naisten tupakointi pysynyt 1980-luvun puolivälin tasolla. Vuonna 2005 miehistä 29 prosenttia ja naisista 45 prosenttia kertoi syövänsä tuoreita kasviksia päivittäin.

Miehistä 40 prosenttia kertoi juovansa rasvatonta tai ykkösmaitoa, ja vastaava osuus naisilla oli 47 prosenttia. Pitkällä aikavälillä tutkimuksessa mitatut ruokatottumukset ovat muuttuneet ravintosuositusten mukaiseen suuntaan. Vuonna 2005 alkoholinkulutus oli edellisen vuoden tasolla, jolloin alkoholinkulutus oli lisääntynyt edellisiin vuosiin verrattuna. Vuonna 2005 miehistä 60 prosenttia ja naisista 68 prosenttia kertoi harrastavansa vapaa-ajan liikuntaa vähintään kaksi kertaa viikossa. Pitkällä aikavälillä vapaa-ajan liikunta on lisääntynyt ja työmatkaliikunta vähentynyt.

Päivittäistupakoinnin koulutusryhmittäiset erot ovat selkeät: korkeimmin koulutetut tupakoivat vähiten ja koulutusryhmien väliset erot ovat kasvaneet. Ravintosuositusten mukaisten ruokatottumusten koulutusryhmittäiset erot taas ovat supistuneet. Miesten alkoholinkulutuksen koulutusryhmittäiset erot ovat jokseenkin hävinneet, kun alkoholin viikkokulutus miesten alimmassa koulutusryhmässä lisääntyi tutkimusjaksolla 2004–2005. Naisilla alkoholin viikkokulutuksen koulutusryhmittäiset erot taas ovat säilyneet: korkeimmin koulutetut naiset ilmoittivat suuremmasta viikkokulutuksesta.

Age Groups

15	24
25	34
35	44
45	54
55	64

Ravitsemuskertomus 2004

Nutrition Report 2004

Project Leader

Project Leader	Marjaana Lahti-Koski and Mervi Sirén
Address	National Public Health Institute
	Mannerheimintie 166
	FIN-00300 Helsinki
	Finland
Executing Institution	Department of health promotion and chronic disease
	prevention, Nutrition Unit
Funding Agency	National Public Health Institute

Project Information

Start of Project	
End of Project	
Start of Data Collection	
End of Data Collection	
URL	http://www.ktl.fi/portal/suomi/osastot/eteo/yksikot/ravitsemus
	yksikko/julkaisut/ravitsemuskertomukset/
Scope	National

Keywords

Abstract (English) Nutrition reports cover the main results of nutritional studies carried out in Finland. These data are presented succinctly, in a readily comprehensible way. The reports are the most important means by which the Finnish National Nutrition Surveillance System (FNNSS) can achieve its objectives, which are to collect, interpret, evaluate, and distribute data on nutrition in Finland, and to assess the need for measures to promote nutrition and health policies. In addition to policy makers and officials, the audience of the FNNSS includes health care professionals, researchers, teachers, journalists, and those working in the food industry, trade, nongovernmental organizations, and largescale catering.

In this report, changes in the health and nutritional status of the Finnish population over the past years are described. The food consumption and nutrition intake of the population are illustrated, mainly by using the results from FINDIET 2002 study. A special topic in this report concerns beverages, the consumption and assortment of which have grown steadily over the past decades. Another special topic concerns meals consumed during office hours. Their prevalence and their implications for nutrition intake are described in a report prepared in a collaborative project between the National Public Health Institute and the Finnish Institute of Occupational Health. In addition, this Nutrition Report presents recently published programmes and recommendations in the field of health and nutrition policy focusing on the publications, which include nutrition as an important means.

The health and functional capacity of working-aged Finns has improved remarkably over the past 20 years. Nevertheless, favorable changes in one of the most important risk factors for cardiovascular diseases, in cholesterol levels, seem to have leveled off. In addition, positive trends in children's dental health dating back to the early 1970s have turned in an adverse direction. Obesity is an increasing problem, especially among adolescents and young adults, in addition to the least educated sectors of the community.

The fat content of the Finnish diet has decreased from the 1970s. However, the most recent results from population surveys show that this positive trend seems to have leveled off. The intake of hard fat has also decreased over the past decades, though no longer in the 2000s. Compared with recommendations, the intake of hard fat is still too high. In contrast, the intake of fiber is too low with the exception of women living in the eastern part of Finland. The intake of sucrose was higher than recommended for women, especially among the youngest ones.

The intake of vitamins and minerals are at recommended levels among men and women. However, the intake of folates could be higher. The folate intake is low especially among young adults, as is the one for thiamin in young women. In addition, Finnish diet in 2002 was poor in vitamin D both for men and women. The total intake of vitamin D was below the recommendation in women. Vitamin D status among Finns is expected to improve because of the fortification of vitamin D in milk products, which commenced in the beginning of 2003.

On the basis of food balance sheets, consumption of rice, wheat, and oats increased, but that of rye decreased between 2001 and 2002. The sugar consumption has been quite stable for a long time, but based on preliminary data for year 2002, the trend seems to have turned upwards. Although vegetable consumption has increased, it is still quite low – especially in men. An increase in fruit consumption seems to have stopped but this is not the case for fruit juices, the consumption of which is higher than ever before. Meat consumption is increasing, too, because of growing popularity of poultry. Fish consumption has been stable, meaning that on average, it is eaten twice a week.

Consumption of beverages has grown remarkably during the past decades. In addition to fruit juices, soft drinks have become more popular. Their consumption has doubled in ten years. About 25% of soft drink consumption are based on drinks that are sweetened artificially. Overall, the variability of beverages has expanded during the past years. In addition to traditional juices, plenty of new types of beverages are currently available, including drinks that are fortified with several vitamins and minerals. Beverages have become a popular target for nutritional fortification. Traditional coffee has kept its status as a popular beverage in Finland, although in younger Finns, there is a growing group of people not drinking coffee. Milk consumption has decreased steadily, and fat-free and low-fat types have substituted for those including more fat. While milk is decreasingly consumed as a drink, consumption of cheese and yogurt has increased.

Trends in alcohol consumption have turned again upwards after a decrease that took place in the early 1990s. Popular types of alcohol have changed to milder products such that most of the ethanol intake is currently covered by beer consumption.

The popularity of ciders and wines has increased, too. The Drinking Habits Survey conducted in 2000 showed that about 10% of men and women aged 15 years or older had not consumed alcohol at all during the past 12 months. In men, the situation has been quite stable, whereas in women the share of those not consuming alcohol has decreased remarkably in less than ten years. The majority of Finns consumes alcohol in moderation. The distribution of consumption is very skewed, so that about half of the total alcohol consumption in Finland is consumed by 10% of the population.

A staff canteen is the most important place for having a lunch for working men. More than third of them eat their lunch there, whereas for women, it is more common to have packed lunch. Almost half of working women report to having a packed lunch at break time. People who live in the capital area and have a higher education are more likely to have a lunch at a staff canteen, when compared with those living elsewhere and those less educated. The size of the working place is related to the usage of staff canteens such that in bigger working places were it is more common to have lunch at a staff canteen, whereas in smaller working places, where it is more common to have a packed lunch or have a lunch at home or elsewhere outside the working area. Those who have lunch at a staff canteen eat more vegetables, fish, and boiled potatoes than others. Having lunch at a staff canteen promotes recommended food choices, and this applies in all educational groups and in all geographical areas. The majority of students on 7th–9th grade visit the school canteen and eat the main course. In contrast, only half of the diners take salad, bread, or milk. Almost half of the students also eat or drink something other than the food served at the school canteen during the school day. Sweets and soft drinks are the most common supplements to the school lunch.

Abstract   (Original   Language) Ravitsemuskertomuksissa   esitetään päätuloksia Suomessa tehdyistä tutkimuksista ja kerätyistä tilastoista help-polukuisessa, tiiviissä muodossa. Ravitsemuskertomukset ovat vuonna 1995 käynnistetyn ravitsemuksen seurantajärjestelmän tärkein väline toteuttaa pää-tarkoitustaan. Seurantajärjestelmän tavoitteena on kerätä, yhdistää, jalostaa ja edelleen välittää suomalaisten ravitsemusta kuvaavaa tietoa ravitsemus- ja terveyspoliittisten ohjelmien ja päätöksenteon tueksi. Viranomaisten ja päättäjien lisäksi ravitsemuskertomukset on tarkoitettu työvälineeksi terveydenhuollossa, elintarviketeollisuudessa ja -kaupassa, ruokapalveluissa, järjestöissä, tutkimus- ja oppilaitoksissa sekä tiedotusvälineissä toimiville.

Tässä ravitsemuskertomuksessa kuvataan ydinkohdittain suomalaisten terveys ja ravitsemusmittareissa viime vuosina tapahtuneita muutoksia. Suomalaisten ruoankulutuksesta ja ravintoaineiden saannista kerrotaan pääasiassa uuden Finravinto-tutkimuksen tulosten perusteella. Tällä kertaa julkaisun yhtenä erityisteemana on juomat, joiden kulutus ja valikoimat ovat kasvaneet rajusti vii-meisten vuosikymmenien aikana. Toinen erityisteema on työaikainen ruokailu, jonka yleisyyttä ja ravitsemuksellista merkitystä tarkastellaan Kansanterveys- ja Työterveyslaitoksen yhteistyönä valmistuneen selvityksen pohjalta. Lisäksi julkaisussa esitellään viime vuosina ilmestyneitä terveys- ja ravitsemuspoliittisia ohjelmia ja hoitosuosituksia, joissa ravitsemushoidolla on merkittävä roolinsa.

Työikäisen väestön terveys ja toimintakyky sekä koettu terveys ovat kohentuneet merkittävästi 20 viime vuoden aikana. Kuitenkin myönteinen kehitys merkittävän sydän- ja verisuonisairauksien riskitekijän, kolesteritasojen, laskussa näyttää pysähtyneen. Samoin 1970-luvun alusta jatkunut lasten suun terveyden paraneminen on kääntynyt huonompaan suuntaan. Lihavuus on yhä kasvava ongelma, etenkin 7. Yhteenveto nuorten ja nuorten aikuisten sekä alempiin koulutusryhmiin kuuluvien joukossa.

Suomalainen ruokavalio on muuttunut vähärasvaisemmaksi 1970-luvulta lähtien. Uusimmat aikuisväestön ruoankäyttötutkimukset kuitenkin osoittavat, että hyvä kehitys näyttää taantuneen. Samoin kovan rasvan saanti on viime vuosikymmeninä vähentynyt, mutta ei enää 2000-luvulle tultaessa, ja on edelleen suositeltua suurempi. Kuidun saanti jää suositusta pienemmäksi itäsuomalaisia naisia lukuun ottamatta. Sakkaroosin saanti ylittää naisilla pienille energian saantitasoille asetetun enimmäissaantisuosituksen, etenkin nuorissa ikäryhmissä.

Vitamiinien ja kivennäisaineiden keskimääräinen saanti on pääosin hyvällä tasolla niin naisilla kuin miehilläkin. Vitamiineista kuitenkin folaattien saanti saisi olla runsaampaa. Erityisen niukkaa saanti on nuorilla aikuisilla, joista naispuolisilla myös tiamiinin saanti jää suositusta pienemmäksi. Ruokavalion laatu kohenisi ja vitamiinien saanti kasvaisi lisäämällä kasvisten, hedelmien ja marjojen sekä täysjyväviljaisten viljavalmisteiden käyttöä ja vähentämällä runsaasti sokeria sisältävien elintarvikkeidenkulutusta. Vuonna 2002 kerätyssä aineistossa ruokavalion D-vitamiinipitoisuus ylsi vaivoin suositukseen sekä miehillä että naisilla. Suositusta pienemmäksi jäi D-vitamiinin kokonaissaanti naisilla. Suomalaisten Dvitamiinitilanteeseen on odotettavissa kohennusta, sillä vuoden 2003 alusta alkaen nestemäisiin maitovalmisteisiin on alettu lisätä tuntuva määrä D-vitamiinia.

Vuoden 2002 ravintotaseiden mukaan viljalajeista riisin, vehnän ja kauran kulutus oli noussut, mutta rukiin kulutus laskenut edellisvuoteen verrattuna. Sokerin kulutus on pitkään pysytellyt tasaisena, mutta näyttää vuoden 2002 ennakkotietojen mukaan kääntyneen lievään nousususuuntaan. Kasviksia suomalaiset syövät enenevässä määrin, mutta silti keskimääräinen kulutus on varsin vähäistä – etenkin miehillä. Hedel mien kulutuksen pitkään jatkunut kasvu näyttää pysähtyneen. Sen sijaan hedelmämehuja juodaan entistä enemmän. Lihan kulutus kasvaa siipikarjanlihan ansiosta. Kalaa syödään entiseen tahtiin – keskimäärin kerran viikossa.

Juomien käyttö on kasvanut runsaasti viimeisten vuosikymmenien aikana. Hedelmämehujen lisäksi entistä enemmän käytettyjä ovat virvoitusjuomat, joiden kulutus on kaksinkertaistunut kymmenessä vuodessa. Nykyään neljännes nautituista virvoitusjuomista on keinotekoisesti makeutettuja. Kaiken kaikkiaan juomien valikoimat ovat laajentuneet kovasti viime vuosina. Perinteiset mehut ovat saaneet rinnalleen joukon uudentyyppisiä juomia, joihin tyypillisesti on lisätty useampia vitamiineja ja kivennäisaineitakin. Juomat on ravitsemuksellisen täydentämisen yhä yleistyvä kohde. Perinteinen kahvi pitää pintansa suomalaisten suosikkijuomana, vaikka nuorempien parissa on kasvava joukko niitä, jotka eivät juo kahvia. Maidon kulutus juoman muodossa on vähentynyt jatkuvasti ja maidon laatu muuttunut rasvapitoisuudeltaan kevyemmäksi. Yhä suurempi osa maidosta nautitaan nykyään juuston ja jogurtin muodossa.

Alkoholin kulutus on kääntynyt uudelleen kasvuun 1990-luvun alussa tapahtuneen notkahduksen jälkeen. Juomalaadut ovat kuitenkin miedontuneet viimeisten vuosikymmenien aikana niin, että suurin osa alkoholista saadaan oluen muodossa. Myös siidereiden ja mietojen viinien suosio on kasvanut. Vuoden 2000 juomatapatutkimuksen mukaan noin joka kymmenes yli 15-vuotias mies tai nainen ei ollut käyttänyt lainkaan alkoholia edellisen vuoden aikana. Miehillä tilanne on pysytellyt samanlaisena, mutta naisilla alkoholia käyttämättömien osuus on pienentynyt selvästi alle kymmenessä vuodessa. Suurin osa suomalaisista käyttää kohtuullisesti tai hyvin vähän alkoholia. Kulutus on jakautunut epätasaisesti niin, että eniten alkoholia käyttävä kymmenys juo noin puolet kaikesta Suomessa käytetystä alkoholista.

Henkilöstöravintola on työssäkäyvien miesten tärkein lounaspaikka. Runsas kolmannes miehistä syö lounaansa henkilöstöravintolassa. Sen sijaan naiset hoitavat yleisimmin lounasruokailunsa eväiden avulla, sillä lähes puolet työssäkäyvistä naisista ilmoittaa syövänsä eväitä lounasaikaan. Pääkaupunkiseudulla asuvat ja korkeammin koulutetut lounastavat henkilöstöravintolassa useammin kuin muualla asuvat ja vähemmän koulutusta hankkineet. Työpaikan koko vaikuttaa henkilöstöravintolan käyttöön siten, että isommilla työpaikoilla lounastetaan useammin henkilöstöravintolassa, pienempien työpaikkojen väki syö useammin eväitä tai ruokailee kotona tai muualla työpaikan ulkopuolella. Henkilöstöravintolassa lounastavat syövät enemmän kasviksia, kalaa ja keitettyä perunaa kuin muuten lounasruokailunsa järjestävät. Henkilöstöravintolassa ruokailun yhteys ravitsemussuositusten mukaisiin ruokavalintoihin on havaittu kaikissa oulutusryhmissä ja kaikilla asuinalueilla.

Yläasteen oppilaista valtaosa käy kouluruokalassa ja nauttii pääruoan. Sen sijaan salaatin, leivän tai ruokajuoman valitsee vain puolet ruokailijoista. Lähes joka toinen oppilaista syö kouluruoan lisäksi jotakin muuta kouluaikana. Yleisimmin kouluruoan lisäksi nautitaan makeisia tai virvoitusjuomia.

Age Groups

School Health Promotion (SHP) Study

Kouluterveyskysely

Project Leader

Project Leader	Minna Pietikäinen
Address	National Research and Development Centre for Welfare and Health (STAKES)
	P.O. Box 220
	00531 Helsinki
	Finland
Executing Institution	National Research and Development Centre for Welfare and Health (STAKES)
Funding Agency	

Project Information

Start of Project	01 /04/2005
End of Project	30/04/2005
Start of Data Collection	01/04/2005
End of Data Collection	30/04/2005
URL	
Scope	National

Keywords

Abstract (English) The aim of the School Health Promotion (SHP) Study, launched in 1995, is to strengthen the planning and evaluation of health promotion activities at the municipality and school levels. While STAKES takes care of the data collection and reporting, the responsibility for the interpretation and practical use of data lies with municipalities and schools.

The first national data are published annually in the end of August, at the School Health Conference in Finland, and reported to the participating municipalities by the end of the year.

Besides the local interests, the School Health Promotion Study also serves national interests. These data are used as material for more detailed studies and, combined with other statistics, for studying the changes in the regional differences in adolescent health and well-being.

The main emphasis is on rapid processing and reporting of the data and further encouraging the municipalities and schools to actively use the knowledge on the basis of the collected data for the purposes of planning and evaluating health promotion.

The questionnaire covers living conditions, school as working environment, health-related behavior (e.g., nutrition, smoking, use of alcohol and drugs, sexual behavior) and health (e.g., diseases and symptoms, depressive mood).

These data are gathered by an anonymous classroom questionnaire in all 8th and 9th grades of secondary schools and 1st and 2nd grades of high schools. These data are gathered biannually in April. The age range of the respondents is 14–18 years. About 90% of the municipalities join in the School Health Promotion Study: even-numbered years: provinces of Southern Finland, Eastern Finland and Lapland odd-numbered years: provinces of Western Finland, Oulu and Åland 158,200 respondents in 2004/2005; 80% of all pupils in comprehensive schools, 69% of all students in high schools.

Abstract (Original Language)

Age Groups

14	16
16	18

The National Findiet 2002 Study

Findiet 2002

Project Leader

Project Leader	Satu Männistö, Marja-Leena Ovaskainen and Liisa Valsta
Address	National Public Health Institute
	Department of Health Promotion and Chronic Disease Prevention
	Mannerheimintie 166
	00300 Helsinki
	Finland
Executing Institution	Department of Health Promotion and Chronic Disease
	Prevention, Nutrition Unit
Funding Agency	

Project Information

Start of Project	01/02/2000
End of Project	01/06/2000
Start of Data Collection	01/02/2000
End of Data Collection	01/06/2000
URL	http://www.ktl.fi/portal/suomi/osastot/eteo/yksikot/ravitsemusyk sikko/julkaisut/finravinto_2002_-tutkimuksen_raportti/
Scope	National

Keywords

Abstract (English) The National FINDIET 2002 Study was carried out as part of the chronic disease risk factor monitoring FINRISK 2002 Study. A random sample involving 13,500 people 25- to 74-years of age and stratified for sex and 10-year age groups was taken from the population register. The participation rate was 65%, i.e., 8,799 subjects. In five areas, 32% of the invited subjects were randomly selected also to the dietary survey. The aim of this National FINDIET 2002 Study was to measure the average food and nutrient intake in early spring 2002. The areas were the same as in 1997: Helsinki and Vantaa (the metropolitan area), the cities of Turku and Loimaa as well as some rural communities in Loimaa, and the provinces of North Karelia, North-Savo, and Oulu. The final sample of the dietary survey was 2007 (63% of those invited).

For the dietary assessment, the participants were interviewed using the 48-h recall. A new interview-based program Finessi was developed for this study for entering and processing the dietary data. Also the National Food Database Fineli® used for the nutrient intake estimations was updated. The dietary intake data consisted of all days of the week except Fridays. Altogether 1,554 different food codes of the National Food Database were used to enter the food consumption data. The diet of the subjects contained on average 25 different foods per day. Nutrient losses caused by food processing were taken into account for vitamins A and C, thiamine, riboflavin, pyridoxine, niacin, vitamin B12, and beta-carotene. The average intake of nutrients in different population groups was evaluated according to the newest Finnish dietary recommendations from 1998.

The average daily diet consisted of six meals including most often one main meal. On working days, the Finnish adults typically had more meals than on days spent at home or on holiday. Two main meals were common on working days both for men (47%) and women (50%). On working days, about every fourth had lunch at the worksite cafeteria, about every fourth ate a packed lunch, and about every fifth had lunch at home. Almost every fourth of the subjects skipped the lunch. About half of the energy was derived from main meals on average, but one third of energy was derived from snacks. There were two energy intake peaks, one at lunch-time and the other at dinnertime (11 a.m. and 5 p.m.).

The diet of almost everyone included cereals, drinks, and milk products. Potato was the most popular side dish among men and women, but rice and pasta were also frequently consumed. Women consumed more frequently vegetables (as fresh vegetables and salads), fruit and berries than men. Men consumed more often meat dishes, potatoes, and sugar than women. The consumption of fish was equally common in men as in women. When adjusted for energy intake, women consumed more vegetables, fruit, berries, and cheese than men, whose diet included more potatoes, milk, meat, and sausages.

According to the National FINDIET 2002 Study, dietary energy intake was 9.2 MJ/day among men and 6.6 MJ/day among women. Among men, dietary energy intake was the highest in the eastern research areas, but there were no regional differences in the energy intake of women. The intake of fat, hard fat (sum of saturated and trans fatty acids), and protein was higher, whereas the intake of carbohydrate and fiber was lower compared with the Finnish nutrition recommendations. The intake of polyunsaturated fatty acids was close to the recommendation and the intake of essential fatty acids and monounsaturated fatty acids was at the recommended level. The fiber recommendation (3 g/MJ) was reached only among women in North Karelia and among women of the oldest age group, 55–64 years of age. The energy adjusted intake of sucrose was higher than recommended among women and highest among the youngest women. Alcohol (ethanol) contributed on average 3.5% of total energy among men and 1.5% of total energy among women. This was not beyond the recommended maximum level (5% of energy). However, alcohol intake was an underestimation, because Fridays were missing from the interview data. Alcohol intake among those who reported consumption of alcoholic beverages was close to double compared with the recommended maximum intake. The diet of men contained more fat and alcohol, but less carbohydrates than the diet of women.

Especially in the youngest age group the intake of vitamin D in women and the intake of folate in both women and men were below the recommendations. The intake of minerals was as recommended except for salt intake (NaCl), which was higher than the recommendations and except for the total daily intake of iron among women, which did not reach the recommendations. The intake of most nutrients varied very little by education. However, men in the highest educational group had the highest intake of vitamin E and C. Women in the lowest educational group had the lowest intake of fiber and vitamin C and the highest intake of saturated fatty acids and selenium. Because of the higher energy intake of men, the daily intake of nutrients, except for vitamin C, was higher among men than among women. The nutrient density of the diets did not differ between men and women for protein, vitamins A, D, B, and selenium. Nutrient density was higher among men for fatty acids, alcohol, salt, and iron. The energy adjusted intake of other nutrients was higher in women compared with men.

One third of energy was derived from bread and other cereal products, and another third was derived from meat dishes and milk products. Meat dishes, sausages, milk, and fat spreads contributed most (about 60–70%) to the dietary fat intake. Meat and sausage dishes (including other ingredients of these dishes), fat spreads, cheese, salty cereal-based foods, and milk products were the main sources of hard fat. Margarines and other vegetable fat spreads were the main sources of essential fatty acids, linoleic, and alpha-linolenic acid. Main sources of cholesterol were meat products and dishes, eggs, and milk products. Bread (especially rye bread) contributed about half of fiber intake. More than half of vitamin C intake was derived from fruit and berries. Similarly, more than half of thiamine was derived from cereals and meat dishes. Other B vitamins were mainly derived from cereals, meat, and milk products. Cereals, meat, and milk were also important food sources of minerals. Bread, other cereals, and meat dishes contributed most to sodium intake.

To ensure an adequate intake of carbohydrates in the diet, increasing the consumption of breads, other cereal products, vegetables, fruit, and berries is recommended. Low fat cereal products and vegetarian dishes should be preferred, because in this study these kinds of foods were also significant sources of fat. To ensure adequate fiber intake, consumption of whole grain bread, porridges, other cereal products, and vegetables is crucial.

The 48-h dietary recall was used in the National FINDIET 2002 Study to assess the average diet of Finnish adults. To validate the 48-h dietary recall, it was compared with the five-day dietary information (48-h recall plus a three-day dietary record) in 146 men and 185 women. Energy and nutrient densities were measured very similarly with both methods. Energy intake by the 48-h dietary recall was 99% of the energy intake obtained by 5-day data among men and women. The only exception was alcohol consumption, which was underestimated, because the dietary data did not include Fridays.

The new methods developed for the National FINDIET 2002 Study functioned well. Also the data collection phase worked out according to the study plan. Only the participation rate (63% of those invited) was lower than in the earlier national dietary surveys, which makes it harder to generalise the results to the whole population. The reasons for the lower participation rate can hardly be related to the FINDIET field study processes, but is most probably related to the general problems of participation, e.g., lack of time.

According to the results of this study, special attention should be paid on the quality of fat as well as the proportion of whole grain cereal products, vegetables, fruit, and berries in men. While the quality of fat turned out to be an issue also in women, the quality of carbohydrates should be equally emphasized. Increase of consumption of whole grain cereals and decrease of consumption of sugar-rich foods would improve the diet especially in the youngest women. The low energy intake of women sets special requirements to the quality of the diet. In addition to the problems caused by alcohol as such, attention should be paid also to the energy obtained from alcoholic beverages in different population groups. The diet of middle-aged and older women has still the best nutritional quality compared with other groups in Finland.

Abstract (Original Language) Finravinto 2002 -tutkimus toteutettiin osana kroonisten sairauksien riskitekijöitä kartoittavaa FINRISKI 2002 –tutkimusta. FINRISKI-tutkimuksen otokseen poimittiin sekä miehistä että naisista 10-vuotisikäryhmittäin satunnaisotos kuuden tutkimusalueen 25–74 -vuotiaasta väestöstä. FINRISKI-tutkimukseen osallistui 65 % kutsutuista, kaikkiaan 8 799 tutkittavaa. Viidellä tutkimusalueella 32 % kutsutuista poimittiin satunnaisesti ravintotutkimukseen. Finravinto-tutkimuksen tavoitteena oli selvittää väestön keskimääräinen ruoankäyttö ja ravintoaineiden saanti kevättalvella 2002. Tutkimusalueet olivat samat kuin vuonna 1997: Helsingin ja Vantaan tutkimusalue, Turun ja Loimaan alue, Pohjois-Savon maakunta, Pohjois-Karjalan maakunta sekä Oulun lääni. Hyväksyttyjä ravintohaastatteluja saatiin 2007 (63 % kutsutuista).

Ruoankäyttö selvitettiin kahden edellisen päivän ruoankäyttöhaastattelun avulla. Haastattelua varten kehitettiin uusi tiedonkeruu- ja laskentaohjelma Finessi ja päivitettiin elintarvikkeiden kansallinen koostumustietokanta Fineli® sekä uudistettiin sen ylläpitojärjestelmät. Kerätty tieto käsitti kaikki muut viikonpäivät paitsi perjantait. Tutkimusaineistoon tallennettiin yhteensä 1554 eri elintarvikkeen käyttötietoja. Tutkittavien ruokavalio sisälsi keskimäärin 25 eri elintarviketta päivässä. Jo laskentavaiheessa otettiin huomioon ravintoaineiden osittainen tuhoutuminen ruoanvalmistuksen aikana A-, ja C-vitamiinien, tiamiinin, riboflaviinin, pyridoksiinin, niasiinin, B12-vitamiinin sekä beetakaroteenin osalta. Ravintoaineiden keskimääräistä saantia eri väestöryhmissä verrattiin uusimpiin, vuoden 1998 suomalaisiin ravitsemussuosituksiin.

Keskimääräinen päivittäinen ruokavalio koostui kuudesta ateriointikerrasta, joista tyypillisimmin yksi oli pääateria. Työpäivinä aterioita oli useampia kuin koti- ja vapaapäivinä. Miehistä 47 % ja naisista 50 % söi työpäivinä kaksi pääateriaa. Työpäivinä noin joka neljäs söi lounaan henkilöstöravintolassa, noin joka neljäs eväinä ja noin joka viides kotona ruokaillen. Lähes joka neljäs tutkittava jätti työpäivinä varsinaisen lounaan syömättä. Noin puolet päivittäisestä energiasta saatiin pääaterioista lounaasta ja päivällisestä. Välipalojen osuus energian saannista oli kolmannes. Energian saannin huiput ajoittuivat suomalaiseen lounas- ja päivällisaikaan (kello 11 ja kello 17).

Lähes kaikkien tutkittavien ruokavalioon kuului viljatuotteita, juomia ja maitovalmisteita. Peruna oli sekä naisilla että miehillä pääasiallinen aterian peruslisäke, mutta riisiä ja pastaa käytettiin myös runsaasti. Naisilla kasvisten (tuoreena ja salaatteina), hedelmien ja marjojen käyttö oli yleisempää kuin miehillä. Miehillä rasvojen, liharuokien, perunoiden ja sokerin käyttö oli yleisempää kuin naisilla. Kalaruokien käyttö oli yhtä yleistä naisilla ja miehillä. Naisten ruokavalio sisälsi energiayksikköä kohden laskettuna enemmän kasviksia, hedelmiä ja marjoja ja juustoja kuin miesten, joiden ruokavalio sisälsi enemmän perunaa, maitoa, lihaa ja makkaraa.

Finravinto 2002 -tutkimuksen mukaan suomalaisten 25–64-vuotiaiden miesten energian saanti oli 9,2 MJ/vrk ja naisten 6,6 MJ/vrk. Miesten energian saanti oli suurin itäisillä tutkimusalueilla. Naisten energian saannissa ei ollut alueellisia eroja. Energiaravintoaineista rasvaa, kovaa rasvaa (tyydyttyneet ja trans-rasvahapot yhteensä) ja proteiinia saatiin yli suositusten, kun taas hiilihydraattien ja kuidun saanti jäi alle suositusten.

Monityydyttymättömien rasvahappojen saanti oli lähes suosituksen mukaista ja välttämättömien rasvahappojen kokonaissaanti ja kertatyydyttymättömien rasvahappojen saanti oli suosituksen mukaista. Energiavakioitu kuidun saanti ylitti suosituksen (3 g/MJ) vain Pohjois-Karjalan naisilla sekä vanhimmilla naisilla (55–64-vuotiaat). Naisten energiavakioitu sakkaroosin saanti ylitti enimmäissuosituksen ja oli runsainta nuorimmassa ikäryhmässä. Alkoholijuomien sisältämästä etanolista miehet saivat keskimäärin 3,5 % kokonaisenergiasta, naiset vastaavasti keskimäärin 1,5 %. Tämä jää alle suositusten enimmäismäärän (5 en%). Tässä tutkimuksessa alkoholin saanti on kuitenkin haastatelluista päivistä johtuen aliarvio. Alkoholijuomia käyttävillä etanolin osuus energiasta oli lähes kaksinkertainen suositusten enimmäismäärään verrattuna. Miesten ruokavalio sisälsi enemmän rasvaa ja alkoholia, mutta vähemmän hiilihydraatteja kuin naisten.

Erityisesti nuorimmissa ikäryhmissä naisten D-vitamiinin, naisten tiamiinin päivittäinen kokonaissaanti ja sekä miesten että nuorten naisten folaatin saanti jäivät alle suositusten. Kivennäisaineiden saannit olivat suositusten mukaisia lukuun ottamatta suolaa (NaCl), jota saatiin noin kaksinkertaisesti suosituksiin nähden sekä naisilla rautaa, jonka päivittäinen kokonaissaanti alitti suosituksen.

Koska yleisesti miesten energian saanti oli suurempi kuin naisten, myös muiden ravintoaineiden absoluuttiset saannit C-vitamiinia lukuun ottamatta olivat suurempia miehillä kuin naisilla. Energiaan suhteutettujen proteiinin, A- ja D-vitamiinin, B-vitamiinien sekä seleenin saannit eivät eronneet tilastollisesti merkitsevästi sukupuolittain. Miesten rasvan, rasvahappojen, alkoholin, suolan ja raudan energiaan suhteutettu saanti oli tilastollisesti merkitsevästi suurempi kuin naisilla. Muiden ravintoaineiden energiaan suhteutetut saannit olivat naisilla suurempia kuin miehillä.

Useimpien ravintoaineiden saanti ei eronnut koulutusryhmittäin. Miehillä ylimpään koulutusryhmään luokiteltujen ruokavalio sisälsi kuitenkin eniten E- ja C-vitamiinia. Naisilla alimpaan koulutusryhmään luokiteltujen ruokavaliossa oli vähiten kuitua ja C-vitamiinia, sekä eniten tyydyttyneitä rasvahappoja ja seleeniä.

Suomalaiset saivat noin kolmasosan ruoan energiasta leivistä ja muista viljavalmisteista ja noin kolmasosan liharuoista ja erilaisista maitovalmisteista. Suurin osa (n. 60 – 70 %) rasvasta saatiin liharuoista, makkaroista, maidosta ja ravintorasvoista. Liha- ja makkararuoat (ruokien kaikki valmistusaineet mukaanlukien), rasvalevitteet, juusto, suolaiset viljapohjaiset ruoat sekä maitovalmisteet olivat keskeiset kovan rasvan lähteet. Kasvirasvalevitteet olivat merkittävin välttämättömien rasvahappojen, linoli- ja alfalinoleenihapon, lähde. Kolesteroli saatiin pääosin liharuoista, kananmunista ja maitovalmisteista. Noin puolet kuidusta saatiin ruis- ja sekaleivistä. Yli puolet C-vitamiinista saatiin hedelmistä ja marjoista, tiamiinin tärkeimmät lähteet olivat viljavalmisteet ja liharuoat. Muita B-vitamiineja saatiin erityisesti vilja- ja maitovalmisteista. Viljavalmisteet, liharuoat ja maito olivat tärkeitä kivennäisaineiden lähteitä. Suolaa saatiin eniten leivästä ja muista viljavalmisteista sekä lihavalmisteista ja –ruoista.

Ruokavalion riittävän hiilihydraattimäärän varmistamiseksi leipien, muiden viljavalmisteiden, kasvisten, hedelmien ja marjojen käytön lisääminen on suositeltavaa. Kuluttajien tulisi valita vähärasvaisia viljavalmisteita ja kasvisruokia, koska tämänkin tutkimuksen mukaan sekä viljavalmisteissa ja kasvisruoissa on myös runsaasti rasvaa sisältäviä ruokalajeja. Kuidun saannin lisäämiseksi tulisi entisestään kasvattaa täysjyväleipien, puurojen ja muiden viljavalmisteiden sekä kasvisten osuutta ruokavaliossa.

Finravinto 2002 –tutkimuksessa käytetyn 48 tunnin ruoankäyttöhaastattelun luotettavuutta tutkittiin suhteessa viiden päivän ruoankäyttötietoihin. Tulokset osoittivat, että energian ja energiaan suhteutettujen ravintoaineiden saannit olivat samansuuruiset kummallakin menetelmällä mitattuna. Haastatteluun perustunut energian saanti oli 99 % viiden päivän ruoankäyttötietoihin perustuneesta energian saannista molemmilla sukupuolilla. Tuloksena saatu alkoholinkulutus oli aliarvio, koska perjantaipäivät puuttuivat haastatteluista.

Finravinto-tutkimuksen menetelmäuudistukset onnistuivat hyvin. Myös kenttä-tutkimus toteutui teknisesti suunnitelmien mukaan. Ainoastaan osallistumisaktiivisuus (63 % kutsutuista) jäi aikaisempiin väestötutkimuksiin verrattuna pienemmäksi, mikä heikentää jonkin verran tutkimustulosten yleistettävyyttä. Syytä tähän ei löydetä Finravinto-tutkimuksen toteutuksesta vaan todennäköisesti yleisestä tutkimuksiin osallistumisen vähentymisestä esim. ajanpuutteen vuoksi.

Tutkimustulosten perusteella tulee kiinnittää erityistä huomiota miehillä ruokavalion rasvan laatuun sekä täysjyväviljan, kasvisten, hedelmien ja marjojen kulutuksen lisäämiseen. Myös naisten tulokset antavat aihetta kiinnittää huomiota ruokavalion rasvan laatuun, mutta vähintään yhtä painokkaasti hiilihydraattien laatuun. Viljavalmisteiden ja erityisesti täysjyväviljan suosiminen ja sokeripitoisten elintarvikkeiden kulutuksen vähentäminen kohentaisi ennen kaikkea nuorimpien ikäryhmien naisten ruokavaliota. Naisten ruokavalion energian niukkuus asettaa erityisvaatimuksia ruokavalion laadulle. Alkoholin aiheuttamien haittojen ohella, alkoholijuomista tulevan energian merkitykseen väestöryhmien ravitsemuksessa tulisi kiinnittää huomiota. Keski-ikäisten ja sitä vanhempien naisten ruokavalio on edelleen ravitsemuksellisesti laadukkain Suomessa.

Age Groups

The National FINRISK 2002 Study

FINRISKI 2002

Project Leader

Project Leader	Erkki Vartiainen,
Address	National Public Health Institute
	Department of Epidemiology and Health Promotion
	Mannerheimintie 166
	00300 Helsinki
	Finland
Executing Institution	Department of Epidemiology and Health Promotion, National Public Health Institute, Finland
Funding Agency	EU and MDECODE (Molecular Diversity and Epidemiology of COmmon DiseasE) program coordinated by the University of Michigan

Project Information

Start of Project	21/01/2002
End of Project	19/04/2002
Start of Data Collection	21/01/2002
End of Data Collection	19/04/2002
URL	
Scope	National

Keywords

Abstract (English) In Finland, the mortality to cardiovascular diseases was among the highest in the world at the end of the1960s. Since then many preventive activities have been carried out in Finland. One important tool in planning and targeting the preventive activities has been continuous monitoring of diseases and risk factors. The cardiovascular disease risk factor levels have been assessed in five-year intervals in Finland since 1972. The main aim of these surveys is to follow the population risk factors trends to serve health policy and prevention planning.

Population risk factor surveys have been carried out first in Eastern Finland in the North Karelia and Kuopio provinces. Later on the surveys have been carried out also in Southwestern Finland, in the capital area and in Northern Finland. A stratified random sample of population aged from 25 to 64 years has been drawn 22 from the population registers. The sample sizes have varied from 8,000 to 13,500 depending on the survey year.

In 2002, the seventh population risk factor survey, the National FINRISK 2002 Study, was carried out in six areas in Finland (Fig. 1). In addition to age group 25–64 years a subsample from elderly population aged 65–74 was also drawn from three survey areas. The total sample size was 13,500 persons (Annex 1). As in earlier years the survey protocol followed closely the WHO MONICA protocol 1 and the later recommendations of the European Health Risk Monitoring project 2. Six teams, with four trained nurses in each, carried out the survey. Survey included a selfadministered questionnaire and a health check, where anthropometric measurements, blood pressure measurements, and blood sampling was carried out. All blood samples were handled with standardized protocol and sent to KTL for analyses. Serum total cholesterol, HDL-cholesterol, triglycerides, GGT, and CRP were analyzed from all the samples.

In this report, the basic results of the survey and comparisons to earlier surveys have been made. The results are mainly presented to the age group 30–59 years, as it is the common age group for most of the surveys. In addition to this report a comprehensive table annex including tables of all the measurements and questions carried out or asked in the survey 3.

The serum cholesterol levels have decreased significantly in Finland from 1972 to 1997 both among men and women. During the last five years from 1997 to 2002, the decrease has leveled off and the serum cholesterol changed among 30- to 59-year-old men from 5.61 mmol/l to 5.69 mmol/l and among women from 5.45 mmol/l to 5.42 mmol/l. Blood pressure levels have decreased significantly both among men and women from 1972 to 2002. Among men both the systolic and diastolic blood pressure decreased statistically significantly between years 1997 and 2002: SBP from 136 to 135 mmHg and DBP from 85 to 82 mmHg. Among women only diastolic blood pressure decreased statistically significantly from 80 to 77 mmHg. Systolic blood pressure level remained unchanged being 130 mmHg. Smoking rates have decreased significantly among Finnish men from 1972 to 1997. Between 1997 and 2002 smoking rate increased among men from 32 to 36% ($p = 0.01$). Among women the smoking rates have increased slightly until 1992. Between 1992 and 1997, the increase in smoking among women leveled off, but between 1997 and 2002 smoking rate has increased again from 20 to 23%.

The average cardiovascular risk factor level has decreased markedly in Finland until 1997. According to the latest risk factor survey in 2002, the trend in risk factor levels is not as favorable any more. Smoking rates are increasing both among men and women and the remarkable decline seen in cholesterol levels among Finnish population has leveled off. However, blood pressure levels are continuously decreasing both among men and women. These results make a great challenge for future health policy as well as disease prevention and health promotion work in Finland.

Abstract (Original Language) Suomalaisten miesten sepelvaltimotautikuolleisuus on laskenut vuodesta 1973 vuoteen 2001 yli 70 % ja naisten yli 75 % (6). Kuolleisuuden lasku on suurelta osin selitettävissä merkittävimpien riskitekijöiden kuten tupakoinnin, seerumin kolesterolin ja verenpaineen laskulla (7). FINRISKI 2002 -tutkimuksen mukaan suomalaisten merkittävimmissä sydän- ja verisuonitautien riskitekijöissä yli 20 vuotta jatkunut lasku näyttää osittain pysähtyneen, jopa kääntyneen nousuun (8). Sekä miesten että naisten tupakointi on lisääntynyt viimeisen viiden vuoden aikana. Kolesterolitasoissa 1970-luvulta alkanut voimakas lasku näyttää pysähtyneen. Miesten ylipaino on merkittävästi lisääntynyt. Myös naisilla vähäistä lisääntymistä on havaittavissa, mutta nousu ei ole tilastollisesti merkitsevä. Myös alkoholinkäytössä on havaittavissa lisääntymistä varsinkin 1990-luvulta alkaen. Verenpainetasoissa on edelleen nähtävissä suotuisa kehitys. Sekä miesten että naisten verenpainetasot ovat laskeneet myös viimeisen viiden vuoden aikana.

Vuonna 2002 miesten seerumin kolesterolin keskiarvo oli sekä miehillä että naisilla yli suositellun 5,0 mmol/l. Miesten kolesterolin keskiarvo (5,58 mmol/l) oli huomattavasti korkeampi kuin naisten (5,38 mmol/l). Yli 65 %:lla 25–64-vuotiaista tutkituista (miehistä 70 %:lla ja naisista 62 %:lla) seerumin kokonaiskolesteroli oli yli 5,0 mmol/l. Myös verenpainetasot olivat miehillä korkeampia kuin naisilla. Naisten systolisen verenpaineen keskiarvo 25–64-vuotiailla alitti 130 mmHg:n rajan, mutta miehillä keskiarvo oli 134 mmHg. Ylipainoisiakin oli miehistä suurempi osuus kuin naisista. Miesten ruumiinpainoindeksin keskiarvo 25–64-vuotiailla oli 27 kg/m2 ja naisten 25,9 kg/m2. Merkittävästi ylipainoisia (BMI yli 30 kg/m2) oli miehistä 20 % ja naisista 18 %. Tärkeimpien riskitekijöiden tasoissa on havaittavissa selviä alueellisia eroja. Seerumin okonaiskolesterolitasot olivat Lapin läänin miehillä korkeampia kuin muilla tutkimusalueilla. Sekä miesten että naisten verenpainetasot olivat selvästi matalampia Helsingissä ja Vantaalla muihin tutkimusalueisiin verrattuna. Samoin painoindeksi oli matalin Helsingissä ja Vantaalla sekä miehillä että naisilla. Sen sijaan tupakoivia miehiä ja naisia oli eniten Lapin läänissä ja elsingissä ja Vantaalla. Suomalaiset kokevat terveydentilansa jatkuvasti kohentuneen. Oman terveydentilansa erittäin tai melko hyväksi kokevien osuus on kasvanut sekä miehillä että naisilla noin 30 %:sta noin 60 %:iin viimeisen 30 vuoden aikana. Lähes kolmasosa tutkituista oli edellisen vuoden aikana käynyt terveystarkastuksessa terveydenhoitajan tai lääkärin vastaanotolla muusta kuin sairaudesta tai oireista johtuvasta syystä. Myös merkittävimpien kansansairauksiemme löytämiseen ja seurantaan tähtääviin mittauksiin osallistumista raportoitiin kohtuullisen paljon.

Lähes kolmannes tutkittavista ilmoitti olleensa kolesterolimittauksessa edeltäneen vuoden aikana. Verenpainetta oli kuluneen vuoden aikana mitattu lähes 60 %:lta miehistä ja yli 70 %:lta naisista. Fyysisesti raskasta työtä tekevien osuus on laskenut 1990-luvulle saakka. Tämän jälkeen fyysisesti raskasta työtä tekevien osuus ei ole juurikaan muuttunut. Miehistä noin 40 % ja naisista noin 25 % raportoi tekevänsä fyysisesti raskasta työtä. Vapaa-aikana liikuntaa harrastavien osuus on kasvanut vuoteen 1997 saakka, mutta tämän jälkeen kasvu näyttää pysähtyneen. Yli 50 % miehistä ja naisista raportoi harrastavansa liikuntaa vapaa-aikanaan vähintään 2 kertaa viikossa.

Kuten terveydentilansa, kokevat suomalaiset myös fyysisen kuntonsa kohentuneen viimeisten 30 vuoden aikana. Yli 40 % sekä miehistä että naisista raportoi fyysisen kuntonsa erittäin tai melko hyväksi. Terveyden edistämistyön kannalta uudet tulokset ovat varsin haastavia.

Tärkeimmissä riskitekijöissä aiemmin tapahtunut merkittävä lasku on pääasiallisesti pysähtynyt, ylipaino ja alkoholin käyttö näyttää lisääntyneen ja liikuntaakaan ei harrasteta enempää kuin 1990-luvun lopulla. Terveydenhuollossa ollaan jo varsin aktiivisia väestön terveydentilan eurannassa ja riskitekijöiden kartoittamisessa. Resursseja tähän ei varmaankaan helposti voida lisätä. Kuitenkin on ilmeistä, että juuri vaaratekijöihin vaikuttaminen on edullisin ja tehokkain tapa vaikuttaa väestömme terveydentilaan tulevaisuudessa. Voimavarojen uudelleen ohjaaminen ja uusien keinojen kehittäminen terveyden edistämiseksi ja sairauksien ehkäisemiseksi on tulevina vuosina entistäkin tärkeämpää.

Age Groups

25	34
35	44
45	54
55	64
65	74

France

Enquête Nutritionnelle en Population Générale à Mayotte

NutriMay

Project Leader

Project Leader	
Address	Institut de Veille Sanitaire (National
Executing Institution	Institute for Public Health Surveillance)
Funding Agency	

Project Information

Start of Project	20/03/2006
End of Project	30/06/2006
Start of Data Collection	20/03/2006
End of Data Collection	20/03/2006
URL	
Scope	National

Keywords

Abstract (English)

Abstract (Original Language)

Age Groups

1	4
5	14
15	49
50	and older

Etude Nationale Nutrition Santé (National Nutrition and Health Survey)

ENNS

Project Leader

Project Leader	Professor Serge Hercberg
Address	Unité de Surveillance et d'Epidémiologie Nutritionnelle (USEN)
	InVS - Université Paris 13 - Cnam
	Porte 136
	74 rue Marcel Cachin
	93 017 Bobigny cedex
	France
Executing Institution	Institut de Veille Sanitaire (National Institute for Public Health Surveillance)
Funding Agency	Institut de Veille Sanitaire (National Institute for Public Health Surveillance)

Project Information

Start of Project	01/02/2006
End of Project	30/09/2007
Start of Data Collection	12/09/2006
End of Data Collection	12/09/2006
URL	
Scope	National

Keywords

Abstract (English)

Abstract (Original Language)

Age Groups

3	17
18	74

Germany

1. Sächsische Verzehrstudie

1. SVS

Project Leader

Project Leader	
Address	Sächsisches Staatsministerium für Umwelt und Landwirtschaft Archivstraße 1 01075 Dresden
Executing Institution	Sächsisches Staatsministerium für Umwelt und Landwirtschaft
Funding Agency	Sächsisches Staatsministerium für Umwelt und Landwirtschaft

Project Information

Start of Project	01/10/1998
End of Project	31/12/2000
Start of Data Collection	01/04/1999
End of Data Collection	14/12/1999
URL	http://www.sachsen.de/de/bf/staatsregierung/ministerien/index_umwelt.html
Scope	National

Keywords East Germany; Population; Attitude; Nutrition; Behaviour; Food; Saxony; Federal Republic of Germany

Abstract (English) The objective of the 1st Saxon Consumption Study was to collect representative data and information about the actual nutrition and consumption behavior of the Saxon population. This representative cross-sectional study collected data of 1,309 persons living in Saxony aged 4–80 years. The study provides information about problems of under nourishment in the Saxon population, the nutritional status as well as information about attitudes and knowledge about nutrition. The results serve as a basis for a more concrete nutrition and consumer information in Saxony.

Abstract (Original Language) Repräsentative Daten und Informationen über das tatsächliche Ernährungs- und Verzehrverhalten der sächsischen Bevölkerung zu ermitteln, war Ziel der ersten sächsischen Verzehrstudie (SVS). Diese repräsentative Querschnittsstudie, in der 1.309 Personen im Alter von vier bis 80 Jahren aus Sachsen befragt wurden, gibt zudem Aufschluss über Probleme der Fehlernährung in der sächsischen Bevölkerung, den Ernährungszustand sowie über Einstellungen und Wissen zum Thema Ernährung. Die Ergebnisse bilden die Basis zur Konkretisierung einer realitäts- und praxisbezogenen Ernährungs- und Verbraucherinformation in Sachsen.

Age Groups

4	80

1. Telefonischer Gesundheitssurvey

1. GSTel03

Project Leader

Project Leader	Dr. Thomas Ziese
Address	Robert Koch-Institut
	Postfach 65 02 61
	D-13302 Berlin
Executing Institution	Robert Koch-Institut
Funding Agency	Bundesministerium für Gesundheit und Soziale Sicherung

Project Information

Start of Project	01/06/2002
End of Project	30/06/2006
Start of Data Collection	01/09/2002
End of Data Collection	31/03/2003
URL	http://www.rki.de/nn_228130/DE/Content/GBE/Erhebungen/
	Gesundheitssurveys/TelSurvey/Cati03__inhalt.html
Scope	National

Keywords

Abstract (English) The Robert Koch Institute has carried out health surveys at irregular intervals since the 1980s. Telephone surveys now supplement these examination surveys.

The Department of Health Reporting at the Robert Koch Institute conducts nationwide telephone health interview surveys since 2002, sponsored by the Federal Ministry of Health and Social Security. The results, for example on health behavior (smoking, physical exercise, etc.) health perception, and living conditions, are important means for the development of planning processes and to improve the health care system in Germany. Health telephone surveys will also serve as a module of a coming health-monitoring system in Germany, which is currently in discussion.

From September 2002 to March 2003, 8,313 German speaking people randomly selected out of the resident population aged 18 years and over were asked on topics like chronic diseases, health behavior, and the extent to which they make use of health care services and others (GSTel03).

Abstract (Original Language) Im Robert Koch-Institut werden Gesundheitssurveys bereits seit den 80er Jahren durchgeführt. Telefonsurveys gehören als Ergänzung zu diesen Untersuchungs- und Befragungssurveys inzwischen auch international zur Routine.

Die damit verbundene kostengünstige und schnelle Art der Datengewinnung ermöglicht es, gesundheitspolitisch zeitnah und flexibel reagieren zu können. Die telefonischen Gesundheitssurveys stellen einen wichtigen Baustein für das aufzubauende Gesundheitsmonitoring-System in Deutschland dar.

Bundesweite telefonische Gesundheitssurveys werden im Fachgebiet Gesundheitsberichterstattung des Robert Koch-Instituts mit Unterstützung des Bundesministeriums für Gesundheit seit 2002 durchgeführt.

Von September 2002 bis März 2003 wurden erstmals 8.313 Personen aus der deutschsprachigen Wohnbevölkerung ab 18 Jahren u.a. zu Krankheiten, zu ihrem Gesundheitsverhalten und zur Inanspruchnahme von Leistungen des Gesundheitswesens befragt (GSTel03).

Age Groups

18	and older

2. Bayerische Verzehrsstudie

BVS II

Project Leader

Project Leader	Prof. Dr. Georg Karg, Ph.D. / Prof. Dr. Günther Wolfram
Address	Technische Universität München
	Fakultät für Wirtschaftswissenschaften
	Lehrstuhl für Betriebswirtschaftslehre
	- Marketing und Konsumforschung -
	Weihenstephaner Steig 17
	85350 Freising-Weihenstephan
Executing Institution	Technische Universität München (Lehrstuhl für Wirtschaftslehre /
	Hochschuldozentur für Huimanernährung u. Krebsprävention)
Funding Agency	Bayerischen Staatsministeriums für Umwelt, Gesundheit und
	Verbraucherschutz

Project Information

Start of Project	01/12/2001
End of Project	
Start of Data Collection	01/09/2002
End of Data Collection	31/07/2003
URL	http://www.wlh.wi.tum.de/Res/BVS2/
Scope	National

Keywords Federal Republic of Germany; Bavaria; Nutrition; Historical development; Food

Abstract (English) A person's psychosocial environment, behavior, state of nutrition, and health are related in a complex way. This has not been sufficiently investigated until present. One aim of the Second Bavarian Consumption Study is to collect current and representative data of the Bavarian population and their nutrition behaviour as well as to define fundamental determinants and health consequences.

Abstract (Original Language) Die psychosoziale Umwelt einer Person, ihr Verhalten und ihr Ernährungs- und Gesundheitszustand stehen in einer komplexen Beziehung, die bislang unzureichend erforscht ist. Ein Ziel der 2. Bayerischen Verzehrsstudie (BVS II) ist es daher, für die bayerischen Bevölkerung aktuelle und repräsentative Daten zum Ernährungsverhalten zu erhalten und dessen wesentliche Determinanten und gesundheitliche Folgen zu bestimmen.

Age Groups

13	80

2. Sächsische Verzehrstudie

2. SVS

Project Leader

Project Leader	
Address	Sächsische Landesanstalt für Landwirtschaft
	August-Böckstiegel-Straße 1
	01326 Dresden
Executing Institution	Sächsische Landesanstalt für Landwirtschaft (LfL)
Funding Agency	Sächsische Staatsministerium für Umwelt und Landwirtschaft

Project Information

Start of Project	01/04/2004
End of Project	28/02/2006
Start of Data Collection	04/11/2004
End of Data Collection	04/11/2005
URL	http://www.sms.sachsen.de; www.landwirtschaft.sachsen.de/lfl
Scope	National

Keywords

Abstract (English) The main objective of the 2. Saxon Consumption Study (SVS) was to update the data about nutrition and consumption behavior of the Saxony's population. Because of the identic study design, which was also used for the 1. SVS, chances in nutrition and consumption behaviour between the two data collections could be described and analysed.

Abstract (Original Language) Hauptziel der 2. SVS war die Aktualisierung der Datensituation zum Ernährungs- und Verzehrverhalten der sächsischen Bevölkerung. Durch das analoge Studiendesign zur 1. SVS konnten Veränderungen im Ernährungs- und Verzehrverhalten zwischen den Erhebungszeiträumen beschrieben und analysiert werden.

Age Groups

4	80

2. Telefonischer Gesundheitssurvey

GSTel04

Project Leader

Project Leader	Dr. Thomas Ziese
Address	Robert Koch-Institut
	Postfach 65 02 61
	D-13302 Berlin
Executing Institution	Robert Koch-Institut
Funding Agency	Bundesministerium für Gesundheit und Soziale Sicherung

Project Information

Start of Project	01/06/2002
End of Project	30/06/2006
Start of Data Collection	01/10/2003
End of Data Collection	31/03/2004
URL	http://www.rki.de/nn_228130/DE/Content/GBE/Erhebungen/ Gesundheitsurveys/TelSurvey/Cati04__inhalt.html
Scope	National

Keywords

Abstract (English) The Robert Koch Institute has carried out health surveys at irregular intervals since the 1980s. Telephone surveys now supplement these examination surveys.

The Department of Health Reporting at the Robert Koch Institute conducts nationwide telephone health interview surveys since 2002, sponsored by the Federal Ministry of Health and Social Security. The results, for example on health behaviour (smoking, physical exercise, etc.) health perception, and living conditions, are important means for the development of planning processes and to improve the health care system in Germany. Health telephone surveys will also serve as a module of a coming health-monitoring system in Germany, which is currently in discussion.

From September 2002 to March 2003, 8,313 German speaking people randomly selected out of the resident population aged 18 years and over were asked on topics like chronic diseases, health behavior, and the extent to which they make use of health care services and others (GSTel03). In addition 7,341 telephone interviews were conducted in a follow-up survey from September 2003 to March 2004 dealing with further aspects of health and illness or health-related behavior (GSTel04).

Abstract (Original Language) Im Robert Koch-Institut werden Gesundheitssurveys bereits seit den 80er Jahren durchgeführt. Telefonsurveys gehören als Ergänzung zu diesen Untersuchungs- und Befragungssurveys inzwischen auch international zur Routine.

Die damit verbundene kostengünstige und schnelle Art der Datengewinnung ermöglicht es, gesundheitspolitisch zeitnah und flexibel reagieren zu können. Die telefonischen Gesundheitssurveys stellen einen wichtigen Baustein für das aufzubauende Gesundheitsmonitoring-System in Deutschland dar.

Bundesweite telefonische Gesundheitssurveys werden im Fachgebiet Gesundheitsberichterstattung des Robert Koch-Instituts mit Unterstützung des Bundesministeriums für Gesundheit seit 2002 durchgeführt.

Von September 2002 bis März 2003 wurden erstmals 8.313 Personen aus der deutschsprachigen Wohnbevölkerung ab 18 Jahren u.a. zu Krankheiten, zu ihrem Gesundheitsverhalten und zur Inanspruchnahme von Leistungen des Gesundheitswesens befragt (GSTel03). In einer Folgeerhebung (September 2003 bis März 2004) sind weitere 7.341 Telefoninterviews realisiert worden (GSTel04).

Age Groups

18	and older

3. Telefonischer Gesundheitssurvey

GSTel05

Project Leader

Project Leader	Dr. Thomas Ziese
Address	Robert Koch-Institut
	Postfach 65 02 61
	D-13302 Berlin
Executing Institution	Robert Koch-Institut
Funding Agency	Bundesministerium für Gesundheit und Soziale Sicherung

Project Information

Start of Project	01/06/2002
End of Project	30/06/2006
Start of Data Collection	01/11/2004
End of Data Collection	30/04/2005
URL	http://www.rki.de/cln_011/nn_228130/DE/Content/GBE/Erhebungen/
	Gesundheitsurveys/TelSurvey/Cati05__inhalt.html
Scope	National

Keywords Health; Quality of life; Health behavior; Prevention; Disability; Usage; Disease; Information; Behaviour; Attitude; Federal Republic of Germany; Health care; Social report; Perception

Abstract (English) The Robert Koch Institute has carried out health surveys at irregular intervals since the 1980s. Telephone surveys now supplement these examination surveys.

The Department of Health Reporting at the Robert Koch Institute conducts nationwide telephone health interview surveys since 2002, sponsored by the Federal Ministry of Health and Social Security. The results, for example on health behavior (smoking, physical exercise, etc.) health perception, and living conditions, are important means for the development of planning processes and to improve the health care system in Germany. Health telephone surveys will also serve as a module of a coming health-monitoring system in Germany, which is currently in discussion.

From September 2002 to March 2003, 8,313 German speaking people randomly selected out of the resident population aged 18 years and over were asked on topics like chronic diseases, health behavior, and the extent to which they make use of health care services and others (GSTel03). In addition 7,341 telephone interviews were conducted in a follow-up survey from September 2003 to March 2004 dealing with further aspects of health and illness or health-related behaviour (GSTel04). To be able to identify changes in the health status and in health-related behaviour at the level of individuals, for the first time in a survey from October 2004 to April 2005, people are recalled, who took part in the first survey and consented to participate in further surveys (GSTel05).

Abstract (Original Language) Im Robert Koch-Institut werden Gesundheitssurveys bereits seit den 80er Jahren durchgeführt. Telefonsurveys gehören als Ergänzung zu diesen Untersuchungs- und Befragungssurveys inzwischen auch international zur Routine.

Die damit verbundene kostengünstige und schnelle Art der Datengewinnung ermöglicht es, gesundheitspolitisch zeitnah und flexibel reagieren zu können. Die telefonischen Gesundheitssurveys stellen einen wichtigen Baustein für das aufzubauende Gesundheitsmonitoring-System in Deutschland dar.

Bundesweite telefonische Gesundheitssurveys werden im Fachgebiet Gesundheitsberichterstattung des Robert Koch-Instituts mit Unterstützung des Bundesministeriums für Gesundheit seit 2002 durchgeführt.

Von September 2002 bis März 2003 wurden erstmals 8.313 Personen aus der deutschsprachigen Wohnbevölkerung ab 18 Jahren u.a. zu Krankheiten, zu ihrem Gesundheitsverhalten und zur Inanspruchnahme von Leistungen des Gesundheitswesens befragt (GSTel03). In einer Folgeerhebung (September 2003 bis März 2004) sind weitere 7.341 Telefoninterviews realisiert worden (GSTel04). Im Rahmen der dritten Erhebung (Oktober 2004 bis April 2005) fand erstmalig eine Wiederbefragung von Teilnehmern des ersten telefonischen Gesundheitssurveys statt. Insgesamt konnten 4.401 Befragte, die sich damals bereit erklärt hatten an weiteren Interviews teilzunehmen, erneut befragt werden (GSTel05).

Age Groups

Persons aged 18 and older

4. Telefonischer Gesundheitssurvey

GSTel06

Project Leader

Project Leader	Dr. Thomas Ziese
Address	Robert Koch-Institut
	Postfach 65 02 61
	D-13302 Berlin
Executing Institution	Robert Koch-Institut
Funding Agency	Bundesministerium für Gesundheit

Project Information

Start of Project	01/06/2002
End of Project	30/06/2006
Start of Data Collection	01/10/2005
End of Data Collection	31/03/2006
URL	http://www.rki.de/cln_011/nn_228130/DE/Content/GBE/ Erhebungen/Gesundheitsurveys/TelSurvey/telsurvey__ node.html__nnn=true
Scope	National

Keywords

Abstract (English) The Robert Koch Institute has carried out health surveys at irregular intervals since the 1980s. Telephone surveys now supplement these examination surveys.

The Department of Health Reporting at the Robert Koch Institute conducts nationwide telephone health interview surveys since 2002, sponsored by the Federal Ministry of Health and Social Security. The results, for example on health behaviour (smoking, physical exercise, etc.) health perception, and living conditions, are important means for the development of planning processes and to improve the health care system in Germany. Health telephone surveys will also serve as a module of a coming health-monitoring system in Germany, which is currently in discussion.

In the meantime the fourth survey has been finalised. From October 2005 to March 2006, 5,600 interviews were conducted. The emphasis this year lies in the collection of factors which contribute to maintaining health. First results will be available at the end of 2006.

Abstract (Original Language) Im Robert Koch-Institut werden Gesundheitssurveys bereits seit den 80er Jahren durchgeführt. Telefonsurveys gehören als Ergänzung zu diesen Untersuchungs- und Befragungssurveys inzwischen auch international zur Routine.

Age Groups

18	and older

Allgemeine Bevölkerungsumfrage der Sozialwissenschaften

ALLBUS 2004

Project Leader

Project Leader	
Address	Zentrum für Umfragen, Methoden und Analysen (ZUMA)
	Abteilung ALLBUS
	Postfach 12 21 55
	68072 Mannheim
Executing Institution	Zentrum für Umfragen, Methoden und Analysen (ZUMA) und
	Zentralarchiv für empirische Sozialforschung (Köln)
Funding Agency	finanziert von Bund und Ländern über die GESIS (Gesellschaft
	sozialwissenschaftlicher Infrastruktureinrichtungen)

Project Information

Start of Project	01/01/1980
End of Project	
Start of Data Collection	01/03/2004
End of Data Collection	12/07/2004
URL	http://www.gesis.org/Dauerbeobachtung/Allbus/index.htm
Scope	National

Keywords ALLBUS; Federal Republic of Germany; Analytical method; Method; Research design; Research object; Health; Sample; Sampling error; Social inequality; Welfare state; National identity; State; Citizen; Internet; Information technology; Communication technology; Microcensus; Questionnaire

Abstract (English) The research programme ALLBUS (German General Social Survey – Allgemeine Bevölkerungsumfrage der Sozialwissenschaften) is to produce high quality data for the empirical social research and to provide them for public use. Like the other Allbus datasets, the survey 2004 contains information on attitudes, behavior, and social structure in Germany. The emphasis of the 2004 study was "social inequality and welfare state." A large part of the items included consists of the replication of the 1984 and 1994 survey, which had the same emphasis. To supplement the emphasis, the topics *health* and *digital divide* are newly included.

Abstract (Original Language) Das Forschungsprogramm ALLBUS (Allgemeine Bevölkerungsumfrage der Sozialwissenschaften) dient dem Ziel, Daten für die empirische Sozialforschung zu erheben und umgehend allgemein bereitzustellen. Wie jeder ALLBUS enthält auch die Umfrage 2004 Informationen zu Einstellungen, Verhaltensweisen und soziostrukturellen Merkmalen der Bevölkerung in Deutschland. Das Schwerpunktthema der Studie ist 'Soziale

Ungleichheit und Wohlfahrtsstaat'. Ein bedeutender Teil des Frageprogramms besteht dabei aus Replikationen der Erhebungen von 1984 und 1994 zum gleichen Thema. Zur Ergänzung des Schwerpunkts neu aufgenommen werden die Unterthemen 'Gesundheit' und 'Digital Divide'.

Abstract (Original Language)

Age Groups

Persons aged 18 and older

Bayerische Verzehrsstudie

BVS

Project Leader

Project Leader	Prof. Dr. Georg Karg, Ph.D.; Dr.oec.troph. Kurt Gedrich
Address	Technische Universität München
	Fakultät für Wirtschaftswissenschaften
	Lehrstuhl für Betriebswirtschaftslehre
	- Marketing und Konsumforschung -
	Weihenstephaner Steig 17
	85350 Freising-Weihenstephan
Executing Institution	Technische Universität München
Funding Agency	Bayerischen Staatsministerium für Ernährung, Landwirtschaft und Forsten

Project Information

Start of Project	01/07/1994
End of Project	31/01/1998
Start of Data Collection	08/05/1995
End of Data Collection	05/12/1995
URL	http://www.wlh.wi.tum.de/Res/BVS1995/index.html
Scope	National

Keywords Federal Republic of Germany; Bavaria; Nutrition; Historical development; Food

Abstract (English) The objective of the research project was an outline of the nutritional situation in Bavaria in 1995. A comparison of these data and data on Bavaria from the National Consumption Study from 1985 to 1989 was intended to serve as a basis for illustrating the development of the nutritional situation in Bavaria for that particular period.

Abstract (Original Language) Ziel des Forschungsprojektes war zum einen, den Stand der Ernährungssituation in Bayern im Jahr 1995 zu erfassen. Zum anderen sollte im Vergleich mit den Daten des bayerischen Teils der Nationalen Verzehrsstudie (NVS-B) aus den Jahren 1985–1989 versucht werden, die Entwicklung der Ernährungssituation in Bayern in diesem Zeitraum darzustellen.

Age Groups

All members of the chosen households (aged 4 and older) were considered in the survey.

Bayerischer Gesundheitssurvey

Project Leader

Project Leader	
Address	Bayerisches Staatsministerium für Umwelt,
	Gesundheit und Verbraucherschutz
	Rosenkavalierplatz 2
	81925 München
Executing Institution	Bayerisches Staatsministerium für Arbeit und Sozialordnung, Familie,
	Frauen und Gesundheit (jetzt: Bayerisches Staatsministerium für
	Umwelt, Gesundheit und Verbraucherschutz)
Funding Agency	Bayerisches Staatsministerium für Arbeit und Sozialordnung, Familie,
	Frauen und Gesundheit

Project Information

Start of Project	
End of Project	
Start of Data Collection	01/03/1998
End of Data Collection	01/04/1999
URL	http://www.rki.de/cln_006/nn_225376/DE/Content/GBE/
	Erhebungen/Gesundheitsurveys/BGSurveys/Bayern/bayern
	__node.html__nnn=true
Scope	National

Keywords State of health; Population; Empirical research; Bavaria; Federal Republic of Germany; Epidemiology; Health policy; Health; Reporting

Abstract (English) The Bavarian Health Survey (1998/1999) is a new element in the Bavarian health reporting system. It was conducted in close connection with the German Health Survey as a combination of a questionnaire and health examination survey with participation of the Bavarian local health offices. On the basis of a random sample of more than 1,800 persons aged 18–79 years, life-prevalence data on diseases of the metabolic system, selected laboratory results, and obesity are reported.

Abstract (Original Language) Der Bayerische Gesundheitssurvey (1998/1999) dient der Fortentwicklung der Gesundheitsberichterstattung in Bayern. Er wurde in enger Anlehnung an die Methodik des Bundes-Gesundheitssurveys als kombinierter Befragungs- und Untersuchungssurvey unter Einbeziehung der bayerischen Gesundheitsämter durchgeführt. Basierend auf einer Zufallsstichprobe von mehr als 1.800 Personen im Alter von 18 bis 79 Jahren werden Lebenszeitprävalenzen chronischer Erkrankungen, ausgewählte Laborbefunde und Prävalenzen von Übergewicht und Adipositas dargestellt.

Age Groups

18	79

Berliner Studie "Gesundheit im Kindesalter"

GIK II

Project Leader

Project Leader	
Address	Robert Koch-Institut
	Postfach 65 02 61
	D-13302 Berlin
Executing Institution	Robert Koch-Institut
Funding Agency	

Project Information

Start of Project	
End of Project	
Start of Data Collection	01/01/1994
End of Data Collection	01/01/1995
URL	http://www.rki.de/cln_011/nn_228116/DE/Content/GBE/
	Erhebungen/WeitereEpiStudien/GIK/gik__node.html__nnn=true
Scope	National

Keywords

Abstract (English) Is a follow up survey about health behaviour and possible determinants on the basis of a two year long-term study conducted in Berlin (West) and Bremen in 1983–85 (GIK I). A total of 5,292 secondary school and grammar school students from grades 7 to 10 took part in the follow up survey in selected schools in Berlin (east and west).

Abstract (Original Language) Die Berliner Studie "Gesundheit im Kindesalter" ist eine Wiederholungsbefragung zum Gesundheitsverhalten und zu möglichen Einfußfaktoren auf der Grundlage einer 1983–85 in Berlin (West) und Bremen durchgeführten zweijährigen Längschnittstudie (GIK I). An der Wiederholungsbefragung in Berlin nahmen 1994–95 insgesamt 5292 Hauptschüler und Gymnasiasten der 7. – 10. Klassen an ausgewählten Berliner Schulen (Ost und West) teil.

Age Groups

Secondary school and grammar school pupils grades 7–10

Bundes-Gesundheitssurvey 1998 (Kernsurvey)

BGS '98

Project Leader

Project Leader	
Address	Robert Koch-Institut
	Abteilung für Epidemiologie und Gesundheitsberichterstattung
	Seestraße 10
	13353 Berlin
Executing Institution	Robert Koch-Institut
Funding Agency	Bundesministerium für Gesundheit

Project Information

Start of Project	
End of Project	
Start of Data Collection	20/10/1997
End of Data Collection	13/03/1999
URL	http://www.rki.de/cln_028/nn_327954/DE/Content/GBE/Erhebungen/
	Gesundheitsurveys/BGSurveys/bgsurveys__node.html__nnn=true
Scope	National

Keywords State of health; Population; Empirical research; Federal Republic of Germany; Medicine; Diagnostic investigation; Epidemiology; Health; Reporting

Abstract (English) The first German Health Survey, a representative study of the health status of the population in unified Germany, was started in October 1997. In this project, which is being carried out by the Robert Koch Institute on behalf of the Federal Ministry of Health, about 7,124 study participants aged between 18 and 79 are going through a medical check-up and are interviewed as to health-relevant issues. The German National Health Survey consists of a core survey and supplementary modules. These modules are, for the most part, carried out in subsamples of the study population. They partially have been designed and co-financed by cooperating institutions of the RKI. This time, the opportunity given to the individual Lander to increase the size of the sample was realized by Bavaria. This practised principle of a modular structure and cofinancing may be regarded as a model and serve as an example for the cost effective implementation of such extensive health surveys. As a result, the German National Health Examination Survey will yield information enabling the RKI to deliver relevant health reports on a federal level and, therefore, to support decisions in health policy. The demand for representative population-based data will be met by supply of survey data as a file for public use.

Abstract (Original Language) Im Oktober 1997 begann der erste gesamtdeutsche Gesundheitssurvey, eine repräsentative Untersuchung zum Gesundheitszustand der Bevölkerung in Deutschland. Im Rahmen dieses Projekts, das vom Robert Koch-Institut im Auftrag des Bundesministeriums für Gesundheit durchgeführt wurde, konnten 7.124 Personen im Alter von 18 bis 79 Jahren zu gesundheitsrelevanten Themen befragt und einer medizinischen Untersuchung unterzogen werden. Die Datenerhebungen einschließlich der Nachfassaktionen waren im März 1999 abgeschlossen.

Mit den Ergebnissen des Bundes-Gesundheitssurveys werden aktuelle Informationen bereitgestellt, die den gesundheitspolitischen Entscheidungsprozeß unterstützen sollen. Darüber wurde ein Public Use File (BGS98) mit bevölkerungsrepräsentativen Daten des Kernsurveys für die epidemiologische Forschung zur Verfügung gestellt.

Age Groups

18	79

Nutritional and Anthropometric Longitudinally Designed-Study

DONALD-Studie

Project Leader

Project Leader	
Address	Forschungsinstitut für Kinderernährung Dortmund
	Heinstück 11
	D-44225 Dortmund
Executing Institution	Forschungsinstitut für Kinderernährung Dortmund (FKE)
Funding Agency	

Project Information

Start of Project	01/01/1985
End of Project	
Start of Data Collection	
End of Data Collection	
URL	http://www.fke-do.de
Scope	National

Keywords Federal Republic of Germany; Nutrition; Child; Youth; Behavior; Food; Trend; Health

Abstract (English)   The Dortmund Nutritional and Anthropometric Longitudinally Designed (DONALD) Study is an open cohort study. Currently, there are over 700 healthy children and adolescents actively participating in this study. They undergo detailed assessments at regular intervals between infancy and young adulthood, to collect information on dietary behaviour, growth, development, metabolism, and health status.

Abstract (Original Language) DONALD (DOrtmund Nutritional and Anthropometric Longitudinally Designed Study) ist eine offene Kohortenstudie, an der zur Zeit über 700 gesunde Kinder und Jugendliche aktiv teilnehmen. Bei den Kindern werden vom Säuglings- bis ins Erwachsenenalter in regelmäßigen Abständen detaillierte Untersuchungsdaten zum Ernährungsverhalten, Wachstum, Entwicklung, Stoffwechsel und Gesundheitsstatus erhoben.

Age Groups

20	22	Participants were considered in the study from infant age from the 3rd/ 4th month of age till the age of 19 years [female] respectively till the age of 22 [male] (corestudy).

Einkommens- und Verbrauchsstichprobe 1993

EVS 1993

Project Leader

Project Leader	
Address	Statistische Bundesamt
	Gustav-Stresemann Ring 11
	65189 Wiesbaden
Executing Institution	Statistisches Bundesamt
Funding Agency	

Project Information

Start of Project	
End of Project	
Start of Data Collection	01/01/1993
End of Data Collection	31/12/1993
URL	http://www.destatis.de
Scope	National

Keywords Federal Republic of Germany; Household; Official statistics; Sample survey of income and expenditure

Abstract (English) The sample survey of income and expenditure (German abbreviation: EVS) serves as a major basis for the production of official statistics on the standards of living of households in Germany. Among other things, it provides statistical information on the households' income, property, and debt situation as well as on their final consumption expenditure. The survey covers households of all social groups to obtain a representative picture of the living standards of nearly the whole population in Germany.

The detailed results on the households' final consumption expenditure for food, beverages, and tobacco are also used for nutritional research projects and are integrated into the Federal Government's Report on Nutrition.

Abstract (Original Language) Die Einkommens- und Verbrauchsstichprobe (kurz: EVS) ist eine wichtige amtliche Statistik über die Lebensverhältnisse privater Haushalte in Deutschland. Sie liefert u.a. statistische Informationen über die Ausstattung mit Gebrauchsgütern, die Einkommens-, Vermögens- und Schuldensituation sowie die Konsumausgaben privater Haushalte. Einbezogen werden dabei die Haushalte aller sozialen Gruppierungen, so dass die EVS ein repräsentatives Bild der Lebenssituation nahezu der Gesamtbevölkerung in Deutschland zeichnet.

Die detaillierten Ergebnisse über die Konsumausgaben für Nahrungsmittel, Getränke und Tabakwaren werden u.a. zu ernährungswissenschaftlichen Forschungsvorhaben herangezogen und fließen in den Ernährungsbericht der Bundesregierung mit ein.

Age Groups

4	6
7	9
10	12
13	14
15	18
19	24
25	50
51	64
65	999

Einkommens- und Verbrauchsstichprobe 1998

EVS 1998

Project Leader

Project Leader	
Address	Statistische Bundesamt
	Gustav-Stresemann Ring 11
	65189 Wiesbaden
Executing Institution	Statistisches Bundesamt
Funding Agency	

Project Information

Start of Project	01/09/1996
End of Project	31/08/2000
Start of Data Collection	01/01/1998
End of Data Collection	31/12/1998
URL	http://www.destatis.de
Scope	National

Keywords Federal Republic of Germany; Household; Official statistics; Sample survey of income and expenditure

Abstract (English) The sample survey of income and expenditure (German abbreviation: EVS) serves as a major basis for the production of official statistics on the standards of living of households in Germany. Among other things, it provides statistical information on the households' income, property, and debt situation as well as on their final consumption expenditure. The survey covers households of all social groups to obtain a representative picture of the living standards of nearly the whole population in Germany.

The detailed results on the households' final consumption expenditure for food, beverages, and tobacco are also used for nutritional research projects and are integrated into the Federal Government's Report on Nutrition.

Abstract (Original Language) Die Einkommens- und Verbrauchsstichprobe (kurz: EVS) ist eine wichtige amtliche Statistik über die Lebensverhältnisse privater Haushalte in Deutschland. Sie liefert u.a. statistische Informationen über die Ausstattung mit Gebrauchsgütern, die Einkommens-, Vermögens- und Schuldensituation sowie die Konsumausgaben privater Haushalte. Einbezogen werden dabei die Haushalte aller sozialen Gruppierungen, so dass die EVS ein repräsentatives Bild der Lebenssituation nahezu der Gesamtbevölkerung in Deutschland zeichnet.

Die detaillierten Ergebnisse über die Konsumausgaben für Nahrungsmittel, Getränke und Tabakwaren werden u.a. zu ernährungswissenschaftlichen Forschungsvorhaben herangezogen und fließen in den Ernährungsbericht der Bundesregierung mit ein.

Age Groups

4	6
7	9
10	12
13	14
15	18
19	24
25	50
51	64
65	and older

Einkommens- und Verbrauchsstichprobe 2003

EVS 2003

Project Leader

Project Leader	
Address	Statistische Bundesamt
	Gustav-Stresemann Ring 11
	65189 Wiesbaden
Executing Institution	Statistisches Bundesamt
Funding Agency	

Project Information

Start of Project	01/10/2001
End of Project	30/06/2005
Start of Data Collection	01/01/2003
End of Data Collection	31/12/2003
URL	http://www.destatis.de
Scope	National

Keywords Federal Republic of Germany; Household; Official statistics; Sample survey of income and expenditure

Abstract (English) The sample survey of income and expenditure (German abbreviation: EVS) serves as a major basis for the production of official statistics on the standards of living of households in Germany. Among other things, it provides statistical information on the households' income, property, and debt situation as well as on their final consumption expenditure. The survey covers households of all social groups to obtain a representative picture of the living standards of nearly the whole population in Germany.

The detailed results on the households' final consumption expenditure for food, beverages, and tobacco are also used for nutritional research projects and are integrated into the Federal Government's Report on Nutrition.

Abstract (Original Language) Die Einkommens- und Verbrauchsstichprobe (kurz: EVS) ist eine wichtige amtliche Statistik über die Lebensverhältnisse privater Haushalte in Deutschland. Sie liefert u.a. statistische Informationen über die Ausstattung mit Gebrauchsgütern, die Einkommens-, Vermögens- und Schuldensituation sowie die Konsumausgaben privater Haushalte. Einbezogen werden dabei die Haushalte aller sozialen Gruppierungen, so dass die EVS ein repräsentatives Bild der Lebenssituation nahezu der Gesamtbevölkerung in Deutschland zeichnet.

Die detaillierten Ergebnisse über die Konsumausgaben für Nahrungsmittel, Getränke und Tabakwaren werden u.a. zu ernährungswissenschaftlichen Forschungsvorhaben herangezogen und fließen in den Ernährungsbericht der Bundesregierung mit ein.

Age Groups

4	6
7	9
10	12
13	14
15	18
19	24
25	50
51	64
65	and older

Ernährungsbericht 1992

Project Leader

Project Leader	Dr. Eva Leschick Bonnet
Address	Deutsche Gesellschaft für Ernährung e. V.
	Godesberger Allee 18
	53175 Bonn
Executing Institution	Deutsche Gesellschaft für Ernährung e.V. (DGE)
Funding Agency	Bundesministerium für Gesundheit; Bundesministerium
	für Ernährung, Landwirtschaft und Forsten

Project Information

Start of Project	
End of Project	
Start of Data Collection	
End of Data Collection	
URL	http://www.dge.de/
Scope	National

Keywords Nutrition survey

Abstract (English) In 1968, the government of the Federal Republic of Germany (FRG) commissioned the German Nutrition Society (DGE) to prepare a report concerning the nutritional status of the German population. This Nutrition Report was well received when it was submitted in June of 1969 because for the first time it provided a wide-ranging overview of data that were available about nutrition in the FRG. As a result the government decided to commission the DGE to prepare a comparable report every 4 years. In addition to an analysis of the nutritional situation in the FRG, the Nutrition Reports from 1972 to 2000 contained reviews of important aspects covering current topics in nutrition. The Nutrition Reports provoked considerable interest both within and outside Germany. From 1984 onwards, summaries of the Nutrition Reports have therefore been translated into English.

The 1992 Report dealt with:

- Development of the nutritional situation in Germany
- Toxicological and microbiological aspects of nutrition
- Selected socio-cultural influences on the nutritional behavior
- Food allergies and food intolerance reactions
- Tumorigenesis – inhibiting and promoting effects of nutritional factors
- Iodine supply and iodine deficiency prophylaxis in Germany

Abstract (Original Language) Der vorgelegte Ernährungsbericht reflektiert die Ernährungssituation in der Bundesrepublik Deutschland. Er soll Grundlage sein für alle, die in der Gesellschaft, im Gesundheitssystem, in Politik und Wirtschaft eine Verantwortung für die Ernährung übernommen haben. Der Bericht reflektiert aber auch Einstellungen und Sorgen der Bevölkerung, die sich auf Ernährungsfragen beziehen. Möge es auf dieser Grundlage gelingen, die Ernährungssituation positiv zu verändern, damit die Bürger mehr Lebensqualität erleben, bis ins hohe Alter weniger an ernährungsabhängigen Krankheiten leiden und ohne übertriebene Skepsis und Bedenken ihr Essverhalten an den Maßstäben einer vollwertigen Ernährung orientieren können.

Aus dem Inhalt:

1. Entwicklung der Ernährungssituation in der Bundesrepublik Deutschland
2. Toxikologische und mikrobiologische Aspekte der Ernährung
3. Ausgewählte sozio-kulturelle Einflüsse auf das Ernährungsverhalten
4. Lebensmittelallergien und -intoleranzreaktionen
5. Tumorentstehung - hemmende und fördernde Ernährungsfaktoren
6. Jodversorgung und Jodmangelprophylaxe in der Bundesrepublik Deutschland

Age Groups

Depending on different studies/data sources used

Ernährungsbericht 1996

Project Leader

Project Leader	Dr. Eva Leschik Bonnet
Address	Deutsche Gesellschaft für Ernährung e. V.
	Godesberger Allee 18
	53175 Bonn
Executing Institution	Deutsche Gesellschaft für Ernährung e.V. (DGE)
Funding Agency	Bundesministerium für Gesundheit; Bundesministerium
	für Ernährung, Landwirtschaft und Forsten

Project Information

Start of Project	
End of Project	
Start of Data Collection	
End of Data Collection	
URL	http://www.dge.de/
Scope	National

Keywords Nutrition survey

Abstract (English) In 1968, the government of the Federal Republic of Germany (FRG) commissioned the German Nutrition Society (DGE) to prepare a report concerning the nutritional status of the German population. This Nutrition Report was well received when it was submitted in June of 1969 because for the first time it provided a wide-ranging overview of data that were available about nutrition in the FRG. As a result the government decided to commission the DGE to prepare a comparable report every 4 years. In addition to an analysis of the nutritional situation in the FRG the Nutrition Reports from 1972 to 2000 contained reviews of important aspects covering current topics in nutrition. The Nutrition Reports provoked considerable interest both within and outside Germany. From 1984 on, summaries of the Nutrition Reports have therefore been translated into English.

The Nutrition Report 1996 dealt with:

- The nutritional situation in Germany
- Institutional feeding in the new Federal Länder (former German Democratic Republic)
- Iodine deficiency prophylaxis in Germany
- Toxicological aspects of nutrition
- Microbiological aspects of nutrition
- Tumorigenesis – inhibiting and promoting effects of nutritional factors
- Significance of phytochemicals for health

- Malnutrition of geriatric patients
- Novel food
- Information provided on food labels as a factor influencing food choice

Abstract (Original Language) Der Ernährungsbericht 1996 stützt sich wieder auf die Ergebnisse mehrerer Forschungsaufträge, die von den Bundesministerien für Gesundheit sowie Ernährung, Landwirtschaft und Forsten gefördert wurden. Mehrere Autoren und Arbeitsgruppen haben durch ihre Forschungsarbeiten und Diskussionsbeiträge zum Gelingen dieses Berichts beigetragen.

Aus dem Inhalt:

I. Zur Entwicklung der Ernährungslage in der Bundesrepublik Deutschland

   1. Ernährungssituation in der Bundesrepublik Deutschland
   2. Entwicklung der Gemeinschaftsverpflegung in den neuen Bundesländern
   3. Jodmangelprophylaxe in der Bundesrepublik Deutschland

II. Zu Risiken und Nutzanwendungen in der Ernährung

   4. Toxikologische Aspekte der Ernährung
   5. Mikrobiologische Aspekte der Ernährung
   6. Tumorentstehung - hemmende und fördernde Ernährungsfaktoren
   7. Gesundheitliche Bedeutung sekundärer Pflanzenstoffe
   8. Mangelernährung geriatrischer Patienten
   9. Neuartige Lebensmittel
  10. Informationsnutzen der Lebensmittelkennzeichnung für deutsche Konsumenten als Entscheidungs-hilfe bei der Lebensmittelauswahl

Age Groups

Depending on different studies/data sources used

Ernährungsbericht 2000

Project Leader

Project Leader	Dr. Eva Leschik Bonnet
Address	Deutsche Gesellschaft für Ernährung e. V.
	Godesberger Allee 18
	53175 Bonn
Executing Institution	Deutsche Gesellschaft für Ernährung e.V. (DGE)
Funding Agency	Bundesministerium für Gesundheit; Bundesministerium
	vfür Ernährung, Landwirtschaft und Forsten

Project Information

Start of Project	
End of Project	
Start of Data Collection	
End of Data Collection	
URL	http://www.dge.de/
Scope	National

Keywords Nutrition survey

Abstract (English) The government of the Federal Republic of Germany commissioned the German Nutrition Society (DGE) in 1968 to prepare a report concerning the nutritional status of the German population. This Nutrition Report was well received when it was submitted in June of 1969, because for the first time it provided an overview of a wide range of data that was available about nutrition in Germany. As a result the government decided to commission the DGE to prepare a comparable report every 4 years. In addition to an analysis of the nutritional situation in the FRG the Nutrition Reports from 1972 to 2000 contained reviews of important aspects covering current topics in nutrition. The Nutrition Reports provoked considerable interest both within and outside Germany. From 1984 on, summaries of the Nutrition Reports have therefore been translated into English.

The Nutrition Report 2000 contains 10 chapters:

- The nutritional situation in Germany
- Breast-feeding and infant nutrition in Germany
- The nutritional situation in day care centers: the Day Care Centers-Nutritional-Situation-Study
- Eating habits and nutritional situation of children and adolescents
- Nutrition of elderly persons
- Toxicological aspects of nutrition
- Microbiological aspects of nutrition
- Technological aspects of food processing
- Influence of nutrition on the intestinal flora
- Prophylaxis of diseases with wholesome nutrition.

Abstract (Original Language)   Die Ernährungsberichte der Deutschen Gesellschaft für Ernährung (DGE), herausgegeben im Auftrag des Bundesministeriums für Gesundheit sowie des Bundesministeriums für Ernährung, Landwirtschaft und Forsten, haben inzwischen eine über 30-jährige Tradition. Der 1. Bericht erschien 1969 und in diesem Jahr wird nun der 9. Bericht vorgelegt. Alle 4 Jahre erfolgt mit dem Ernährungsbericht eine Darstellung verschiedener ernährungsrelevanter Themen sowie die Aufzeichnung der Ernährungssituation der Bevölkerung, um Ernährungsrisiken, aber auch positive Veränderungen aufzuzeigen. Zusammen mit den ebenfalls neu erstellten Referenzwerten für die Nährstoffzufuhr können außerdem Mittlerkräfte – ob im Bildungsbereich, in öffentlich geförderten Institutionen, in der Beratung, in den Medien oder in der Wirtschaft – qualifiziert aufklärend, informierend oder gezielt beratend tätig werden.

Der neunte Ernährungsbericht der DGE befasst sich in 10 Kapiteln mit folgenden Themen:

Teil I: Zur Entwicklung der Ernährungslage in Deutschland

1. Ernährungssituation in Deutschland
2. Stillen und Säuglingsernährung in Deutschland - die "SuSe-Studie"
3. Ernährungssituation in Kindertagesstätten: Die Kindertagesstätten-Ernährungs-Situations-Studie "KESS"
4. Essverhalten und Ernährungszustand von Kindern und Jugendlichen - eine Repräsentativerhebung in Deutschland
5. Ernährung älterer Menschen

Teil II: Zu Risiken und Nutzanwendungen in der Ernährung

6. Toxikologische Aspekte der Ernährung
7. Mikrobiologische Aspekte der Ernährung
8. Aspekte der Lebensmittelverarbeitung
9. Beeinflussung der Darmflora durch Ernährung
10. Krankheitsprophylaxe mit vollwertiger Ernährung

Age Groups

Depending on different studies/data sources used

Ernährungsbericht 2004

Project Leader

Project Leader	Dr. Eva Leschik Bonnet
Address	Deutsche Gesellschaft für Ernährung e. V.
	Godesberger Allee 18
	53175 Bonn
Executing Institution	Deutsche Gesellschaft für Ernährung e.V. (DGE)
Funding Agency	Bundesministerium für Verbraucherschutz,
	Ernährung und Landwirtschaft

Project Information

Start of Project	
End of Project	
Start of Data Collection	
End of Data Collection	
URL	http://www.dge.de/
Scope	National

Keywords Nutrition survey

Abstract (English) The government of the Federal Republic of Germany commissioned the German Nutrition Society (DGE) in 1968 to prepare a report concerning the nutritional status of the German population. This Nutrition Report was well received when it was submitted in June of 1969, because for the first time it provided an overview of a wide range of data that was available about nutrition in Germany. As a result the government decided to commission the DGE to prepare a comparable report every 4 years. The Nutrition Reports provoked considerable interest both within and outside Germany. From 1984 on, summaries of the Nutrition Reports have therefore been translated into English.

The Nutrition Report 2004 dealt with:

- Nutritional situation in Germany
- Toxicological aspects of nutrition
- Microbiological aspects of nutrition
- Vitamin and mineral content of vegetable food
- Tumorigenesis – inhibiting and promoting nutritional factors
- Nutritional influence on the intestinal flora
- Influence of phytochemicals on health
- Representation and effect of nutritional information on television
- Enrichment of food and new products

Abstract (Original Language) Die in Abständen von 4 Jahren veröffentlichten Ernährungsberichte bieten jeweils aktuelle Daten aus Erhebungen zur Ernährungssituation und werden durch Übersichten, Analysen und Berichte von Studien zu aktuellen Problemen der Ernährung ergänzt und durch deren Bewertungen abgerundet. Diese Inhalte sind auf zwei Abschnitte verteilt:

I. Zur Entwicklung der Ernährungslage in Deutschland

   1. Ernährungssituation in Deutschland

II. Zu Risiken und Nutzanwendungen in der Ernährung

   2. Toxikologische Aspekte der Ernährung
   3. Mikrobiologische Aspekte der Ernährung
   4. Vitamin- und Mineralstoffgehalt pflanzlicher Lebensmittel
   5. Tumorentstehung - hemmende und fördernde Ernährungsfaktoren
   6. Beeinflussung der Darmflora durch Ernährung
   7. Einfluss sekundärer Pflanzenstoffe auf die Gesundheit
   8. Darstellung und Wirkung von Ernährungsinformationen im Fernsehen
   9. Anreicherung von Lebensmitteln und neue Produktkonzeptionen

Age Groups

Depending on different data sources used

Ernährungsstudie als KiGGS-Modul

EsKiMo

Project Leader

Project Leader	
Address	Robert Koch-Institut
	Postfach 65 02 61
	D-13302 Berlin
	Universität Paderborn
	Fakultät für Naturwissenschaften
	Department Sport und Gesundheit
	Ernährung und Verbraucherbildung
	Warburger Str. 100
	D-33098 Paderborn
Executing Institution	Robert Koch-Institut in Zusammenarbeit
	mit der Universität Paderborn, Fachgruppe
	für Ernährung und Verbraucherbildung
Funding Agency	Bundesministerium für Ernährung, Landwirtschaft
	und Verbraucherschutz

Project Information

Start of Project	01/01/2003
End of Project	31/12/2006
Start of Data Collection	01/01/2006
End of Data Collection	31/12/2006
URL	http://www.rki.de/cln_012/nn_744100/
	DE/Content/GBE/Erhebungen/
	Gesundheitsurveys/Eskimo/
	eskimo__node.html__nnn=true
Scope	National

Keywords

Abstract (English) EsKiMo is a study that investigates nutrition of children and adolescents in Germany. The study was commissioned by the Federal Ministry of Food, Agriculture, and Consumer Protection to gather information about children's intake of food and drinks. These details are important as the offer of available food has been extended over the last years, and children's nutrition habits have changed accordingly.

Abstract (Original Language) EsKiMo ist eine Studie, die die Ernährung von Kindern und Jugendlichen in Deutschland untersucht. Das Bundesministerium für Ernährung, Landwirtschaft und Verbraucherschutz hat diese Studie in Auftrag gegeben, um Erkenntnisse darüber zu gewinnen, was Kinder essen und trinken. Diese Informationen sind wichtig, weil sich in den letzten Jahren das Lebensmittelangebot ständig erweitert hat und Kinder dementsprechend anders essen als noch vor einigen Jahren.

Age Groups

6	17

Ernährungssurvey 1998 als Modul des Bundes-Gesundheitssurveys

Ernährungssurvey 1998

Project Leader

Project Leader	
Address	Robert Koch-Institut
	Abteilung für Epidemiologie
	und Gesundheitsberichterstattung
	Seestraße 10
	13353 Berlin
Executing Institution	Robert Koch-Institut
Funding Agency	

Project Information

Start of Project	
End of Project	
Start of Data Collection	03/11/1997
End of Data Collection	13/03/1999
URL	http://www.rki.de/cln_028/
	nn_327954/DE/Content/
	GBE/Erhebungen/Gesundheitsurveys/
	BGSurveys/Ernaehrungsmodul/
	ernaehrungsmodul__node.html__nnn=true
Scope	National

Keywords Health; Nutrition questions; Survey; Computer; Programme; Comparison; FRG; East Germany

Abstract (English) Nutrition plays an important role in the genesis and course of many civilisation diseases. Latest representative data on nutrition behavior in Germany base on surveys that were already conducted at the end of the 1980s. This does not allow for valid statements on the current nutritional status. Therefore, in a subsample of the German Health Survey, 4,000 persons were asked in detail about their nutrition behavior in the last four weeks. The collected data are valuable for analyses on different aggregation levels (nutrients, foods, etc.) and could be connected with the health data of the main survey.

Abstract (Original Language) Die Ernährung spielt eine wichtige Rolle bei Entstehung und Verlauf vieler Zivilisationskrankheiten. Die aktuellsten repräsentativen Daten zum Ernährungsverhalten in Deutschland basieren auf Untersuchungen, die bereits Mitte bis Ende der 80er Jahre durchgeführt wurden. Valide Aussagen zum derzeitigen Ernährungszustand sind auf dieser Grundlage nicht möglich. Deshalb wird in einer Unterstichprobe des Bundes-Gesundheitssurveys von insgesamt 4000

Personen das Ernährungsverhalten der vergangenen 4 Wochen ausführlich erfragt. Dies geschieht mit der eigens entwickelten Computer-Software "DISHES 98", die die Ernährung nach der Dietary-History-Methode erfasst. Parallel hierzu läuft eine Validierungsstudie mit 150 Personen, in der die Dietary-History-Methode sowohl mit 3-Tage-Ernährungsprotokollen als auch mit 24-Stunden-Recalls verglichen wird. Die erhobenen Daten sind geeignet für Auswertungen auf verschiedenen Aggregationsebenen (Nährstoffe, Lebensmittel etc.) und können mit den Gesundheitsdaten des Hauptsurveys in Verbindung gebracht werden.

Age Groups

18	79

Ernährungsverhalten außer Haus

EVA 1998

Project Leader

Project Leader	Prof. Dr. Georg Karg
Address	Technische Universität München
	Fakultät für Wirtschaftswissenschaften
	Lehrstuhl für Betriebswirtschaftslehre
	- Marketing und Konsumforschung -
	Weihenstephaner Steig 17
	85350 Freising-Weihenstephan
Executing Institution	Technische Universität München, Fak. für
	Wirtschaftswissenschaften, Lehrstuhl für
	Wirtschaftslehre des Haushalts,
	Konsumforschung und Verbraucherpolitik
Funding Agency	Bundesministerium für Gesundheit und Soziale Sicherung

Project Information

Start of Project	01/11/1996
End of Project	01/03/1999
Start of Data Collection	01/01/1998
End of Data Collection	31/12/1998
URL	http://www.wzw.tum.de/wdh
Scope	National

Keywords Federal Republic of Germany; Nutrition; Behaviour

Abstract (English) To evaluate the situation of food supply away-from-home in Germany, a representative survey "Nutritional habits away-from-home" was carried out in 1998. Food supply away-from-home consumption was defined as foods and beverages that are consumed outside the own home, but not taken along from home.

For the EVA-Study 3,000 participants at the minimum age of 15 years were recruited from a citizen register with the help of a two-stage sampling and were asked about their away-from-home consumption. A short questionnaire and a one-day open nutrition record were applied.

Abstract (Original Language) Zur Situation des Außer-Haus-Verzehrs in Deutschland wurde 1998 eine repräsentative Verzehrserhebung "Ernährungsverhalten außer Haus" (EVA) durchgeführt. Dabei wurde als Außer-Haus-Verzehr definiert, was jeweils außerhalb der eigenen Wohnung gegessen und/oder getrunken, aber nicht von zu Hause mitgenommen wird. Für die EVA-Studie wurden nach einem 2-stufigen Stichprobenverfahren ca. 3.000 Personen ab einem Alter von 15 Jahren aus den Einwohnermelderegistern ausgewählt und zu ihrem Außer-Haus-Verzehr befragt. Als Erhebungsinstrumente kamen ein Kurzfragebogen und ein 1-tägiges offenes Ernährungsprotokoll zum Einsatz.

Age Groups

15   and older

Gesundheit in Deutschland

Gesundheitsbericht 2006

Project Leader

Project Leader	Cornelia Lange (RKI)
Address	Robert Koch-Institut
	Nordufer 20
	13353 Berlin
Executing Institution	Robert Koch-Institut in
	Zusammenarbeit mit dem
	Statistischen Bundesamt
Funding Agency	Bundesministerium für Gesundheit

Project Information

Start of Project	
End of Project	
Start of Data Collection	
End of Data Collection	
URL	http://www.gbe-bund.de/
Scope	National

Keywords

Abstract (English) Life expectancy is rising and the general health situation is good, but the number of people who smoke, are too fat, take too little exercise and/or drink too much alcohol is still too high. These are the main conclusions of the health report entitled "Health in Germany," which has just been published as part of Federal Health Reporting (GBE) by the Robert Koch Institute on behalf of the Federal Ministry of Health. In six chapters and 220 pages, it provides an easy-to-read overview of the population's health and Germany's health service, and records developments over the last ten years: How good is our health? What are the factors affecting health? What is the health service doing in the fields of prevention and health promotion? How have supply and demand in healthcare changed? How much do we spend on our health? How can patients obtain information and take part in decisions?

The generally positive health trends over the last few years are being qualified by demographic change. The incidence of many diseases increases with age: this applies not only to cancer, but also illnesses such as diabetes mellitus, osteoporosis, stroke, and dementia. Hence, on the one hand, Germans can expect a long life spent for the most part in good health; on the other hand, the increasing number of older people with chronic diseases will need good treatment and care in the future. The aging of society is, therefore, one of the health system's greatest challenges.

Abstract (Original Language) Steigende Lebenserwartung und gute Gesundheit, aber: immer noch zu viele Menschen rauchen, sind zu dick, bewegen sich zu wenig und trinken zu viel Alkohol. Das sind die Kernaussagen des

Gesundheitsberichts "Gesundheit in Deutschland", den das Robert Koch-Institut im Auftrag des Bundesministeriums für Gesundheit jetzt im Rahmen der Gesundheitsberichterstattung des Bundes (GBE) veröffentlicht hat. Sechs Kapitel auf insgesamt 220 Seiten bieten einen allgemeinverständlichen Überblick über die gesundheitliche Situation der Bevölkerung und das Gesundheitswesen in Deutschland und zeichnen Entwicklungen der letzten zehn Jahre auf: Wie steht es um unsere Gesundheit, welche Faktoren beeinflussen die Gesundheit, was leistet das Gesundheitswesen für Prävention und Gesundheitsförderung, wie haben sich Angebot und Inanspruchnahme in der Gesundheitsvorsorgung verändert, wie viel geben wir für unsere Gesundheit aus, wie können sich Patientinnen und Patienten informieren und an Entscheidungen beteiligen? Die wesentlichen Datenquellen, auf die sich der Bericht stützt, werden online im Gesundheitsinformationssystem der Gesundheitsberichterstattung (http://www.gbe-bund.de) für ergänzende Analysen und Recherchen zur Verfügung gestellt.

Die insgesamt positiven Gesundheitstrends der letzten Jahre relativieren sich aber durch den demografischen Wandel. Nicht allein Krebserkrankungen, sondern auch Leiden wie Diabetes mellitus, Osteoporose, Schlaganfall und Demenz nehmen mit steigendem Lebensalter zu. So können die Deutschen zwar mit einem langen – und über lange Zeit in Gesundheit verbrachten – Leben rechnen. Gleichzeitig aber werden zukünftig immer mehr ältere Menschen mit chronischen Krankheiten eine gute Behandlung und Pflege benötigen. Die Alterung der Gesellschaft ist daher eine der größten Herausforderungen des Gesundheitssystems.

Age Groups

Depending on different data sources used

Gesundheitsbericht für Deutschland

Gesundheitsbericht 1998

Project Leader

Project Leader	Ulrich Hoffmann
Address	Statistisches Bundesamt
	Gustav-Stresemann-Ring 11
	65189 Wiesbaden
Executing Institution	Statistisches Bundesamt
Funding Agency	Bundesministerium für Bildung,
	Wissenschaft, Forschung und Technologie;
	Bundesministerium für Gesundheit

Project Information

Start of Project	01/01/1994
End of Project	01/12/1998
Start of Data Collection	
End of Data Collection	
URL	http://www.gbe-bund.de/
Scope	National

Keywords Germany ; Health reporting; History 1980–1995

Abstract (English) This Health Report presents the first overall picture of the complex health care system that has developed in Germany. The focus is on major trends, current problems, and connections. Anyone interested may consult the Health Report for a wealth of information, which otherwise is dispersed over many different sources and in many cases is difficult to access. These data concern 100 subject fields, any one of which has been condensed into just a few pages. At the same time, the Report is a reference book especially for those who, for professional or personal reasons, wish to acquire information on specific aspects of the health care system. This is why the individual contributions are not intended as technical reports that would be comprehensible to experts only; instead, emphasis is placed on presenting the information in the overall context of our health care system.

Contents:

1. Health Monitoring: Objectives and Operation
2. Framework Conditions of the Health Care System
3. Health Status
4. Behavioral and Risk Aspects of Health
5. Diseases
6. Resources of the Health Care System
7. Production and Consumption of Health Care Services
8. Expenditures for and Costs and Financing of Health Care

Abstract (Original Language) Der Gesundheitsbericht zeichnet erstmals ein Gesamtbild des in Deutschland gewachsenen komplexen Gesundheitswesens. Die wichtigsten Entwicklungen, aktuellen Problemlagen und Zusammenhänge stehen im Mittelpunkt der Betrachtung. Der Gesundheitsbericht bietet der interessierten Öffentlichkeit in mehr als 100 Themenfeldern – jeweils auf wenigen Seiten komprimiert – eine Fülle von Informationen, die sonst nur verstreut vorliegen und oft schwer zugänglich sind. Der Bericht ist zugleich Nachschlagewerk insbesondere für diejenigen, die sich aus beruflichen oder privaten Gründen vorab über Teilaspekte des Gesundheitswesens informieren möchten. Deshalb wollen die Einzelbeiträge keine nur noch Spezialisten verständlichen Berichte sein, sondern legen jeweils Wert auf eine Darstellung im Gesamtzusammenhang unseres Gesundheitssystems.

Inhaltsverzeichnis:

Age Groups

Depending on different data sources used

Gesundheitssurvey Ost

OW 91

Project Leader

Project Leader	
Address	Robert Koch-Institut
	Postfach 65 02 61
	D-13302 Berlin
Executing Institution	Robert Koch-Institut
Funding Agency	Bundesministerium für Gesundheit

Project Information

Start of Project	
End of Project	
Start of Data Collection	01/09/1991
End of Data Collection	30/06/1992
URL	http://www.rki.de/cln_011/
	nn_228118/DE/Content/GBE/
	Erhebungen/Gesundheitsurveys/
	SurveyOst/surveyost_node.html_nnn=true
Scope	National

Keywords

Abstract (English) The Health Survey East was conducted at almost the same time as the third wave of the National Health Surveys in 1991/1992. The outcomes of the first standardized data collection in East Germany closed gaps in research and information on state of health in the New Laender. The Health Survey East additionally provided a basis for a comparison with the Old Laender and the harmonisation of health care in both parts of Germany. It laid at the same time, the foundation for health monitoring, i.e., the long-term monitoring of developments in the state of health. Within the frame of the Health Survey East an Environmental Survey of the Federal Environmental Agency was also conducted.

Abstract (Original Language) Der Gesundheitssurvey Ost wurde etwa zeitgleich mit dem 3. Durchgang des Nationalen Untersuchungssurveys (NUST2) in den Jahren 1991/1992 durchgeführt. Mit dieser ersten standardisierten Erhebung im Ostteil Deutschlands wurden Erkenntnislücken über den Gesundheitszustand in den neuen Bundesländern geschlossen, ein Vergleich mit den alten Bundesländern ermöglicht und eine wesentliche Voraussetzung zur Angleichung der gesundheitlichen Versorgung in beiden Teilen Deutschlands geschaffen. Gleichzeitig entstand damit eine Basis für ein

Gesundheitsmonitoring, d.h. die längerfristige Überwachung der Entwicklung des Gesundheitszustandes.

Im Rahmen des Gesundheitssurvey Ost wurde ein Umweltsurvey des Umweltbundesamtes (Teilstichprobe) durchgeführt.

Age Groups

18	79

Gießener Senioren Langzeitstudie

GISELA

Project Leader

Project Leader	Prof. Dr. Monika Neuhäuser-Berthold
Address	Justus-Liebig-Universität Gießen
	Institut für Ernährungswissenschaft
	Professur Ernährung des Menschen
	Goethestrasse 55
	35390 Gießen
Executing Institution	Justus-Liebig-Universität Gießen, Institut für Ernährungswissenschaft, Professur Ernährung des Menschen
Funding Agency	

Project Information

Start of Project	01/01/1994
End of Project	
Start of Data Collection	
End of Data Collection	
URL	http://www.uni-giessen.de/ fbr09/human-nutrition/
Scope	National

Keywords Nutrition and health status throughout ageing; References for nutrient intake in elderly

Abstract (English) The GISELA-Study is a prospective cohort study about the nutrition and health status of approximately 500 seniors during the course of their ageing period. The study also covers factors which have an impact on the nutrition and health status. Inclusion criteria for study participation were a minimum age of 60 years as well as physical mobility. The study started in 1994. Till now 430 participants were recruited.

Abstract (Original Language) Die GISELA-Studie ist eine prospektiv angelegte Kohortenstudie zum Ernährungs- und Gesundheitsstatus von ca. 500 Senioren im Verlauf des Alterns. Mit der Studie werden auch solche Faktoren erfaßt, die Einfluß auf den Ernährungs- und Gesundheitsstatus nehmen. Einschlusskriterien für die Teilnahme an der Studie sind ein Mindestalter von 60 Jahren sowie körperliche Mobilität. Mit der Studie wurde 1994 begonnen. Bisher wurden 430 Studienteilnehmer rekrutiert.

Age Groups

60	and older

Kinder- und Jugendgesundheitssurvey

KiGGS

Project Leader

Project Leader	
Address	Robert Koch-Institut
	Postfach 65 02 61
	D-13302 Berlin
Executing Institution	Robert Koch-Institut
Funding Agency	Bundesministerium für Gesundheit;
	Bundesministerium für Bildung und
	Forschung; Bundesministerium für
	Ernährung, Landwirtschaft
	und Verbraucherschutz

Project Information

Start of Project	01/01/2003
End of Project	31/12/2006
Start of Data Collection	01/05/2003
End of Data Collection	01/05/2006
URL	http://www.kiggs.de/
Scope	National

Keywords

Abstract (English) As there have been no representative data on the health and development of children and adolescents in Germany, the Robert Koch Institute, Berlin, was commissioned by the Federal Ministry of Health to develop a health examination survey approach to fill this information gap.

Against this background KiGGS was designed as a representative nationwide health survey of children and adolescents from 0 to 17 years. In total, 18,000 participants will be examined from May 2003 to May 2006 in 167 randomly chosen study locations all over Germany. These data collected at an individual level include objective measures of physical and mental health as well as self-reported information regarding subjective health status, health behavior, health care services use, social and migrant status, living conditions, and environmental determinants of health.

First results will be available at the end of 2006.

Abstract (Original Language) Die derzeit verfügbaren Informationen über die Verbreitung von Krankheiten, gesundheitsbeeinflussende Verhaltensweisen und umweltbedingte Belastungen der Bevölkerung unter 18 Jahren sind unzureichend und lassen keine bundesweit vergleichbaren Aussagen zum Gesundheitszustand zu.

Dieser Mangel soll durch die Studie beseitigt werden. Sie wird erstmalig in Deutschland durchgeführt und soll zu Beginn des 21. Jahrhunderts wichtige Informationen zur gesundheitlichen Lage im Kindes- und Jugendalter liefern.

Mit Hilfe der Ergebnisse können zeitliche und regionale Entwicklungen der Häufigkeit von Krankheiten sowie Schadstoffbelastungen aufgezeigt werden. Die Ergebnisse der Untersuchung sollen zu gezielten Präventionsmaßnahmen und gesundheits- sowie umweltpolitischen Entscheidungen führen, die allen zugute kommen.

Age Groups

Kindertagesstätten-Ernährungs-Situations-Studie

KESS

Project Leader

Project Leader	Dr. Wolfgang Sichert-Hellert
Address	Forschungsinstitut für Kinderernährung
	Dortmund (FKE)
	Heinstück 11
	44225 Dortmund
Executing Institution	Forschungsinstitut für Kinderernährung
	Dortmund (FKE)
Funding Agency	Bundesministerium für Gesundheit

Project Information

Start of Project	01/11/1996
End of Project	31/05/1999
Start of Data Collection	01/04/1997
End of Data Collection	01/03/1998
URL	http://www.fke-do.de
Scope	National

Keywords Nutrition questions; Day care center; Health promotion; Research; Method; Lunch; Menu

Abstract (English) In the Day Care Centers-Nutritional-Situation-Study, the food provision, the nutritional education and the food supply in day care centres with all-day care (at least 6 hours of care, including a warm-meal lunch) for children over 3 years of age were representatively investigated nation-wide for the first time. Of the 10 million children aged 3–14 in Germany, about every tenth child is attended to in a day care center according to the above-mentioned definition. Special attention was paid to the location of the day care centers in the new (49%) or the old (59%) states, the differing provision systems and possibilities of improving the food supply. Of the 493 randomly chosen day care centers that fulfilled the conditions of participation, 301 day care centers took part in the study between April 1997 and March 1998. These 301 day care centers take care of 14,324 children at kindergarten and after-school care center age that were on average cared for 9.9 h/day between 6 a.m. and 6 p.m.

Abstract (Original Language) In der Kindertagesstätten-Ernährungs-Situations-Studie (KESS) wurden die Nahrungsversorgung, die Ernährungserziehung und das Verpflegungsangebot in Tageseinrichtungen mit Ganztagsbetreuung (mindestens 6 Stunden Betreuung einschließlich einer warmen Mittagsmahlzeit) für Kinder über 3 Jahre erstmals bundesweit repräsentativ untersucht. Von den 10 Mio. Kindern im Alter von 3 bis 14 Jahren in Deutschland wird derzeit etwa jedes 10. Kind in einer Kindertagesstätte im oben definierten Sinn ganztags betreut. Besondere Berücksichtigung fanden die Lage der Kindertagesstätten in den neuen (49%) oder alten (51%) Ländern, die verschiedenen Verpflegungssysteme und Verbesserungsmöglichkeiten der Ernährungsversorgung. Von April 1997 bis März 1998 nahmen von 493 zufällig ausgewählten Kindertagesstätten, die die Teilnahmebedingungen erfüllten, insgesamt 301 Kindertagesstätten, in denen 14.324 Kinder im Kindergarten- und Hortalter an durchschnittlich 9,9 Stunden pro Tag zwischen 6 bis 18 Uhr betreut wurden, an der Studie teil.

Age Groups

Landesgesundheitssurvey Nordrhein-Westfalen

Landesgesundheitssurvey NRW

Project Leader

Project Leader	
Address	Wissenschaftliches Institut
	der Ärzte Deutschlands e.V. -WIAD-
	Godesberger Allee 54
	D-53175 Bonn
Executing Institution	Wissenschaftliches Institut der Ärzte
	Deutschlands e.V. -WIAD-
Funding Agency	Land Nordrhein-Westfalen, Ministerium
	für Frauen, Jugend, Familie und Gesundheit;
	Landesinstitut für den Öffentlichen
	Gesundheitsdienst des Landes Nordrhein-Westfalen -LÖGD-

Project Information

Start of Project	01/01/1999
End of Project	01/12/2001
Start of Data Collection	09/05/2000
End of Data Collection	30/10/2000
URL	http://www.wiad.de
Scope	National

Keywords

Abstract (English) The German Health Survey, which was completed in 1999, admits representative analyses about the health status of the adult resident population in Germany at the age of 18–79. However, the analysis of the German Health Survey data at the Federal State level is because of the sample size not or only with relevant restrictions possible.

Therefore, the Ministry for Women, Youth, Family, and Society of North Rhine-Westphalia used the opportunity – as before Bavarian – to extend the NRW subsample out of the German Health Survey. As a result, for the Federal State NRW exists with the State Health Survey North Rhine-Westphalia a representative survey. Thus, for the first time representative survey data about health and disease of the adult population are available.

The State Health Survey North Rhine-Westphalia provides up to date information about the health situation as well as harmful and constitutional impacts on the life of our citizen in NRW.

Abstract (Original Language) Die im Jahre 1999 abgeschlossenen Erhebungen zum aktuellen Bundesgesundheitssurvey erlauben repräsentative Analysen zum Gesundheitszustand der erwachsenen Wohnbevölkerung in Deutschland im Alter von 18 bis 79 Jahren. Eine Darstellung auf der Ebene einzelner Bundesländer aber ist infolge der jeweiligen Stichprobengröße und -anlage mit den Daten des Bundes-Gesundheitssurvey nicht oder allenfalls mit erheblichen Einschränkungen zulässig.

Das Ministerium für Frauen, Jugend, Familie und Gesundheit (MFJFG) des Landes Nordrhein-Westfalen hat sich daher – wie zuvor bereits der Freistaat Bayern – entschieden, die günstige Konstellation zu nutzen und die bereits vorhandenen Daten aus der auf NRW entfallenden Teilstichprobe aus dem Bundes-Gesundheitssurvey so aufzustocken, dass hieraus ein für das Land repräsentativer Survey entsteht: der Landesgesundheitssurvey Nordrhein-Westfalen.

Somit liegen jetzt erstmals für dieses Bundesland repräsentative Surveydaten zu Gesundheit und Krankheit der Erwachsenenbevölkerung vor.

Der Landesgesundheitssurvey Nordrhein-Westfalen liefert aktuelle Informationen über die gesundheitliche Situation sowie über gesundheitsgefährdende und gesundheitsfördernde Einflüsse auf das Leben der Bürgerinnen und Bürger in diesem Lande.

Age Groups

18	79

Lebensstile und ihr Einfluss auf Gesundheit und Lebenserwartung (Lebenserwartungssurvey)

Lebenserwartungssurvey

Project Leader

Project Leader	Karla Gärtner
Address	BiB - Bundesinstitut für
	Bevölkerungsforschung beim
	Statistischen Bundesamt
	Postfach 5528
	Friedrich-Ebert-Allee 4
	65180 Wiesbaden
Executing Institution	Bundesinstitut für Bevölkerungsforschung
	(Federal Institute for Population Research)
Funding Agency	Bundesinstitut für Bevölkerungsforschung

Project Information

Start of Project	01/01/1995
End of Project	31/12/2003
Start of Data Collection	01/01/1998
End of Data Collection	31/12/1998
URL	http://www.bib-demographie.de/index_projekte.html
Scope	National

Keywords Lifestyle; Health; Life expectancy; Life situation; Family; Federal Republic of Germany; Behavior; Old person; Threat

Abstract (English) During the last decades, chronic and cardiovascular diseases as well as malignant growth have become increasingly important as causes of death. New analyses show that most of these diseases are caused by personal attitudes, lifestyles, and environmental conditions and are therefore in many cases preventable. Unhealthy lifestyles also complicate successful and active ageing. To investigate the current life situation and changes in life circumstances and their impacts on the former, current, and future state of health, the Federal Institute for Population Research commissioned I+G Gesundheitsforschung (Health Research) to carry out a survey entitled "Life + Health in Germany" in 1998. The survey was conducted as follow up of the National Health Surveys, which was carried out in Western Germany in 1984/1986 and in Eastern Germany in 1991/1992. Fundamental parts of the new questionnaire with regard to the object of investigation concerned the retrospective collection of events, which took place between the beginning and end of data collection as well as a more detailed collection of the respondents' family situation. Therefore, it did not include medical questions. The results of the study are intended to at least partly fill information gaps and gaps in research. This is especially relevant with regard to increasing life expectancy and the growing proportion of elderly, who are more vulnerable to health threats. The survey was conducted to contribute to health reporting.

Abstract (Original Language) Im Verlauf der letzten Jahrzehnte gewannen chronische Krankheiten, Herz-/ Kreislauferkrankungen und bösartige Neubildungen als Todesursachen immer mehr an Bedeutung. Wie neuere Analysen zeigen, sind viele dieser Erkrankungen durch persönliche Verhaltensweisen, Lebensformen und Umweltbedingungen beeinflusst und damit auch häufig "vermeidbar". "Ungesunde" Verhaltensweisen erschweren auch das erfolgreiche, aktive Altern. Um die derzeitige Lebenssituation und einen Wechsel der Lebensumstände mit ihren Auswirkungen auf den früheren, derzeitigen und erwarteten Gesundheitszustand untersuchen zu können, wurde 1998 von der I + G Gesundheitsforschung eine Erhebung durchgeführt, die als Wiederholungsbefragung der 1984/1986 in West- und 1991/1992 in Ostdeutschland durchgeführten Nationalen Gesundheitssurveys angelegt war. Wesentliche Bestandteile des neuen Fragebogens im Hinblick auf den Untersuchungsgegenstand war die retrospektive Erfassung von Ereignissen, die zwischen den zeitlich sehr weit auseinanderliegenden Erhebungszeitpunkten aufgetreten sind sowie eine detailliertere Erfassung der familiären Situation. Dafür wurde auf rein medizinische Fragen verzichtet. Die Ergebnisse sollen derzeit noch bestehende Informations- und Forschungslücken zumindest teilweise schließen, was insbesondere im Hinblick auf die weiterhin steigende Lebenserwartung und den wachsenden Anteil älterer und damit auch gesundheitlich gefährdeter Menschen von Bedeutung ist. Der Survey versteht sich auch als Beitrag zur Gesundheitsberichterstattung.

Age Groups

45	and older	Participants born in 1952 and earlier

Mikrozensus-Zusatzerhebung "Fragen zur Gesundheit" 2005

Project Leader

Project Leader	
Address	Statistische Bundesamt
	Gustav-Stresemann Ring 11
	65189 Wiesbaden
Executing Institution	Statistisches Bundesamt
Funding Agency	

Project Information

Start of Project	
End of Project	
Start of Data Collection	01/01/2005
End of Data Collection	31/12/2005
URL	http://www.destatis.de/
	themen/d/thm_mikrozen.htm
Scope	National

Keywords

Abstract (English) In addition to the annual German Microcensus survey, there is a set of questions, which is collected only in four-year intervals. Health questions are part of this set. In 2005, 1% of the population (390,000 households with about 830,000 persons) were asked health questions. Participation was voluntary. The following topics were included: "state of health" (invalid and casualty), "disease risks" (smoking attitude) as well as "body measures" (height, weight, body-mass-index). The questions concerning the state of health included all diseases and accident injuries participants had suffered from on the day of and in the four weeks prior to data collection.

Abstract (Original Language) Neben dem jährlichen Grundprogramm des Mikrozensus gibt es eine Reihe von Merkmalen, die nur im Abstand von vier Jahren zu erheben sind. Dazu zählt das Zusatzprogramm "Fragen zur Gesundheit". Die Fragen zur Gesundheit wurden 2005 an 1% der Bevölkerung (390.000 Haushalte mit rund 830.000 Personen) gerichtet. Ihre Beantwortung war freiwillig. Es werden die Themenkomplexe "Gesundheitszustand (Kranke und Unfallverletzte)", "Krankheitsrisiken (Rauchgewohnheiten)" sowie "Körpermaße (Größe, Gewicht, Body-Mass-Index)" abgedeckt. Bei den Fragen zum Gesundheitszustand werden entsprechend all jene Krankheiten und Unfallverletzungen erfasst, unter denen die Befragten am Erhebungstag und in den davor liegenden vier Wochen gelitten haben.

Age Groups

18	20
20	25
25	30
30	35
35	40
40	45
45	50
50	55
55	60
60	65
65	70
75	and older

Motorik-Modul zur KiGGS-Studie

MoMo

Project Leader

Project Leader	Prof. Dr. Klaus Bös, Dr. Annette Worth
Address	Universität Karlsruhe
	Institut für Sport und Sportwissenschaft
	76128 Karlsruhe
Executing Institution	Instituts für Sport und Sportwissenschaft der Universität Karlsruhe
Funding Agency	Bundesministerium für Familie, Senioren, Frauen und Jugend

Project Information

Start of Project	01/01/2003
End of Project	31/02/2006
Start of Data Collection	01/05/2003
End of Data Collection	01/05/2006
URL	http://www.motorik-modul.de/
Scope	National

Keywords

Abstract (English) Currently, the Children and Youth Health Survey (KIGGS) is conducted by the Robert Koch-Institute (Berlin) throughout the Federal Republic of Germany. This study collects for the first time representative data on the health situation of children and adolescents in Germany. One part of the study is data acquisition on motor functions and sport behavior of adolescents. The ability to be physically active is besides health behavior, nutrition, injuries, existential orientation, environmental, and psychosocial factors one important health aspect.

Abstract (Original Language) Am Robert Koch-Institut (Berlin) wird derzeit der bundesweite Kinder- und Jugendgesundheitssurvey (KIGGS) durchgeführt, mit dem erstmals repräsentative Daten zur gesundheitlichen Situation von Kindern und Jugendlichen in Deutschland erhoben werden. Ein Teilbereich der Studie ist die Erfassung von Motorik und Sportverhalten der Heranwachsenden. Die sportlich-körperliche Leistungsfähigkeit ist u.a. neben dem Gesundheitsverhalten, der Ernährung, Unfällen, der Befindlichkeit, Umweltdaten und psycho-sozialen Faktoren ein wichtiger Gesundheitsaspekt.

Age Groups

4	17

Nationale Verzehrsstudie II

NVS II

Project Leader

Project Leader	Dr. Christine Brombach
Address	Bundesforschungsanstalt für Ernährung und Lebensmittel (BfEL)
	Standort Karlsruhe
	Haid-und-Neu-Straße 9
	D-76131 Karlsruhe
Executing Institution	Bundesforschungsanstalt für Ernährung und Lebensmittel (BfEL)
Funding Agency	Bundesministerium für Ernährung, Landwirtschaft und
Verbraucherschutz	

Project Information

Start of Project	01/11/2003
End of Project	
Start of Data Collection	03/11/2005
End of Data Collection	
URL	http://www.was-esse-ich.de/
Scope	National

Keywords

Abstract (English) Food choices as well as nutrition habits have changed dramatically in the last 10–20 years. Therefore, food consumption and subsequently nutrient supply probably has shifted in the German population. However, the dimension of these alterations is not clear.

The Federal Ministry of Consumer Protection, Food, and Agriculture commissioned the Federal Research Center for Nutrition and Food in Karlsruhe to conduct a nationwide National Consumption Study. The first representative National Consumer Study dates back almost 20 years and concerned only the old western German States. Current, reliable, and valid data for Germany are urgently needed to evaluate and update programmes for prevention, nutrition recommendations, and consumer education.

To implement continuous coverage of the nutritional situation, a monitoring system is planned as follow up to the actual National Consumer Study.

Abstract (Original Language) Das Lebensmittelangebot und unsere Ernährungsgewohnheiten haben sich in den letzten Jahren deutlich gewandelt. Es ist zu erwarten, dass sich mit dem Lebensmittelverzehr auch die Nährstoffversorgung der in Deutschland lebenden Menschen verändert hat. Keiner weiß das jedoch genau.

Daher hat das Bundesministerium für Verbraucherschutz, Ernährung und Landwirtschaft die Bundesforschungsanstalt für Ernährung und Lebensmittel in Karlsruhe beauftragt, die Nationale Verzehrsstudie II durchzuführen. Die letzte repräsentative Erhebung liegt fast 20 Jahre zurück und betraf nur die alten Bundesländer. Aktuelle, für das Bundesgebiet repräsentative Informationen sind dringend erforderlich für Präventionsprogramme, die Verbraucheraufklärung sowie konkrete Empfehlungen für Risikogruppen.

Es ist für eine fortlaufende Ernährungsberichterstattung in Deutschland geplant, in regelmäßigen Abständen repräsentative Verzehrsdaten zu erheben.

Age Groups

14	80

Nationaler Gesundheitssurvey T2

NUST2

Project Leader

Project Leader	
Address	Robert Koch-Institut
	Postfach 65 02 61
	D-13302 Berlin
Executing Institution	Robert Koch-Institut
Funding Agency	Bundesministerium für
	Forschung und Technologie

Project Information

Start of Project	
End of Project	
Start of Data Collection	01/04/1990
End of Data Collection	01/05/1991
URL	http://www.rki.de/cln_006/nn_744100/
	DE/Content/GBE/Erhebungen/
	Gesundheitsurveys/NationaleGesundheitssurveys/
	nationalgessurvey__node.html__nnn=true
Scope	National

Keywords

Abstract (English) The German Cardiovascular Prevention Study was conducted as a community oriented, multicenter intervention study with the aim to reduce cardiovascular risk circumstances as well as cardiovascular mortality (ICD 9: 410–414 and 430–438) over a period of eight years. The evaluation of the success of the intervention programmes was carried out at the German resident population aged between 25 and 69 years with the help of adequate national reference samples. These health surveys were conducted as cross section studies at the beginning of the study (t0: 1984–1986), at halftime (t1: 1987–1989) and at the end of the study (t2: 1990–1992).

Within the National Health Surveys representative samples of the German population went through a medical check-up and were interviewed as to health-relevant issues.

Abstract (Original Language) Die Deutsche Herz-Kreislauf-Präventionsstudie (DHP) war eine gemeindeorientierte, multizentrische Interventionsstudie mit dem Ziel der Reduktion der kardiovaskulären Risikofaktoren und der Herz-Kreislauf-Mortalität (ICD 9: 410–414 und 430–438) über einen Zeitraum von 8 Jahren. Die Evaluation des Erfolges der Interventionsprogramme wurde an der deutschen Wohnbevölkerung im Alter von 25–69 Jahren mit Hilfe entsprechender nationaler Referenzerhebungen vorgenommen. Diese Gesundheitssurveys fanden als Querschnittserhebungen zu Beginn der Studie (t0: 1984–86), zur Studienmitte (t1: 1987–89) und zum Studienende (t2: 1990–92) statt. Sie unterteilten sich in folgende Bereiche:

– Die Regionalen Untersuchungssurveys (RUS) in den Interventionsregionen mit einer Soll-Fallzahl von 1.800 Probanden je Region in t0 und einer Soll-Fallzahl von 1.400 Probanden in t1 und t2
– Die Nationalen Untersuchungssurveys (NUS) mit einer Soll-Fallzahl von 5.000 Probanden zu den drei Zeitpunkten als Referenzstichproben

Age Groups

25	69

Stillen und Säuglingsernährung in Deutschland

SuSe-Studie

Project Leader

Project Leader	PD Dr. Mathilde Kersting
Address	Forschungsinstitut für Kinderernährung
	an der Universität Witten-Herdecke
	Heinstück 11
	D-44225 Dortmund
Executing Institution	Forschungsinstitut für Kinderernährung Dortmund (FKE)
Funding Agency	Bundesministerium für Gesundheit

Project Information

Start of Project	01/12/1996
End of Project	31/08/1998
Start of Data Collection	01/02/1997
End of Data Collection	01/06/1998
URL	http://kunden.interface-medien.de/fke/
Scope	National

Keywords Breastfeeding; Determinants of breastfeeding; Baby feeding

Abstract (English) Breastfeeding and infant nutrition in Germany were first investigated in the SuSe-Study (February 1997 to June 1998). Attention focussed on breastfeeding conditions in maternity clinics and breastfeeding habits of women on the one hand, and nutrition of infants as a whole in the first year of life on the other hand. In total, 1,717 mother child pairs (participation rate 54.3%) from 177 maternity clinics (82% from the old states) took part in this study. Breastfeeding conditions were assessed according to the recommendations of the German National Committee on Breastfeeding.

Abstract (Original Language) In der SuSe-Studie wurden das Stillen und die Säuglingsernährung in Deutschland erstmals repräsentativ untersucht (Februar 1997 bis Juni 1998). Im Zentrum des Interesses standen einerseits die Stillbedingungen in den Geburtskliniken und die Stillpraxis der Frauen, andererseits die Gesamternährung der Säuglinge im 1. Lebensjahr. 1.717 Mutter-Kind-Paare (Teilnahmequote 54.3%) aus 177 Geburtskliniken (82% aus den alten Ländern) nahmen an der Studie teil. Die Beurteilung der Stillbedingungen in den Kliniken erfolgte anhand der Empfehlungen der Nationalen Stillkommission.

Age Groups

Mother-Child-Pairs

Verbundstudie "Jod-Monitoring 1996"

Project Leader

Project Leader	Prof. Dr. med. Friedrich Manz
Address	Forschungsinstitut für Kinderernährung an der Universität Witten-Herdecke Heinstück 11 D-44225 Dortmund
Executing Institution	Forschungsinstitut für Kinderernährung Dortmund (FKE)
Funding Agency	Bundesministerium für Gesundheit

Project Information

Start of Project	01/10/1995
End of Project	30/06/1998
Start of Data Collection	12/03/1995
End of Data Collection	25/03/1996
URL	http://kunden.interface-medien.de/fke/index.php
Scope	National

Keywords Germany; Iodine absence; Prevention; Monitoring

Abstract (English) Germany is still endemic in terms of iodine deficiency. To assess the present state as well as the regional differences of iodine supply and to elucidate the possibilities of improving iodine deficiency prophylaxis in Germany, the integrated study "Iodine Monitoring 1996" was carried out.

Abstract (Original Language) Deutschland ist nach wie vor ein Jodmangelgebiet. Um den aktuellen Jodversorgungszustand der Bevölkerung und dessen regionale Ausprägung zu erfassen und um Möglichkeiten einer Verbesserung der Jodmangelprophylaxe in Deutschland zu eruieren, wurde die Verbundstudie "Jod-Monitoring 1996" durchgeführt.

Age Groups

16	46
17	21
50	70

Verzehrsstudie zur Ermittlung der Lebensmittelaufnahme von Säuglingen und Kleinkindern für die Abschätzung eines akuten Toxizitätsrisikos durch Rückstände von Pflanzenschutzmitteln

VELS

Project Leader

Project Leader	Prof. Dr. Helmut Heseker
Address	Universität Paderborn
	Fakultät für Naturwissenschaften
	Department Sport und Gesundheit
	Ernährung und Verbraucherbildung
	Warburger Straße 100
	D–33098 Paderborn
Executing Institution	Universität Paderborn, Department Sport und Gesundheit, Ernährung und Verbraucherbildung
Funding Agency	Bundesministerium für Verbraucherschutz, Ernährung und Landwirtschaft

Project Information

Start of Project	01/01/2001
End of Project	01/01/2003
Start of Data Collection	01/06/2001
End of Data Collection	30/09/2002
URL	http://fb6www.uni-paderborn.de/evb/index.html
Scope	National

Keywords

Abstract (English) Children consume different kinds and quantities (related to their weight) of food in comparison to adults. They are accounted as especially sensitive population group considering potential toxic effects from residues of pesticide in food. Detailed food consumption data do not exist in Germany until now. Study objectives:

- Collection of nurslings' and infants' kind and quantity of consumed food and beverages in Germany
- Breakdown the consumed foods and meals into their elementary substances

Abstract (Original Language) Kinder verzehren andere Arten und Mengen (bezogen auf ihr Körpergewicht) von Lebensmitteln als Erwachsene.

Sie werden hinsichtlich der möglichen toxischen Effekte von Pflanzenschutzmitteln in Lebensmitteln als besonders empfindliche Bevölkerungsgruppe angesehen.

Detaillierte Lebensmittel-Verzehrsdaten liegen in Deutschland bislang nicht vor. Ziele der Studie:

- Erfassung der Art und Menge der verzehrten Lebensmittel und Getränke von Säuglingen und Kleinkindern in Deutschland
- die Aufschlüsselung der verzehrten Lebensmittel und Speisen in ihre Grundbestandteile

Age Groups

Nursling and babies in the age of 6 month till 5 years

Zeitbudgeterhebung 1991/1992

Project Leader

Project Leader	
Address	Statistisches Bundesamt
	Zweigstelle Bonn
	Graurheindorfer Strasse 198
	53117 Bonn
Executing Institution	Statistisches Bundesamt
Funding Agency	Bundesministeriums für Familie und Senioren

Project Information

Start of Project	
End of Project	
Start of Data Collection	01/10/1991
End of Data Collection	31/07/1992
URL	http://www.destatis.de
Scope	National

Keywords Federal Republic of Germany; Official statistics; Time expenditure; Household; Time budget

Abstract (English) Data from time use surveys provide information on the time use of persons belonging to different population groups and household types. Unpaid work such as housework and childcare, voluntary work or help provided to neighbours is of particular interest here. However, information is gathered also on education and leisure activities, for instance the use of media. The results can be used in particular as valuable basic material for the discussion of and research into issues of women and family politics. As the complete 24-h day is covered, time use surveys also provide information on a wide variety of other subjects. These may be topics as different as the time use of elderly people, the use of means of transport and mobility or working time arrangements.

Abstract (Original Language) Die Daten von Zeitbudgeterhebungen geben Aufschluss über die Zeitverwendung von Personen in unterschiedlichen Bevölkerungsgruppen und Haushaltstypen. Dem Umfang unbezahlter Arbeit, wie zum Beispiel Hausarbeit und Kinderbetreuung, Ehrenamt oder Nachbarschaftshilfe, gilt hierbei besonderes Interesse. Aber auch Angaben über Bildungs- oder Freizeitaktivitäten, beispielsweise die Mediennutzung, werden erhoben. Die Ergebnisse bieten sich vor allem als Grundlagenmaterial für frauen- und familienpolitische Diskussions- und Forschungsbereiche an. Da der vollständige Tagesablauf über 24 Stunden erfasst wird, liefern Zeitbudgeterhebungen aber auch Erkenntnisse zu einer Vielzahl anderer Themenschwerpunkte, beispielsweise zu so unterschiedlichen Bereichen wie die Zeitverwendung älterer Menschen, Verkehrsverhalten und Mobilität oder zu Arbeitszeitarrangements.

Age Groups

12	and older

Zeitbudgeterhebung 2001/2002

Project Leader

Project Leader	
Address	Statistisches Bundesamt
	Zweigstelle Bonn
	Graurheindorfer Strasse 198
	53117 Bonn
Executing Institution	Statistisches Bundesamt
Funding Agency	Bundesministeriums für Familie, Senioren, Frauen und Jugend

Project Information

Start of Project	
End of Project	
Start of Data Collection	01/04/2001
End of Data Collection	31/03/2002
URL	http://www.destatis.de
Scope	National

Keywords Federal Republic of Germany; Official statistics; Time expenditure; Household; Time budget

Abstract (English) Data from time use surveys provide information on the time use of persons belonging to different population groups and household types. Unpaid work such as housework and childcare, voluntary work, or help provided to neighbors is of particular interest here. However, information is gathered also on education and leisure activities, for instance the use of media. The results can be used in particular as valuable basic material for the discussion of and research into issues of women and family politics. As the complete 24-h day is covered, time use surveys also provide information on a wide variety of other subjects. These may be topics as different as the time use of elderly people, the use of means of transport, and mobility or working time arrangements.

The first time use survey was carried out in Germany in 1991/1992; ten years later, in 2001/2002, another study was conducted. The new survey does not only show the present time use of the population but makes it possible to describe changes when compared with the results of the first survey. The design chosen for the survey meets the methodological requirements set for European time use surveys by the Statistical Office of the European Communities, Eurostat. Thus comparisons can be made with other European countries.

Abstract (Original Language) Die Daten von Zeitbudgeterhebungen geben Aufschluss über die Zeitverwendung von Personen in unterschiedlichen Bevölkerungsgruppen und Haushaltstypen. Dem Umfang unbezahlter Arbeit, wie zum Beispiel Hausarbeit und Kinderbetreuung, Ehrenamt oder Nachbarschaftshilfe, gilt hierbei besonderes Interesse. Aber auch Angaben über Bildungs- oder Freizeitaktivitäten, beispielsweise die Mediennutzung, werden erhoben. Die

Ergebnisse bieten sich vor allem als Grundlagenmaterial für frauen- und familienpolitische Diskussions- und Forschungsbereiche an. Da der vollständige Tagesablauf über 24 Stunden erfasst wird, liefern Zeitbudgeterhebungen aber auch Erkenntnisse zu einer Vielzahl anderer Themenschwerpunkte, beispielsweise zu so unterschiedlichen Bereichen wie die Zeitverwendung älterer Menschen, Verkehrsverhalten und Mobilität oder zu Arbeitszeitarrangements.

1991/1992 fand in Deutschland die erste Zeitbudgeterhebung statt; 2001/2002 wurde nach 10 Jahren eine neue Studie durchgeführt. Die neue Erhebung zeigt nicht nur die aktuelle Zeitverwendung der Bevölkerung auf, sondern erlaubt auch, Veränderungen gegenüber den Ergebnissen der ersten Befragung darzustellen. Gleichzeitig wurde ein Untersuchungsdesign gewählt, das die methodischen Anforderungen erfüllt, die vom Statistischen Amt der Europäischen Gemeinschaften, Eurostat, an europäische Zeitbudgeterhebungen gestellt werden. Damit wird auch ein Vergleich zu anderen europäischen Ländern ermöglicht.

Age Groups

10	and older

Greece

Ageing of Population and Health: Emphasis on Cardiovascular Disease and on Mental Disorders

Project Leader

Project Leader	Dr. Haris Symeonidou
Address	Mesogeion Avenue 14–18
	115 27 Athens
	Greece
Executing Institution	The National Center for Social Research
Funding Agency	

Project Information

Start of Project	01/01/2005
End of Project	30/12/2005
Start of Data Collection	23/05/2005
End of Data Collection	30/06/2005
URL	
Scope	National

Keywords

Abstract (English) The aims of the study are presented below. In the course of the research information was selected on physical activity

- To present the demographic developments in Greece, emphasizing the issue of population ageing and to present population forecasts up to the year 2020, emphasizing predictions on the developments of population ageing
- To investigate the self-reported morbidity and mortality "profile" of the elderly and the future elderly in Greece, targeting on self reported risk factors and the incidence of cardiovascular disease and of mental disorders
- To record the current use of healthcare services (primary, hospital and medicinal care) by Greek elderly and future elderly individuals, particularly focusing on the correlation of the frequency of use with parameters like healthcare demand, insurance coverage, certain socioeconomic and demographic factors, healthcare service access indicators, etc.
- To estimate the impact of the ageing Greek population on out of hospital prescription drug use by age, gender, disease, and other socio-demographic variables
- To record drug consumption patterns and to assess whether these patterns are actually linked with the increase in pharmaceutical expenditures
- To develop a model for assessing the impact of demographic ageing on the population self-reported morbidity, the use of healthcare services and the health expenditure for the next ten years

Concerning physical activity the following were found:

Physical exercise, another important factor affecting population health status, does not seem to be very popular among the respondents: about two thirds of them do not practice any physical exercise, while from the remaining one third, about 50% had physical exercise at least three times per week, and the other 50% less than three times per week. Among the 2,440 respondents who answered the questions about their height and weight, the body mass index (BMI) equals to 25–30 for the 1,109: almost half of them (45%) suffered from overweight. Even worse, (BMI > 30) were 451 of the respondents, i.e., almost one fifth of the total sample (18.5%) suffered from obesity, while only 880 of the respondents (36%) had normal weight (BMI < 25).

Abstract (Original Language)

Age Groups

40	85

Geographical Distribution of Socio Economic Factors in the Attica Region in Relation to Levels of Pollution

Project Leader

Project Leader	Associate Professor Klea Katsougianni
Address	Mikras Asias 75
	115 27 Athens
Executing Institution	Department of Hygiene and Epidemiology
Funding Agency	

Project Information

Start of Project	01/01/1997
End of Project	30/06/1998
Start of Data Collection	
End of Data Collection	
URL	
Scope	National

Keywords

Abstract (English) The study was designed to examine socio economic factors in the Attica region in relation to levels of environmental pollution. The questionnaire used in the survey included questions on levels of physical exercise.

Abstract (Original Language)

Age Groups

All ages

Health and Nutrition Survey

ATTICA STUDY

Project Leader

Project Leader	
Address	Demosthenes B. Panagiotakos, DrMedSci, FESC, MACE
	Lecturer in Biostatistics - Epidemiology
	Department of Nutrition - Dietetics
	70 E. Venizelou st., 17671
	Harokopio University
	Athens
	Greece
Executing Institution	First Cardiology Clinic, School of Medicine, Universirty of Athens
	& Department of Nutrition – Dietetics, Harokopio University,
	Greece
Funding Agency	Hellenic Society of Cardiology

Project Information

Start of Project	31/12/2001
End of Project	30/12/2002
Start of Data Collection	01/05/2001
End of Data Collection	30/12/2002
URL	
Scope	National

Keywords

Abstract (English) In an attempt to evaluate the levels of several cardiovascular risk factors in Greece a population-based health and nutrition survey was conducted, the "ATTICA study." The survey was conducted from May 2001 to December 2002 among 1,514 adult men and 1,528 adult women, stratified by age – gender (census 2000), from the greater area of Athens. More than 300 demographic, lifestyle, behavioral, dietary, clinical, and biomedical variables have been recorded. The prevalence of the common cardiovascular risk factors in our population seems high.

Abstract (Original Language)

Age Groups

18	89

Household Budget Surveys

Project Leader

Project Leader	Mr Giorgos Ntouros
Address	Pireos 46 & Eponiton Str. GR 185 10
	Pireas
	Greece
Executing Institution	National Statistical Service of Greece
Funding Agency	

Project Information

Start of Project	
End of Project	
Start of Data Collection	
End of Data Collection	
URL	http://www.statistics.gr
Scope	National

Keywords

Abstract (English) This research project describes changes in consumption of specific types of food from 1974 to 2004. These data are derived from the Household Budget Surveys from 1974 and 2004/2005.

Abstract (Original Language)

Age Groups

All members of a household

National Nutrition and Health Survey

Project Leader

Project Leader	
Address	Lecturer in Biostatistics - Epidemiology
	Department of Nutrition - Dietetics
	70 E. Venizelou st., 17671
	Harokopio University
	Athens
	Greece
Executing Institution	Department of Nutrition – Dietetics, Harokopio University, Greece
	& First Cardiology Clinic, School of Medicine, Universirty of Athens
Funding Agency	

Project Information

Start of Project	01/09/2004
End of Project	30/11/2004
Start of Data Collection	01/09/2004
End of Data Collection	30/11/2004
URL	
Scope	National

Keywords

Abstract (English) The study aimed at investigating the prevalence of self-reported hypercholesterolaemia and its relation to dietary habits in Greek adults. A representative nationwide sample of an adult Greek population were interviewed by trained personnel using a standard questionnaire. Differences between people with and without hypercholesterolaemia are analysed.

Abstract (Original Language)

Age Groups

18	74

Physical Activity & Health

Project Leader

Project Leader	Dr Avgerinos Andreas
Address	Department of Physical Education and Sports Science, Democritus University of Thrace
	7? Km Komotinis – Xanthis
	Xanthi, 69100
Executing Institution	Democritus University of Thrace
Funding Agency	

Project Information

Start of Project	
End of Project	
Start of Data Collection	
End of Data Collection	
URL	
Scope	National

Keywords

Abstract (English) The relationship between physical activity and health for children and adults is well established. However, the sedentary lifestyle is widespread among Western societies and Greece is no exception. Data on physical activity were selected as part of a needs assessment for an experimental intervention aimed at promoting physical activity among students. A cross-sectional sample of 950 students answered the "Lifestyle Questionnaire" in order to depict the profile of students' physical activity patterns and habits related to health. Results revealed that physical activity level was below that recommended for good health in a large proportion of the sample especially among girls.

Abstract (Original Language)

Age Groups

Students aged 11, 14 and 17

Physical Exercise and Health

Project Leader

Project Leader	Mr Christoforos Vernardakis
Address	17, Lycavittou Str. GR-106 72
	Athens
	Greece
Executing Institution	VPRC Private Opinion Poll Company
Funding Agency	

Project Information

Start of Project	04/12/1998
End of Project	14/01/1999
Start of Data Collection	04/12/1998
End of Data Collection	14/01/1999
URL	
Scope	National

Keywords

Abstract (English)

Abstract (Original Language)

Age Groups

18	and older

The Health Profile of the city of Patras

Project Leader

Project Leader	Professor Aris Sissouras
Address	MEAD
	University of Patras,
	26500 Rio Patra
Executing Institution	Department of Operational Research and Management
Funding Agency	

Project Information

Start of Project	01/01/2005
End of Project	15/06/2006
Start of Data Collection	01/06/2005
End of Data Collection	15/07/2005
URL	
Scope	National

Keywords

Abstract (English) The study examined the health profile of the city of Patras through a questionnaire that measured among other items the level of physical active citizens of Patras engaged in as well as their eating and other nutritional habits.

Abstract (Original Language)

Age Groups

18	and older

Hungary

Hungarostudy 2002

Project Leader

Project Leader	Dr. Mária Kopp
Address	H-1089 Budapest
	Nagyvárad tér 4.
	Hungary
Executing Institution	Semmelweis University, Institute of Behavioral Sciences
Funding Agency	National Research and Development Fund, Ministry of Education

Project Information

Start of Project	01/01/2002
End of Project	30/06/2002
Start of Data Collection	01/01/2002
End of Data Collection	30/06/2002
URL	http://www.behsci.sote/hungarostudy2002
Scope	National

Keywords Health survey; Health status; Mental health

Abstract (English) THE HUNGAROSTUDY 2002 national representative health survey assessed the populations' physical and mental well-being, needs, and problems with health care services and the psycho-social risk factors. The interviewers, who were the members of the National Nursing Service, visited 12,643 inhabitants in their home between January and June 2002. The sample represented the Hungarian population above age 18 according to sex, age, county. The survey contains questions on socio-economic variables, work, family, somatic illnesses, mental state, smoking, alcohol use, physical exercise, use of and satisfaction with health care services, health insurance. The results help to study the changes in the physical-mental health status of the population and the role of social, mental, and behavioral factors behind it. Hungarostudy is a cross-sectional study that follows the earlier Hungarostudy surveys in 1983, 1988, and 1995.

Abstract (Original Language) A HUNGAROSTUDY 2002. országos reprezentatív egészségfelmérés a lakosság testi-lelki egészségi állapotát, az egészségüggyel kapcsolatos problémáit és igényeit, a pszichoszociális rizikófaktorok átfogó vizsgálatát valósította meg. 2002. január-június között 12643 lakost kerestek fel otthonában a kérdezobiztosok, akik a Védonoi Szolgálat munkatársai voltak. A megkeresett lakossági minta reprezentatív volt, azaz nemek, korcsoportok, megyék és településnagyság szerint megfelelt a teljes magyar lakosság arányainak. A használt kérdoívben részletesen szerepelnek a társadalmi és gazdasági helyzettel, munkával, családdal kapcsolatos változók, a szomatikus betegségek elofordulása, a lelkiállapot mutatói, a dohányzás, alkoholfogyasztás, testmozgás, valamint az egészségüggyel, a betegség-biztosítással kapcsolatos kérdések. Az eredményekbol következtetni lehet a magyar társadalom különbözo csoportjainak testi és lelki egészségi állapotára. Meghatározhatók a legfontosabb szomatikus és pszichés betegségek elofordulási aránya. Hasonlóan fontosak a betegségek háttértényezoire vonatkozó adatok, amelyekbol következtetni lehet a betegségek kialakulásának folyamataira. A Hungarostudy keresztmetszeti vizsgálat, amely a korábbi Hungarostudy felméréseket, 1983, 1988, 1995, követi.

Age Groups

18	and older

National Health Interview Survey Hungary 2000 (Országos Lakossági Egészségfelmérés 2000)

OLEF2000

Project Leader

Project Leader	Dr. Zoltán Vokó, dr. József Vitrai
Address	H 1097 Budapest IX.ker. Gyáli út 2-6; H 1966 Bp. Pf.64
	Tel.központ: (+36-1) 476-1100
	Fax: (+36-1) 476-1226
Executing Institution	Research Institute for Health Development. From 2001: Johan Béla National Center for Epidemiology
Funding Agency	Ministry of Health, Hungary

Project Information

Start of Project	01/05/1999
End of Project	01/07/2002
Start of Data Collection	16/10/2000
End of Data Collection	10/12/2000
URL	http://www.oek.hu/oek.web?to=8,712&nid=204&pid=1&lang=hun
Scope	National

Keywords Health survey

Abstract (English) The design and implementation of the National Health Interview Survey was commissioned by the Ministry of Health between 1999 and 2001 in the frame of the Hungarian Health Monitoring Program launched in 1999. The development of the questionnaire was based on WHO recommendations and other recognized international standards. The questionnaire design process was supported by a scientific committee with experts from the CDC and Hungary. The questionnaire had an interviewer and a self-administered part. A stratified, two-steps sampling method was used. The sample consisted of 7,000 noninstitutionalized inhabitants, addresses received from the Central Registry and Election Offices, being 18 years and over. The survey was implemented between October and December of 2000. Response rate was nearly 80% ($N = 5503$). High response rate was due to excessive PR preceding the survey. The results are representative for the entire Hungarian population. Topics covered in the questionnaire: functionality, chronic diseases, health behavior including alcohol consumption, smoking, physical activity, eating habits, access and use of health care, health care expenditures, social-economic-demographic background variables.

Abstract (Original Language) Az OLEF2000 tervezését és megvalósítását az Egészségügyi Minisztérium megbízásából 1999 és 2001 között végezték. A tervezést felkért hazai és amerikai szakemberek (CDC), illetve neves szakmai vezetokbol álló tanácsadó testület támogatta. Az OLEF kérdoívet a WHO által javasolt illetve a fejlett országokban használt kérdoívek alapján lett kialakítva. Az érzékenynek tekintett kérdésekre ún. önkitöltos kérdoívben adtak választ a kérdezettek. A kérdoív felvételéhez a Központi Nyilvántartó és Választási Hivatal nyilvántartásából 7000, véletlenül kiválasztott, 18 éves vagy idosebb lakost kerestek fel a Magyar Gallup Intézet kérdezoi az ország 440 településén. A kérdezendok kiválasztása úgy történt, hogy minden településnagyság és megye arányosan képviselve legyen a mintában. A kérdezés 2000. október közepén kezdodött és december elején fejezodött be. A mintába került felnottek mintegy 80%-ával, 5503 fovel sikerült felvenni a kérdoívet. A visszautasítás aránya a lakosok érdeklodése és a megfelelo elokészítés következtében alacsony volt. A válaszadók így a teljes magyar felnott lakosságot képviselik, azaz az eredmények a teljes felnott lakosságra általánosíthatók.Témakörök: funkcionalitás, betegségek, alkoholfogyasztás, dohányzás, egészségügyi ellátás igénybevétele, egészséggel kapcsolatos kiadások, testmozgás, táplálkozás, társadalmi-gazdasági, demográfiai háttértényezok.

Age Groups

| 18 | and older |

National Health Interview Survey Hungary 2003 (Országos Lakossági Egészségfelmérés 2003)

OLEF2003

Project Leader

Project Leader	Dr. József Vitrai
Address	Gyáli út 2-6.
	1097 Budapest
	Hungary
Executing Institution	Johan Béla National Center for Epidemiology
Funding Agency	Ministry of Health, Hungary

Project Information

Start of Project	15/07/2002
End of Project	30/12/2005
Start of Data Collection	30/10/2003
End of Data Collection	19/12/2003
URL	http://www.oek.hu/oek.web?to=836,8,711&nid=203 &pid=1&lang=hun
Scope	National

Keywords Health survey

Abstract (English) The National Health Interview Survey 2003 (NHIS2003) was commissioned by the Ministry of Health and implemented by the National Center for Epidemiology and the National Food Research Institute. NHIS2003 supplied baseline data to monitor the Hungarian National Public Health Program. The questionnaire used in the survey was developed in line with the recommendations of relevant international professional forums – the WHO and EUROSTAT among others – and relied also on existing national surveying experience such as the NHIS2000. Furthermore, the design for the NHIS2003 questionnaire ensured that the data collected provides comparison with the results of both the NHIS2000 and surveys carried out in other countries. The questionnaire had four parts: an interviewer administered, a self-administered, a 24-h food recall, a 3-day food consumption diary. A random sample of 7,000 noninstitutionalized individuals, citizens of Hungary, aged 18 and over, from 447 settlements of the country, was selected from the registry of the national Registry and Election Office. The respondents of the survey are representative of the entire Hungarian adult population by age, gender, and place of residence (more precisely by county of residence and by the size of their community). Data collection took place between 30 October and 19 December 2003. The response rate was 72% ($N = 5,072$). Although this figure is somewhat lower than the response rate achieved by NHIS2000 (78%), it is still a favorable result compared with national and international averages. Topics surveyed: Functionality: self-care, mobility, vision, hearing, diseases, conditions, body weight, health behavior (physical exercise, alcohol consumption, tobacco smoking, use of health services, gratuity, social-economic-demographic background variables, and specially this year detailed food consumption survey.

Abstract (Original Language) A 2003. évi Országos Lakossági Egészségfelmérést az Egészségügyi, Szociális és Családügyi Minisztérium megbízásából végezte a Johan Béla Országos Epidemiológiai Központ (OEK) és az Országos Élelmezés- és Táplálkozástudományi Intézet (OÉTI). A felmérés egyik kiemelt célja volt, hogy kiindulási adatokat szolgáltasson az Egészséges Nemzetért Népegészségügyi Programhoz az egészségproblémák elofordulási gyakoriságáról, azok kialakulását, lefolyását és kimenetelét befolyásoló legfontosabb fizikális, pszichológiai, környezeti és társadalmi tényezokrol, az igénybevett egészségügyi szolgáltatásokról, az egészséggel kapcsolatos lakossági kiadásokról. Az OLEF2003 közvetlen elozménye a 2000-ben lezajlott OLEF2000, amely módszereiben és tematikájában közel azonos volt az OLEF2003-mal. A felmérésben használandó kérdoív többek között az Egészségügyi Világszervezet, az EUROSTAT ajánlásai és az eddigi hazai tapasztalatok, így az OLEF2000 - tapasztalatai alapján készült. Az OLEF2003 kérdoívét úgy lett kialakítva, hogy mind az OLEF2000-rel, mind külföldi vizsgálatokkal összehasonlítható legyen. A kérdoív négy részbol állt, egyéni kérdoív, önkitöltos kérdoív, 3 napos táplálkozási napló. A fovizsgálat 2003. október 30. és december 19. között zajlott le. A felmérés során az ország 447 településén, tudományos szempontok alapján, véletlenszeruen kiválasztott 7000 felnott korú lakost kerestek fel otthonukban. A részvételre felkért személyeket úgy választották ki, hogy legfontosabb jellemzoiket illetoen, összességükben az egész magyar lakosságot jelenítsék meg. A kérdezés során a válaszarány 72%-os (N=5072) volt, ami hazai és nemzetközi összehasonlításban még így is nagyon kedvezonek mondható. A felmért területek: funkcionalitás: önellátás, mobilitás, látás, hallás, betegségek, életmód, egészségügyi ellátás igénybevétele, hálapénz, társas, társadalmi, gazdasági háttérváltozók, és speciális ebben az évben részletes táplálkozási felmérés.

Age Groups

18	and older

Ireland

Survey of Lifestyle, Attitudes, and Nutrition 2003

SLAN 2003

Project Leader

Project Leader	
Address	Department of Health Promotion
	Clinical Science Institute
	National University of Ireland, Galway
	University Road
	Galway
	Ireland
Executing Institution	Health Promotion Unit, National University of Ireland, Galway
Funding Agency	Department of Health and Children

Project Information

Start of Project	
End of Project	
Start of Data Collection	
End of Data Collection	
URL	http://www.healthpromotion.ie/uploaded_docs/Slan03(PDF).pdf
Scope	National

Keywords

Abstract (English) Cross-sectional study of the population of Ireland to ascertain health and lifestyle

Abstract (Original Language)

Age Groups

15	19
20	24
25	29
30	34
35	39
40	44
45	49
50	54
55	59
60	64
65	69

Italy

"IN & OUT della new generation a tavola": i risultati dell'indagine COLDIRETTI-INRAN

Project Leader

Project Leader	
Address	INRAN – Instituto Nazionale di Ricerca per gli Alimenti e la Nutrizione Via Ardeatina 546 - 00178 Roma
Executing Institution	INRAN – Instituto Nazionale di Ricerca per gli Alimenti e la Nutrizione
Funding Agency	

Project Information

Start of Project	
End of Project	
Start of Data Collection	
End of Data Collection	
URL	http://www.inran.it/inran/stampa_e_relazioni_esterne/comunicati_stampa/comunicato_6
Scope	National

Keywords

Abstract (English)

Abstract (Original Language)

Age Groups

14	19

Antioxidants and Physical Performance in Elderly Persons: the Invecchiare in Chianti (InCHIANTI) Study

InCHIANTI

Project Leader

Project Leader	Matteo Cesari
Address	Sticht Center on Aging, Wake Forest University Health Sciences, 1 Medical Center Boulevard, Winston-Salem, NC 27157
Executing Institution	Sticht Center on Aging, Wake Forest University Health Sciences, Winston-Salem, NC
Funding Agency	Supported by Bristol-Myers Squibb Company (Princeton, NJ) and by an unrestricted grant from BRACCO Imaging SpA, Italy. The InCHIANTI study was supported as a "targeted project" (ICS 110.1/ RS97.71) by the Italian Ministry of Health

Project Information

Start of Project	
End of Project	
Start of Data Collection	01/09/1998
End of Data Collection	30/03/2000
URL	http://intl.ajcn.org/cgi/content/full/79/2/289#T1
Scope	National

Keywords Antioxidants; Dietary intake; Physical performance; Elderly

Abstract (English) *Background:* Muscle strength and physical performance in old age might be related to the oxidative damage caused by free radicals.

Objective: The objective was to assess the correlation of plasma concentrations and daily dietary intakes of antioxidants with skeletal muscle strength and physical performance in elderly persons.

Design: This study is part of the Invecchiare in Chianti (InCHIANTI) study, which was conducted in 986 Italians aged 65 years. Physical performance was assessed on the basis of walking speed, ability to rise from a chair, and standing balance. Knee extension strength was assessed with a hand-held dynamometer. The European Prospective Investigation into Cancer and Nutrition (EPIC) questionnaire was used to evaluate the daily dietary intakes of vitamin C, vitamin E, ß-carotene, and retinol. Plasma and tocopherol concentrations were measured. Adjusted linear regression analyses were used to calculate regression coefficients per SD increase in plasma concentrations and daily dietary intakes.

Results: In adjusted analyses, plasma–tocopherol was significantly correlated with knee extension ($\beta = 0.566$, $P = 0.003$) and the summary physical performance score ($\beta = 0.044$, $P = 0.008$). Plasma-tocopherol were associated only with knee extension strength ($\beta = 0.327$, $P = 0.04$). Of the daily dietary intake measures, vitamin C and β-carotene were significantly correlated with knee extension strength, and vitamin C was significantly associated with physical performance ($\beta = 0.029$, $P = 0.04$).

Conclusions: Plasma antioxidant concentrations correlate positively with physical performance and strength. Higher dietary intakes of most antioxidants, especially vitamin C, appear to be associated with higher skeletal muscular strength in elderly persons.

Abstract (Original Language)

Age Groups

65	and older

Association between Social Class and Food Consumption in the Italian EPIC Population

Project Leader

Project Leader	Francesca Vannoni
Address	Servizio di Epidemiologia ASL 5
	Via Sabaudia 164
	10065, Grugliasco (Turin)
	Italy
Executing Institution	Social Epidemiology Unit, Department of Epidemiology, Piedmont Region, Grugliasco (Turin)
Funding Agency	Piedmont Region. Associazione Italiana per la Ricerca sul Cancro (AIRC, Milan). The European Union.

Project Information

Start of Project	
End of Project	
Start of Data Collection	01/01/1993
End of Data Collection	31/03/1998
URL	http://www.istitutotumori.mi.it/int/rivistatumori/pdf/pdf2003_06/11_Vannoni(669_678).pdf
Scope	National

Keywords Diet; Educational level; Italian EPIC population; Social class; Socio-economic data validation

Abstract (English) *Aims and background:* The objectives of the present study were to validate the social stratification variables adopted by the European Prospective Investigation into Cancer and Nutrition (EPIC) by comparing them with data from another independent source and to evaluate the geographic and social distribution of eating habits in the Italian EPIC population.

Methods: The validation of the socioeconomic data collected by the EPIC study was performed with the Turin Longitudinal Study as gold standard and using Cohen's kappa statistics to evaluate the concordance between the studies. We then analyzed food groups on the basis of the consumption of meat and fats, carbohydrates, sweets and alcohol, and on an index of the Mediterranean diet. The standardized scores for each food group were subdivided into quartiles, which were used to compare persons in the extreme quartiles. The analysis of the differences in eating habits by center and by educational level was conducted separately for men and women, calculating the prevalence rate ratios and controlling for age, area of birth, and body mass index.

Results: Concordance between the two data sources was high for educational level and low for the social-class index on the basis of occupation. Most of the eating habits considered to be potentially harmful (high consumption of meat or fats and alcohol and low consumption of olive oil and fish) were more frequent in Northern than in Southern Italy. These habits were inversely correlated with educational level, especially in the south.

Conclusions: A significant improvement in health could be obtained in the Italian population if culturally and socioeconomically disadvantaged individuals were to abandon their diet rich in meat and fats, as done by more advantaged persons. In the absence of preventive interventions specifically addressed to disadvantaged groups, it is quite likely that social inequalities in mortality and morbidity will increase.

Abstract (Original Language)

Age Groups

35	64

Diet in the Italian EPIC Cohorts: Presentation of Data and Methodological Issues

Project Leader

Project Leader	Valeria Pala
Address	Epidemiology Unit, National Cancer Institute
	Via Venezian 1
	20133 Milan
	Italy
Executing Institution	UO Epidemiologia, Istituto Nazionale per lo Studio e la Cura dei Tumori, Milan;
Funding Agency	Associazione Italiana per la Ricerca sul Cancro (AIRC, Milan). At the international level, EPIC has been supported by the European Union.

Project Information

Start of Project	
End of Project	
Start of Data Collection	01/01/1993
End of Data Collection	31/03/1998
URL	http://www.ncbi.nlm.nih.gov/entrez/query.fcgi?cmd=Retrieve&db=PubMed&list_uids=14870824&dopt=Abstract
Scope	National

Keywords Cohort studies, Diet, Dietary questionnaire, Italy, 24-h dietary recall

Abstract (English) One of the aims of the EPIC study is to produce accurate descriptions of the dietary habits of the participants recruited in the 27 EPIC centers of ten European countries. To do this, different dietary assessment instruments were developed and applied to capture the wide range of diets characterizing the different European populations. Three different food frequency questionnaires were developed for Italy: one for the centers of Varese, Turin, and Florence, one for Ragusa, and one for Naples. These inquired about eating habits over the previous year and were completed by 46,839 Italian EPIC participants. Specially developed software analyzed the responses and linked them to food composition tables to provide a nutritional breakdown of individual and collective diets. A further aim of EPIC was to develop a method of rendering data from different dietary questionnaires comparable. To do this, dietary data were collected from a sample of about 8% of the Italian EPIC cohort, using a standardized computer-driven 24-h dietary recall interview, and then compared with the dietary data collected by the questionnaires.

This paper provides an extensive description of the technical features and performance of the food frequency questionnaires and the 24-h recall interview, including a comparison of estimates of the intake of different food groups provided by the two instruments. From this comparison, the repeatability and reliability of consumption estimates was assessed, resulting in indications for improving data comparability.

The paper also presents food frequency questionnaire estimates of the daily intake of foods and nutrients by center, sex, and age group, as well as information on dietary habits such as place and time of intake, and food preparation and preservation methods as provided by the 24-h recall interview. The picture that emerged is that Italian eating habits are undergoing marked changes, with a tendency to less healthy eating. Documentation of these changes in relation to age, sex, and region provides an essential starting point for investigating the influence of diet on the development of cancer and other chronic diseases.

Abstract (Original Language)

Age Groups

35	64

Extra-Curricular Physical Activity and Socioeconomic Status in Italian Adolescents

Project Leader

Project Leader	Giuseppe La Torre
Address	University General Hospital "Agostino Gemelli" – Largo Agostino Gemelli 8
	00168 Rome
	Italy
Executing Institution	Institute of Hygiene, Catholic University Rome, Italy
Funding Agency	

Project Information

Start of Project	
End of Project	
Start of Data Collection	01/10/2002
End of Data Collection	30/05/2003
URL	http://www.biomedcentral.com/1471-2458/6/22
Scope	National

Keywords

Abstract (English) *Background:* The relationship between physical activity and health status has been thoroughly investigated in several studies, while the relation between physical activity and socio-economic status (SES) is less investigated. The aim of this study was to measure the extracurricular physical activity of adolescents related to the socio-economic status (SES) of their families.

Methods: The survey was carried out by submitting an anonymous questionnaire to junior high school students in the following Regions: Lazio, Abruzzo, Molise, Campania, Puglia, during the school year 2002–2003. Extracurriculum physical activity was evaluated considering whether or not present and hours of activity weekly conducted, and 2,411 students agreed to participate in the study.

Results: Participants were 1,121 males (46.5%) and 1,290 females (53.5%), aged between 11 and 17 years (median age: 12 years). 71.1% of the students reported to practice extracurricular physical activity. Parents' educational levels and work activities play an important role in predicting students' physical activity, with the more remunerative activities and higher educational levels being more predictive.

Conclusion: These results confirm the relationship between adolescents' physical activity and their families' SES. In particular, a positive relationship between participation in extracurricular physical activity and their families high SES was found.

These data will be useful for school administrators and for politicians to reduce the gap between adolescents from the least and most disadvantaged families.

Abstract (Original Language)

Age Groups

11	17	Parents

Physical Activity in the EPIC-Italy

Project Leader

Project Leader	Simonetta Salvini
Address	Molecular & Nutritional Epidemiology Unit
	CSPO
	Scientific Institute of Tuscany
	Via di San Salvi 12
	50135 Florence
	Italy
Executing Institution	Molecular & Nutritional Epidemiology Unit, CSPO, Scientific Institute of Tuscany, Florence
Funding Agency	Associazione Italiana per la Ricerca sul Cancro (AIRC, Milan). At the international level, EPIC has been supported by the European Union

Project Information

Start of Project	
End of Project	
Start of Data Collection	01/01/1993
End of Data Collection	31/03/1998
URL	http://www.ncbi.nlm.nih.gov/entrez/query.fcgi?cmd=Retrieve&db=PubMed&list_uids=14870829&dopt=Abstract
Scope	National

Keywords Prospective cohort study; Physical activity; Life-style questionnaire; Energy expediture

Abstract (English) The European Prospective Investigation into Cancer and nutrition offers the opportunity to explore patterns of physical activity in a large series of healthy adults enrolled in the different local cohorts of the Italian section of the European EPIC project. Physical activity is considered one of the means by which chronic disease could be prevented. Subjects in the EPIC study completed a life-style questionnaire, with a section dedicated to the assessment of physical activity at work and during leisure time. Time spent in the various activities was transformed into an index of physical activity (physical activity level, PAL) and an activity index that includes intense activity (PAL; intense activity included). Quintiles of these indexes were computed to observe the distribution of subject characteristics according to levels of physical activity.

In general, the population was characterized by low levels of physical activity at work, with more than 50% of the sample reporting sedentary occupations. During leisure time, only a small percentage of subjects compensated for the inactivity at work by engaging in energy-consuming activities. In particular, organized fitness activities were reported by a small percentage of people, whereas walking was the most common sort of physical activity. Specific types of activity seemed to characterize subjects in the different areas of the country, reflecting local traditions or specific living situations. Detailed information about physical activity habits, together with a description of other characteristics, could help in designing physical activity promotion programmes in different Italian populations and age groups.

Abstract (Original Language)

Age Groups

35	64

Progressi delle Aziende Sanitarie per la Salute in Italia

Passi

Project Leader

Project Leader	
Address	Istituto Superiore di Sanità
	Viale Regina Elena 299
	00161 - Roma (I)
Executing Institution	Istituto superiore di sanità (Iss)
Funding Agency	

Project Information

Start of Project	01/11/2004
End of Project	31/12/2005
Start of Data Collection	01/04/2005
End of Data Collection	30/06/2005
URL	http://www.epicentro.iss.it/passi/
Scope	National

Keywords

Abstract (English)

Abstract (Original Language) The following is a presentation of the project made by the leading institution.

Effettuare una sorveglianza sullo stato di salute della popolazione italiana, grazie a un monitoraggio delle abitudini, degli stili di vita e dei programmi di intervento che il Paese sta realizzando per modificare i comportamenti a rischio. È questo lo scopo di Passi (Progressi delle Aziende Sanitarie per la Salute in Italia), lo studio di popolazione affidato al gruppo Profea del Centro nazionale di epidemiologia, sorveglianza e promozione della salute (Cnesps) dell'Istituto superiore di sanità (Iss).

Gli argomenti scelti per lo studio includono: attività fisica, fumo, alimentazione, consumo di alcol, sicurezza stradale, ipertensione e ipercolesterolema, screening del cancro della mammella, del collo dell'utero e del colon retto. Inoltre saranno raccolti dati su alcune variabili demografiche e sulla percezione dello stato di salute.

Lo studio Passi si inserisce nell'ambito delle attività politiche e sanitarie intraprese in Italia per promuovere la prevenzione. L'adozione di stili di vita non corretti oggi viene infatti considerata una vera e propria emergenza sanitaria, che comporta l'aumento di rischio di malattie cardiovascolari, tumori e diabete: le principali cause di mortalità e morbilità nella popolazione adulta. Il Piano sanitario nazionale 2003–2005 affronta il tema della prevenzione sanitaria e della promozione della salute, dedicando un'apposita sezione agli stili di vita sani e all'importanza di sottoporsi a periodici controlli e test di screening. Anche il Centro nazionale per il controllo e la prevenzione delle malattie (Ccm), recentemente istituito dal ministero della Salute, riconosce tra i propri obiettivi strategici quello di sostenere il Paese per l'adozione di stili di vita sani attraverso l'individuazione dei modelli operativi più efficaci e la verifica del raggiungimento degli obiettivi di salute relativi.

Lo studio Passi vuole sperimentare una forma di monitoraggio dei comportamenti a rischio associati con le principali cause di mortalità e morbilità e dei possibili interventi effettuati dai medici o da altro personale sanitario e delle attività da intraprendere per modificarli. Inoltre, si propone di stimare quante persone abbiano ricevuto informazioni sullo screening del cancro e quante lo abbiano effettivamente intrapreso. Oltre a fornire dati utili alle Regioni e alle Asl partecipanti, l'esperienza maturata verrà utilizzata per la pianificazione di un sistema di monitoraggio a lungo termine dei comportamenti a rischio.

Age Groups

18	69

Statistiche culturali anni 2003–2004 (Cultural statistics 2003–04)

Project Leader

Project Leader	Fabrizio Maria Arosio
Address	Istat - Istituto Nazionale di Statistica
	Via Cesare Balbo 16 00184 - Roma
Executing Institution	ISTAT- National Institute of Statistics
Funding Agency	

Project Information

Start of Project	
End of Project	
Start of Data Collection	01/09/2003
End of Data Collection	31/10/2004
URL	http://www.istat.it/dati/catalogo/20060628_01/
Scope	National

Keywords

Abstract (English)

Abstract (Original Language) La pubblicazione propone i principali dati statistici relativi alla produzione e distribuzione di cultura e alla partecipazione culturale nel nostro Paese, fornendo un panorama dei fenomeni e delle tendenze che caratterizzano il settore culturale. I dati presenti si riferiscono agli anni 2003 e 2004. Ogni capitolo corrisponde a ciascuna delle aree tematiche definite a livello europeo per le statistiche culturali. In particolare, nel volume vengono presentate le principali informazioni relative a: patrimonio culturale, archivio di Stato, editoria e stampa, biblioteche, spettacolo dal vivo, audiovisuale (cinema, radio e televisione) e sport.

Age Groups

6	13
14	24
25	44
45	64
65	and older

Stili di Vita e Condizioni di Salute (Lifestyle and Health Conditions)

Project Leader

Project Leader	Sante Orsini
Address	Istat – Istituto Nazionale di Statistica
	Via Cesare Balbo 16 00184 – Roma
Executing Institution	ISTAT – National Institute of Statistics
Funding Agency	

Project Information

Start of Project	
End of Project	
Start of Data Collection	01/10/2003
End of Data Collection	31/10/2003
URL	http://www.istat.it/salastampa/comunicati/non_calendario/
	20051118_00/
Scope	National

Keywords

Abstract (English)   There is no abstract. It is a National multiscope survey.

Abstract (Original Language)   A partire dal dicembre del 1993 l'Istat ha avviato il nuovo corso delle Indagini multiscopo sulle famiglie. Alla fine di ogni anno vengono rilevati gli aspetti fondamentali della vita quotidiana della popolazione e il livello di soddisfazione dei cittadini rispetto al funzionamento dei servizi di pubblica utilità. I principali contenuti informativi dell'indagine sono: famiglia, abitazione, zona in cui si vive, istruzione e formazione, lavoro domestico ed extra-domestico, spostamenti quotidiani, tempo libero e partecipazione sociale, stili di vita e condizioni di salute, consumo di farmaci e utilizzo dei servizi sanitari, funzionamento dei servizi di pubblica utilità.

Il volume contiene i dati dell'indagine condotta ad ottobre 2003. Il campione è a due stadi con stratificazione delle unità di primo stadio (comuni). Sono state intervistate 20.574 famiglie, per un totale di 53.708 individui. Per una parte dei quesiti le informazioni sono state raccolte per intervista diretta. Nei casi in cui l'individuo non era disponibile all'intervista per particolari motivi, le informazioni sono state fornite da un altro componente la famiglia. Per un'altra parte dei quesiti è stata prevista l'autocompilazione diretta da parte del rispondente. Anticipazioni di risultati sono già state pubblicate nell'Annuario Statistico Italiano, edizione 2004.

Le modalità di diffusione dei dati dell'Indagine multiscopo sulle famiglie "Aspetti della vita quotidiana" prevedono la pubblicazione ogni anno di quattro volumi brevi, ciascuno dedicato ad un particolare aspetto della vita quotidiana:

- "Stili di vita e condizioni di salute";
- "Famiglia, abitazione e zona in cui si vive";
- "Cultura, socialità e tempo libero";
- "I servizi pubblici e di pubblica utilità: utilizzo e soddisfazione".

Il sistema di Indagine multiscopo prevede che ogni anno, accanto all'indagine "Aspetti della vita quotidiana", si affianchino, a cadenza quinquennale, altre indagini che approfondiscono tematiche particolari, e un'indagine continua a cadenza trimestrale su "Viaggi e vacanze".

Age Groups

3	5
6	10
11	14
15	17
18	19
20	24
25	34
35	44
45	54
55	59
60	64
65	74
75	and older

Lithuania

Lithuanian Nutrition Survey

LNS

Project Leader

Project Leader	Dr. Roma Bartkeviciute
Address	Kalvariju 153
	LT-26000, Vilnius
	Lithuania
Executing Institution	National Nutrition Center
Funding Agency	State budget

Project Information

Start of Project	01/02/2002
End of Project	01/12/2002
Start of Data Collection	01/03/2002
End of Data Collection	01/11/2002
URL	
Scope	National

Keywords 24-h recall; National survey; Nutrients; Region

Abstract (English) The main objective of the surveys was to provide national representative information on several aspects of food patterns and lifestyle behaviors, including food and nutrient intake, food beliefs, and knowledge. The national random sample of 3,000 inhabitants has been taken from the National Population Register. 24-h recall was used for dietary assessment. Common sets of household measures and photographs of commonly used foods were shown to the participants to help them to estimate food portion sizes. Height and weight of the respondents have been measured. Mean values and standard deviations of different nutrients were calculated.

Abstract (Original Language)

Age Groups

20	64

Physical activity of school-children in the largest Lithuanian cities

PASC

Project Leader

Project Leader	Assoc.Prof. Vida Volbekiene
Address	Sporto 6
	LT-44221 Kaunas
	Lithuania
Executing Institution	Lithuanian Academy of Physical Education
Funding Agency	

Project Information

Start of Project	01/01/2001
End of Project	31/12/2001
Start of Data Collection	01/01/2001
End of Data Collection	31/12/2001
URL	
Scope	National

Keywords IPAQ; Schloochildren; Cities

Abstract (English) In 2001, the survey was conducted in five largest cities of Lithuania, in 14 secondary schools. The target population was schoolchildren aged 11–18 years. About 1,074 schoolchildren from the largest cities partcipated in the study. These data were collected by interview using IPAQ questionnaire.

Abstract (Original Language)

Age Groups

11	18

Macedonia

Health and Nutritional Status of the Elderly in the Republic of Macedonia

HNSERM

Project Leader

Project Leader	Andrea Seal, Francesco Branca
Address	Mirka Ginova 17
	Skopje
	+389 2 3063 710
Executing Institution	World Health Organization (WHO) office Skopje, Macedonia, UNICEF
Funding Agency	UNICEF, WHO

Project Information

Start of Project	01/09/1999
End of Project	01/11/1999
Start of Data Collection	15/09/2006
End of Data Collection	15/09/2006
URL	http://www.who.org, www.unicef.org
Scope	National

Keywords BMI; Elderly men and women; Nutrition habits; Macedonia

Abstract (English) A household survey of men and women, 65 years of age or more, was conducted in the Republic of Macedonia in September 1999. Households were selected using a cluster sampling methodology with one urban and one rural stratum, each containing 30 clusters. Eleven elderly men and eleven women, from 1,015 households were selected at random from each cluster and invited to take part in the survey. The population's mean BMI was 26.89 with men having a mean 25.48 and women significantly higher figure of 28.36. The BMI was also higher in urban than in rural areas with a mean of 27.59 compared with 26.19.

Abstract (Original Language) Оваа студија ја даде првата национална слика за здравствената и нутритивна состојба на старите лица во РМ и обезбеди корисна база за идентификација на проблемот на оваа популациона група во однос на преваленцата на дијагнозираните заболувања помеѓу урбаното и руралното население, нутритивниот статус и исхраната на старите лица. Оваа студија опфатила мажи и жени од 65г. и постари, од 1015 домаќинства кои биле избрани рандомизирано од секој кластер. Биле собрани податоци од 1287 луѓе. Утврдени се екстремни варијации на БМИ што значително ги компромитирале дневните активности. Процентот на гојазни мажи бил значително понизок (14.4%) во однос на гојазноста кај жените (36.3%). Преваленцата на анемија била 14.9% (повисока кај мажите) а коскено-зглобните и кардиоваскуларните болести биле две најчести утврдени состојби. Спроведен е и посебн Прашалник за животните навики-стилови и посебно исхраната. Мерките кои се предлагаат за подобрување на јавното здравство и квалитетот на животот кај старите луѓе во Македонија се: да се направат напори да се зголеми приходот и безбедноста на храната вклучувајќи разновидна исхрана, подобрување на здравствената едукација и други мерки кои би ја намалиле преваленцата од пушење, промоција на здрави животни стилови, контрола на ризичните фактори од дебелина, подобрување на снабдубањето со вода и канализација особено во руралните средини, ефективен третман и контрола од ТБ.

Age Groups

The study involved families from age of 65 and more

Influence of obesity to acceleration of growing up

IOAGU

Project Leader

Project Leader	Bojic-Milicevic G, Mikov M, Milicevic B.
Address	
Executing Institution	Institute of Public Health, Novi Sad, Serbia
	Department of Pharmacology and Toxicology, Serbia
Funding Agency	Institute of Public Health, Novi Sad, Serbia
	Department of Pharmacology and Toxicology, Serbia

Project Information

Start of Project	
End of Project	
Start of Data Collection	
End of Data Collection	
URL	
Scope	National

Keywords Acceleration; Obesity; Growing up

Abstract (English) The aim of this study is to investigate correlation between obesity in school-aged children and acceleration of growing up. Determined values of bone age were compared with chronological bone age for certain age and sex. The results indicate the presence of advanced bone age in obese children compared with the chronological age. This investigation has determined acceleration of growing up in obese children with respect to the chronological bone age.

Abstract (Original Language)

Age Groups

6	18

Nutrition, Physical Possibility of Young Persons from Age 18–20, Before and After 6 Months Intensive Physical Activity

NPHPBAPHA

Project Leader

Project Leader	Atanasovski A, Ivanovska P, Hadzi-Naumov J.
Address	Voena Bolnica
	bul. Partizanski odredi bb
	Skopje
	Macedonia
Executing Institution	Military Hospital, Skopje, Macedonia
Funding Agency	Military Hospital, Skopje, Macedonia

Project Information

Start of Project	
End of Project	
Start of Data Collection	
End of Data Collection	
URL	
Scope	National

Keywords Nutritional status; Young; Physical activity

Abstract (English) The aim of this survey is to investigate the situation of nutrition and physical activity of young persons of age 18–20 in a period of 6 months and to verify whether planned nutrition is in line with the planned activity. In this study anthropometrically are interviewed 100 persons on random principle. The measures have been realized before and after 6 months activity. The results show that planned nutrition was in positive correlation with the intensive activity, which means that with such nutrition and activity giving the best results of BMI.

Abstract (Original Language)

Age Groups

18	20

Nutritional Status of the Population Aged 2–18 years in Macedonia

NSPM

Project Leader

Project Leader	Zlatka Dimitrovska, Gordana Ristovska, Vladimir Kendrovski,
Address	National Public Health Institute, Skopje Macedonia
	50 Divizija bb
	Skopje
	Macedonia
Executing Institution	National Public Health Institute, Skopje Macedonia
Funding Agency	National Public Health Institute

Project Information

Start of Project	01/04/1999
End of Project	01/01/2003
Start of Data Collection	
End of Data Collection	
URL	http://www.rzzz.org.mk
Scope	National

Keywords Nutritional status; Young; Overweight

Abstract (English) Assessment of the nutritional status in participants aged 2–18 years from the population in Macedonia. Participants were at age 2–5 years (675); 6–14 (1,543); 15–18 years (753). Anthropometrical measurements performed were body weight, body height, and relative body weight for nutritional status assessment. Results: 60.7–73.7% of participants aged 2–5 years had normal nourishing, 5.7–10% of this group were underweight and obese. Participants aged 6–14 years had normal nourishing in 52.6–60.7%; underweight was assessed in 19.8–26.8% from this study group.

Data analysis showed that one half of participants had normal nourishing; overweight and obesity were assessed in approximately 30% of the participants. Participants had in greater proportion overweight and obesity compared with underweight. Only school children aged 6–14 had equal distribution of underweight and overweight and obesity.

Abstract (Original Language)

Age Groups

2	18

Obesity, Dyslipidemia, and Other Risk Factors in Adults

ODRHA

Project Leader

Project Leader	Z.Dimitrovska, I.Spiroski, D.Gudeva-Nikovska
Address	National Public Health Institute, Skopje Macedonia
	50 Divizija bb
	Skopje
	Macedonia
Executing Institution	National Public Health Institute, Skopje Macedonia
Funding Agency	

Project Information

Start of Project	01/01/1999
End of Project	01/01/1999
Start of Data Collection	
End of Data Collection	
URL	
Scope	National

Keywords Obesity; BMI; Dyslipidemia; CVD; Diabetes

Abstract (English) Early detection of obesity, dyslipidemia (risk values of total holestorol and lipoprotein components), and other risk conditions in adult population as a cause for development of noncommunicable diseases.

Results: 18.1% participants are classified as Class I obesity, 5.1% as Class II, and 31.9% of women are classified as at high risk for developing CVD. Cholesterol values range from min 1.38 mmol/L to max 8.1 mmol/L, SD = 1,6489. High risk cholesterol levels (>6.71 mmol/L) was identified in 6.8% of the participants. 10.6% of them have also moderately increased fasting blood glucose level while 1.5% have high blood glucose levels. Systolic blood pressure was above the risk border line of more than 165 mmHg in 23.2% of the participants; 15.5% have moderate levels and 7.7% systolic blood pressure significantly higher than borderline.

Abstract (Original Language)

Age Groups

20	60

Overweight and Obesity and It's Association with Other Cardiovascular Risk Factors in Adults

OOAWCVDIA

Project Leader

Project Leader	Zlatka Dimitrovska, Gordana Ristovska, Vladimir Kendrovski
Address	National Public Health Institute, Skopje
	50 Divizija bb
	Skopje
	Macedonia
Executing Institution	National Public Health Institute, Skopje, Macedonia
Funding Agency	National Public Health Institute, Skopje

Project Information

Start of Project	
End of Project	
Start of Data Collection	
End of Data Collection	
URL	
Scope	National

Keywords CVD; Obesity; Risk factors; Adults

Abstract (English) Cardiovascular diseases are the major cause for morbidity and serious health problems in Macedonia. It is very important to prevent cardiovascular risk factors and their impact on human health.

Objective: To assess the association of BMI with levels of total plasma cholesterol, lipoprotein content with diastolic pressure.

Abstract (Original Language)

Age Groups

35	55

The Importance of the Prevention of Children's Obesity

OPC

Project Leader

Project Leader	Stanislevic E
Address	Medical Center Ohrid
	Macedonia
Executing Institution	Department for Children in Medical Center - Ohrid
Funding Agency	Medical Center Ohrid

Project Information

Start of Project	01/05/2001
End of Project	01/07/2001
Start of Data Collection	01/05/2001
End of Data Collection	01/05/2001
URL	
Scope	National

Keywords Obesity; Children

Abstract (English) Importance of discovering the children's obesity, with possibility not to spread out the diseases, which will be showed up in adults, to explore the diseases/factors that are causing the obesity, to recommend healthy lifestyle, and to change the habits of children and their families. This is the survey to show the number of children with obesity in age of 6–7 years. The results show a high percentage of obesity of children in the sample. It shows that 22% of the children have higher weight for their age.

Abstract (Original Language)

Age Groups

6	7

Norway

A Youth Study in Hedmark and Oppland 2001–2002

UNGOPPHED

Project Leader

Project Leader	Linn Kristin Stölan
Address	Norwegian Institute of Public Health
	PO Box 4404 Nydalen
	N-0403 Oslo
	Norway
Executing Institution	Norwegian Institute of Public Health
Funding Agency	

Project Information

Start of Project	01/03/2001
End of Project	30/06/2002
Start of Data Collection	01/03/2001
End of Data Collection	30/06/2002
URL	http://www.fhi.no/artikler/?id=28289
Scope	National

Keywords

Abstract (English) The population-based OPPHED (Oppland and Hedmark) Health Study was conducted in 2000–2001. All men and women in selected age groups were invited to participate.

The objectives were in principle the same as for the Oslo Health Study.

All men and women in Oppland and Hedmark counties in five different age groups (born in 1925, 1940, 1955, 1960, and 1970) were invited to participate. The OPPHED Health Study participants provided standard blood samples and measurements, and answered the mutual CONOR questionaire that covered the same main topics as for the Oslo Health Study.

In addition to the original invitation, nonresponders received two reminders. Of the 22,000 invited, 12,400 individuals (56%) participated in the survey and provided a blood sample. Two 6 ml full blood samples are stored at −80°C. A 2 ml aliquot is reserved for CONOR.

A cohort including all 15- and 16-year olds in Oppland and Hedmark will be asked to complete two questionnaires at school. They will not be invited to the clinical examination and no blood samples will be collected.

Abstract (Original Language) Ungdomsundersøkelsen i Oppland og Hedmark foregikk i 2001–2002 og ble gjennomført i de samme fylkene som det ble kjørt helseundersøkelser for voksne (OPPHED). Undersøkelsen besto av hovedundersøkelse samt flere tilleggsundersøkelser/delprosjekter.

Vi spør ungdommene om ulike temaer slik som for eksempel sykdom og helse, kosthold, idrett, nærmiljø, og hvordan de har det. Vi bruker to ulike skjemaer, et hovedskjema som er likt for alle fylkene, samt ett tilleggsskjema som varierer noe. Ungdommene ble bedt om å fylle ut spørreskjemaer i en dobbelt skoletime. Biologiske prøver inngikk ikke i undersøkelsen, og data for høyde og vekt er selvrapportert.

Vi henvendte oss til ungdom som hadde fylt 15 år og som gikk i 10. klasse i grunnskolen. De fleste av disse ungdommene var 15 eller 16 år. Svarprosenten ble 88 i Hedmark og 90 i Oppland, etter en purring.

Selv om så mange av ungdommene svarte på undersøkelsen, vil det nok være en viss skjevhet i datamaterialet, som skyldes at det sannsynligvis ikke er tilfeldig hvem som ikke var tilstede da undersøkelsen pågikk. Det kan være større sykelighet blant ungdommene som ikke deltok, eller en overhyppighet av andre problemer.

Den høye svarprosenten vil likevel sikre god representativitet, og undersøkelsen vil derfor gi et relativt godt bilde av ungdommenes helse og leveforhold i år 2001–2002 i Oppland og Hedmark. Undersøkelsen ble gjennomført våren 2001 i Hedmark og våren 2002 i Oppland.

Vi har valgt å gi tall for kommuner og regioner som har minst 50 deltakere for hvert kjønn. Dette er gjort slik at den statistiske usikkerheten i tallene som publiseres ikke skal være for stor.

Det betyr at vi kan presentere tall på fylkesnivå og for regionene i Oppland og Hedmark, der flere kommuner er slått sammen (se nedenfor). I tillegg presenterer vi tall for de største kommunene i begge fylker. Dette er Lillehammer, Gjøvik, Østre Toten, Vestre Toten og Gran i Oppland, og Kongsvinger, Hamar, Ringsaker, Stange og Elverum i Hedmark.

I alle statistiske analyser forekommer to typer feil: Tilfeldige feil som skyldes at vi har et begrenset antall personer med i undersøkelsene våre og systematiske skjevheter som kan oppstå ved at de fremmøtte skiller seg fra de ikke fremmøtte. Noen steder i teksten skriver vi at forskjellene kan være statistisk sikre eller usikre. Forskjeller som her betegnes som statistisk sikre, har en p-verdi på 0,05 eller mindre.

Resultater i tabellene blir presentert som hele prosenter, uten desimaler. Når for eksempel tallet 0 angis i tabellen, betyr dette at verdien ligger et sted mellom 0,0 og 0,049. Tall fra slike undersøkelser er alltid beheftet med en viss usikkerhet, og angivelse av desimaler gir dermed liten mening.

Age Groups

15	16

Romsås in Motion Study

MoRo

Project Leader

Project Leader	Roald Bahr
Address	Norwegian Institute of Public Health
	PO Box 4404 Nydalen
	N-0403 Oslo
	Norway
Executing Institution	Norwegian Institute of Public Health
Funding Agency	

Project Information

Start of Project	01/03/2000
End of Project	31/05/2003
Start of Data Collection	01/03/2000
End of Data Collection	31/05/2003
URL	http://www.fhi.no/artikler/?id=56624
Scope	National

Keywords Physical activity; Psycho-social factors; Intervention; Diabetes prevalence; Cardiovascular disease; Cardiovascular risk factors; Socio-economic status; Immigrant status; Adiposity; Ethnicity; Diabetes prevalence (type 2); Sex; South-Asians

Abstract (English) The Romsås in Motion study (MoRo) is an interventional study with three-years' follow-up. Romsås is a low-income district in Oslo, Norway, with 6,700 inhabitants of multiethnic origin.

All individuals 30–67 years of age were invited by letter to the baseline health survey, and as controls an age-matched population-based sample from a similar population in a neighboring district (Furuset) was used.

The intervention district had the highest mortality rates of all the 25 administrative districts in Oslo, and was the most disadvantaged by measures of socioeconomic status, such as education.

The National Health Screening Service collected data from questionnaires, conducted a physical examination, and collected blood samples according to protocols in mobile units in each district between March and May 2000, with follow-up surveys in 2003 (MoRo I and II).

The invitation contained brief information in the languages of the main immigrant groups, and the questionnaires were translated (English, Urdu, Turkish, Vietnamese, Tamil). The attendees signed an informed consent form and were offered counseling while completing the questionnaire.

A total of 2,950 persons (48% of the invited cohort) were examined at baseline, 22% of non-western origin. On the basis of demographic and socioeconomic variables, the attendees were fairly representative of the invited cohort. Attendees consenting to follow-up contact and future use of their data and still living in the Oslo area were invited for the follow-up tests ($N = 2,644$). The Regional Ethics Committee and the Norwegian Data Inspectorate approved the study protocol.

Abstract (Original Language) Det har lenge vært store forskjeller i helse og levealder i Oslo. Disse helsemessige ulikhetene har sammenheng med tilsvarende forskjeller i sosioøkonomiske forhold, levekår og risikofaktorer for sykdom. Oslo fremstår som en delt by, med ugunstige forhold øst for Akerselva. Også andelen fysisk inaktive er høyere her enn i Oslo vest. Det foreligger i dag omfattende dokumentasjon på at regelmessig fysisk aktivitet gir redusert risiko for hjerte- og karsykdom og type 2 diabetes. Det er likevel stor mangel på kunnskap om hvordan man best går frem for å tilrettelegge for og stimulere til økt aktivitet i brede befolkningsgrupper.

Forskere har de senere årene understreket behovet for intervensjonsstudier med teoribaserte, sammensatte strategier med tiltak på flere nivåer. Tidligere forskning tyder på at intervensjonstiltak bør ta sikte på å påvirke såkalte mediatorer (mellomliggende faktorer) for fysisk aktivitet. Psykososiale forhold som støtte fra familie og venner for å være aktiv, holdninger til fysisk aktivitet og mestringsforventninger knyttet til fremtidig aktivitetsdeltakelse, er eksempler på slike mediatorer. Økt fysisk aktivitet antas å være lettere å utløse om slike faktorer blir styrket. Også tilpasning av tiltak til den enkeltes psykologiske forutsetning - eller psykososiale beredskap - for endring av aktivitetsnivå, og tilgang til fysisk aktivitetsarenaer, er dokumentert å være av betydning, samt det å involvere lokale aktører. Intervensjonen i MoRo-prosjektet er basert på denne kunnskapen. Prosjektet ble gitt navnet MoRo, etter forslag fra et medlem i den lokale ressursgruppe (se s. 20), som en forkortelse for Mosjon på Romsås, og for å signalisere målsetningen om å fremheve og gi erfaringer med morsom og lystbetont fysisk aktivitet.

Målet for MoRo-prosjektet var å gjennomføre og evaluere tiltak for å fremme fysisk aktivitet og positive holdninger til fysisk aktivitet blant voksne i bydel Romsås, for derigjennom å redusere risikofaktorer for hjerte- og karsykdom og diabetes. Den fysisk aktivitetsfremmende intervensjonen skulle pågå i bydel Romsås i tre år (2000–2003).

Evalueringen av intervensjonstiltakenes effekt skulle bygge på:

- data om status før intervensjonen, basert på en tverrsnittsundersøkelse våren 2000 av personer bosatt i Romsås bydel i alderen 31–67 år, samt et kontrollutvalg med tilsvarende alders-, kjønns- og befolkningssammensetning fra Furuset bydel
- data fra oppfølgingsundersøkelsen av det samme utvalget våren 2003, og vurdering av endringer fra 2000 til 2003.
- erfaringer fra intervensjonen i Romsås bydel Tverrsnittsundersøkelsene i 2000 og 2003 besto av helseundersøkelse, samt ett spørreskjema om egen helse og levevaner og ett om vaner og holdninger knyttet til fysisk aktivitet. Befolkningsi

ntervensjonen ble utviklet i tråd med anbefalinger fra forskningslitteraturen og besto av fire typer tiltak:

- strategiske (forankring av prosjektet i bydelens planer, involvering av eksisterende strukturer og nettverk i lokalsamfunnet)
- informasjonsrettede (informasjon om fysisk aktivitet og helse og om prosjektets aktivitetstiltak formidlet via lokal presse, rundskriv, plakater, stands osv.)
- fysisk aktivitetsrettede (gågrupper, trimgrupper, dansekurs, test av fysisk form)
- strukturelle (opprettelse av merkede stier, økt gatebelysning samt snømåking og strøing om vinteren).

Hovedfunn ved første tverrsnittsundersøkelse (2000). Av de 6140 som ble invitert til tverrsnittsundersøkelsen i år 2000, møtte 2950 personer (48 %). Andelen med ikke-vestlig bakgrunn var 21,3 %. Vi fant en betydelig høyere forekomst av diabetes sammenlignet med tidligere norske data, i det 9 % av mennene og 5,1 % av kvinnene hadde diabetes. Hele 39% av disse tilfellene ble oppdaget via undersøkelsen. For nordmenn var forekomsten noe lavere (7,2% av menn og 3,3% blant kvinner) men den var betydelig høyere i enkelte innvandrergrupper (14,3% blant menn og 27,5% blant kvinnene fra det indiske subkontinent i aldersgruppen 30–59 år). En tredel av de fremmøtte var fysisk inaktive, betydelig flere menn enn kvinner. Mer enn 50% av innvandrerne av begge kjønn var inaktive. Disse funn dokumenterte behovet for å styrke det helsefremmende arbeid i bydelen, og at prosjektets målsetning om å satse på å fremme fysisk aktivitet var fornuftig. Resultatene viste forholdsvis gunstige verdier når det gjaldt den psykososiale beredskapen for økning i fysisk aktivitetsnivå, spesielt blant kvinnene. Dette indikerte at potensialet for atferdsendring som følge av intervensjonstiltak syntes å være til stede.

Intervensjonseffekter (endring fra 2000 til 2003). Den forskningsmessige evaluering er ikke sluttført, men vi har funnet å kunne presentere noen hovedresultater allerede nå. De 2644 deltakerne i 2000 som fortsatt bodde i de to bydelene eller i Oslo-distriktet ble re-invitert I 2003. Av disse møtte 1766 personer (67% i begge bydeler), herav 18% ikke-vestlige.

- Andel inaktive fra bydel Romsås var ved oppfølgingsundersøkelsen redusert med ca 9 %, en relativ reduksjon på 25 %, mens det kun var beskjedne endringer på Furuset.
- Romsås bydel hadde en gunstig utvikling på alle mål knyttet til psykososial beredskap for endring i fysisk aktivitet, mens Furuset bydel viste enten negativ utvikling eller tilnærmet ingen endring.
- Økningen i gjennomsnittlig kroppsvekt var betydelig mindre i bydel Romsås sammenlignet med bydel Furuset. En betydelig lavere andel av befolkningen gikk opp i vekt, og en høyere andel gikk ned i vekt på Romsås i forhold til Furuset. Beskyttelsen i forhold til vektøkning var særlig tydelig hos de gruppene som har høyest risiko for diabetes og hjerte- karsykdom: menn, personer > 50 år og ikkevestlige innvandrere, og ble funnet hos personer med høyt og lavt utdanningsnivå.
- Gjennomsnittsverdiene for hvilepuls, fettstoffer i blodet og glukose viste en gunstigere utvikling på Romsås enn på Furuset for menn. Slike forandringer som kan ses ved økning i fysisk aktivitet, og understøtter de selvrapporterte

endringene i aktivitetsnivå. For kvinner på Romsås var disse endringene mindre, men gikk i gunstig retning.

- Flere sluttet å røyke i bydel Romsås (6,3%) enn i bydel Furuset (3,4%). For kvinner <50 år var bydelsforskjellene størst, ettersom 7% flere sluttet å røyke på Romsås I forhold til Furuset.
- Analyser basert på data fra et spørreskjema om eksponering for og erfaring med intervensjonstiltakene viste at en stor andel av personer i intervensjonsgruppen la merke til prosjektet (93,2%) og dets ulike tiltak (29%-88,7%). Andelen som deltok I de ulike tiltakene var en del lavere, og varierte sterkt fra tiltak til tiltak (1,1%-45,5%).

En meget høy andel stilte seg positive til prosjektet (82,7%), mente at prosjektet hadde ført til at de selv (44,1%) og folk generelt på Romsås (55,5%) var blitt mer positive til fysisk aktivitet, at de selv (24,4%) og folk generelt på Romsås (49,6%) var blitt mer fysisk aktive, at de hadde snakket mer om fysisk aktivitet med andre (45,4%), samt at de hadde fått mer støtte for å være fysisk aktive (29,5%). Erfaringer fra prosjektet. Våre erfaringer fra intervensjonen er meget positive. Prosjektet fikk stor grad av legitimitet i lokalmiljøet, og det lyktes å involvere og samarbeide med lokale aktører. Disse aktørenes kjennskap til lokalmiljøets og befolkningens verdier, preferanser, behov, ressurser og barrierer har vært av uvurderlig betydning for utviklingen av prosjektets innhold. Når det gjelder de informasjonsrettede tiltak, antar vi at bruken av lokale informasjonskanaler og eksisterende strukturer i lokalmiljøet har vært viktige. Medarbeiderne fikk mange positive tilbakemeldinger om ulike fysisk aktivitetsrettede tiltak, spesielt gå- og trimgruppene. At disse ble utformet som "lavterskel"-tilbud (lokalisert i nærmiljøet, gratis, enkle aktiviteter av lav til moderat intensitet, ingen krav til tøy og utstyr) og fokuserte på trivselsaspektet, ser ut til å ha vært avgjørende for den gode oppslutningen. Videreføring av aktivitetstiltakene ble tidlig etterspurt. Tilretteleggingen for mer fysisk aktivitet på gangveiene på Romsås så ut til å gi ønsket effekt, da det stadig ble rapportert om økning i antall turgåere i nærområdet. Vårt inntrykk underveis var at tiltakene skapte mer positive holdninger til fysisk aktivitet og mobiliserte flere til fysisk aktivitet blant de voksne på Romsås, noe som også ble bekreftet av "eksponerings- og evalueringsspørreskjemaet" ved undersøkelsen i 2003.

Ovennevnte positive funn knyttet både til den vitenskapelige og den erfaringsbaserte evalueringen tyder på at de strategier og tiltak som inngikk i intervensjonen var effektive. Det å basere intervensjonen på den valgte flerteoretiske modell og å gi prosjektet en sterk lokal forankring, mener vi har vært de to viktigste suksessfaktorene. Ved overføring av denne typen intervensjon til andre lokalmiljøer vil det likevel være avgjørende å tilpasse tiltak og strategier til lokale kulturelle og sosiale forhold.

Age Groups

30	39
40	49
50	59
60	67

The Hordaland Health Study

HUSK

Project Leader

Project Leader	Kari Juul
Address	HUSK - Project Center
	University of Bergen
	The Department of Public Health
	and Primary Health Care
	Section for Preventive Medicine
	Kalfarveien 31
	N - 5018 Bergen
	Norway
Executing Institution	University of Bergen
Funding Agency	

Project Information

Start of Project	03/11/1997
End of Project	24/06/1999
Start of Data Collection	03/11/1997
End of Data Collection	24/06/1999
URL	http://www.fhi.no/artikler/?id=28287
	AND http://www.uib.no/isf/husk/
Scope	National

Keywords

Abstract (English) The Hordaland Health Study 1997–1999 (HUSK) was conducted during 1997–1999. The study population included all individuals in Hordaland County born 1953–1957 (29,400).

A total of 8,598 men and 9,983 women participated in the study, yielding a participation rate of 57% for men and 70% for women. The study also included 2,291 men and 2,558 women born 1950–1951 and 1,868 men and 2,470 women born 1925–1927 and who had participated in an earlier study in 1992–1993 (the Hordaland Homocysteine Study, referred to as the Homocysteine cohort). Participation rates in these groups were 73%, 81%, 79%, and 76%, respectively.

In addition to the standard measurements of CONOR, baseline measurements included serum creatinine. Self-administered questionnaires included open-ended questions regarding occupation and industrial affiliation as well as use of medicinal and dietary supplements.

HUSK includes a total of 1.5–2 ml full blood stored in two vials from 25,583 participants. In addition, there is serum from 23,151 participants. For the Homocysteine cohort, there is plasma from 7,053 persons. In addition there is stored blood from approximately 18,000 persons who participated in the Homocysteine study in 1992/1993.

Ancillary projects addressed psychiatric disorders, psychosocial factors, social support, and social stress, while several projects were related to occupation, health-related quality of life, as well as standard questionnaires on sleeping behavior. In addition to the survey components included for the youngest cohort, the homocysteine cohort included ancillary studies on plasma homocysteine, serum measurements of B-vitamins and related genetic polymorphisms (methylene tetra hydroxy folate reductase, factor V Leiden, apo E and folate reductase), a quantitative food frequency questionnaire, measurements of bone mineral density (total body and hip), and spirometry. The oldest cohort (born 1925–1927) also participated in a 30-min interview on cognitive function.

Abstract (Original Language)

Age Groups

The Nord-Trøndelag Health Study

HUNT

Project Leader

Project Leader	
Address	HUNT forskningssenter
	Neptunvn. 1
	7650 Verdal
Executing Institution	HUNT forskningssenter
Funding Agency	The Ministry of Health, through The National
	Institute of Public Health and The National
	Health Screening Service (SHUS)

Project Information

Start of Project	01/01/1984
End of Project	31/12/1997
Start of Data Collection	01/01/1984
End of Data Collection	31/12/1997
URL	http://www.hunt.ntnu.no/index.php?
	side= AND http://www.fhi.no/artikler/?id=28286
Scope	National

Keywords Health survey; Methods; Participation; Epidemiology; Cardiovascular disease; Hypertension; Diabetes; Lung disease; Osteoporosis; Depression; Anxiety; Hemochromatosis; Hearing loss; Headache; Migraine; Prostate; Women's health

Abstract (English) HUNT is a database of personal and family medical histories, collected in two intensive studies, HUNT 1 (1984–1986), including 75,000 individuals 20 years and older (88%), and HUNT 2 (1995–1997) including 74,000 individuals 13 years and older (70%). Health information relevant to individuals and families, includes:

Disease status of individuals, and progressions, obtained from questionnaires including information on subjective health, diabetes, lung, cardiovascular, thyroid, muscle and skeletal diseases, and mental diseases, especially anxiety and depression, quality of life measures, migraine and other headache, physical and mental dysfunction, prostate complaints, urine incontinence, female reproductive data i.e., on menarche, pregnancies, hormone consumption, and gynaecological diseases. Personal environmental information is obtained from questionnaires, like residence, size of household, education, occupation, and in-house environment. Personal habits information, such as food intake, drug consumption, alcohol and tobacco consumption, physical activities and family medical histories, are also obtained from questionnaires. Clinical assessments, including measurement of height, weight, waist, hip, blood pressure, heart rate, lung function, bone mass, hearing and vision, are also obtained. Blood tests include measurement of total cholesterol, HDL, triglycerides, glucose, creatinin, ferritin, TSH. Urine analyses on microalbuminuria.

The population in Nord-Trøndelag County is stable, with a net out migration of 0.3 % per year (1996–2000), and homogeneous (less than 3% non-Caucasian), making it suitable for genetic epidemiology. The unique 11-digit personal identification number allows cross-reference of individuals in both HUNT databases and other regional and national health registries in Norway. Cross-referenced registries at regional level are being developed, such as registries on radial and hip fractures, venous thrombosis, lung embolism, ischemic heart disease, and stroke.

The HUNT database is also linked to endpoint registries at national level, for instance the Cancer Registry, The Medical Birth Registry, and The National Health Insurance Register. Additionally, Statistics Norway has provided The Population Census Register and a Family Registry, making a genealogical database.

Blood samples from 65,000 individuals aged 20 and above, consisting of serum (1.5 ml) and full blood samples, are stored at −70°C. From 33,000 subjects, clots (from 7 ml full blood) were stored, while EDTA full blood (3–4 ml) was stored from 32,000 individuals.

Abstract (Original Language) *HUNT 1 (1984 – 86)*: HUNT 1 var den første helseundersøkelsen i Nord-Trøndelag. HUNT 1 besto i hovedsak av fire delstudier hvor temaene var blodtrykk, diabetes, lungesykdommer og livskvalitet. Formålet med undersøkelsen var å finne prevalenser av høyt blodtrykk og diabetes, samt å evaluere livskvalitet hos personer med høyt blodtrykk, personer med diabetes og perso ner med tuberkulose. I denne undersøkelsen ble deltakernes blodtrykk målt, høyde og vekt ble registrert og det ble også foretatt en skjermbildeundersøkelse. Hver deltaker fylte ut to spørreskjema. I tillegg ble ikke-fastende blodsukker målt hos alle deltakere over 40 år. Om resultatet av denne undersøkelsen indikerte diabetes, fikk deltakeren tilbud om en klinisk undersøkelse i tillegg. Det ble ikke tatt blodprøver i denne undersøkelsen. 74,599 personer som var 20 år og eldre deltok (88,1%). En omfattende frafallsstudie ble også gjennomført. I dag er databasen en verdifull kilde til epidemiologisk forskning, både innenfor hjerte-kar sykdommer, diabetes og livskvalitet. Studier av kreft og sosialmedisin har også blitt gjennomført på dette materialet, og det pågår fortsatt forskning på data fra HUNT 1 *HUNT 2 (1995–97)*: HUNT 2 var en oppfølging av HUNT 1, ved at spørsmål og vurderinger av høyt blodtrykk, diabetes og livskvalitet var identiske eller like spørsmålene i HUNT 1. HUNT 2 var imidlertid en langt større undersøkelse, med et større aldersspenn (fra 13 år og oppover), et bredere spekter av emner, samt at mer data ble samlet inn for hver deltaker. Det var et nært samarbeid mellom ulike institusjoner som gjorde en så omfattende undersøkelse mulig; først og fremst Folkehelseinstituttet (tidligere Folkehelsa og SHUS), HUNT forskningssenter og Det medisinske fakultet, NTNU. Omkring 70 000 personer deltok i HUNT 2 (ca 70%), hvorav 45 000 også hadde deltatt i HUNT 1. Klinisk oppfølging, databehandling og kvalitetskontroller ble utført etter at datainnsamlingen var avsluttet, og fra og med høsten 1998 har datafilene vært tilgjengelig for forskersamfunnet. I tillegg til spørreskjemadata og kliniske målinger ble det i HUNT 2 tatt en venøs blodprøve fra alle deltakere over som var 20 år eller eldre (totalt ca 65 000 personer), og etter foreløpige analyser ble både serumprøver og fullblodprøver frosset ned. Disse oppbevares i dag på minus 70°C. Også koagler er oppbevart i nedfrosset tilstand. Blodprøvene er en kilde til genetisk informasjon, og har dermed et stort potensiale for forskning innen genetisk epidemiologi; eller den relative betydningen av genetiske og miljømessige årsaker til sykdom, f.eks. innen hjerte-kar sykdommer, lungesykdommer, osteoporose, kreftsykdommer, hodepine, stoffskiftesykdommer, m.fl. Det arbeides med å ekstrahere DNA fra prøvene, og flere studier som involverer analyser av biomateriale har startet opp.

De store datamengdene i HUNT har potensiale for mange typer studiedesign (f.eks. kohortstudier, case-control studier, tverrsnittsstudier, endepunktstudier og prospektive studier) og mer enn 100 forskere arbeider i dag med dataene. Likevel er deler av databasen lite benyttet, og det er fortsatt stort potensiale for videre forskning.

Age Groups

20	29
30	39
40	49
50	59
60	69
70	79
80	89

The Norwegian Mother and Child Cohort Study

MoBa

Project Leader

Project Leader	Per Magnus, Principal Investigator
Address	Norwegian Institute of Public Health
	P. O. Box 4404 Nydalen,
	NO-0403 Oslo
	Norway
Executing Institution	Norwegian Institute of Public Health
Funding Agency	The Ministry of Health

Project Information

Start of Project	13/11/2006
End of Project	13/11/2006
Start of Data Collection	01/01/1999
End of Data Collection	
URL	http://www.fhi.no/artikler/?id=51488
Scope	National

Keywords Automation; Biobank; Birth Cohort Study; DNA; Plasma; Quality Control; Predictors; Pregnancy; Folic acid; Supplements

Abstract (English) To achieve better health for mothers and children in the future, we wish to test specific hypotheses about the causes of a number of serious diseases by recruiting 100,000 pregnant women to a cohort study. Possible causal factors will be linked to information obtained from questionnaires, blood samples from mother, father, and child, and urine sample from mother and medical registries. The Norwegian Mother and Child Cohort Study has multiple endpoints. Primarily those associated with adverse pregnancy outcomes will be studied, as well as diseases affecting mother, father, or child. Endpoints will be taken from questionnaires and medical registries. The study will be carried out nationally and researchers with relevant questions will be welcome to participate. No interventions will be undertaken, which means that any conditions that may, potentially, expose the families to disease will not be modified. Both basic and applied research will be undertaken, with projects.

Abstract (Original Language)

Age Groups

Pregnant women of all ages

The OPPHED Health Study

OPPHED

Project Leader

Project Leader	Wenche Nystad
Address	Norwegian Institute of Public Health
	PO Box 4404 Nydalen
	N-0403 Oslo
	Norway
Executing Institution	Norwegian Institute of Public Health
Funding Agency	

Project Information

Start of Project	01/01/2001
End of Project	31/12/2002
Start of Data Collection	01/01/2001
End of Data Collection	31/12/2002
URL	http://www.fhi.no/ artikler/?id=28289
Scope	National

Keywords

Abstract (English) The population-based OPPHED (Oppland and Hedmark) Health Study was conducted in 2000–2001. All men and women in selected age groups were invited to participate.

The objectives were in principle the same as for the Oslo Health Study.

All men and women in Oppland and Hedmark counties in five different age groups (born in 1925, 1940, 1955, 1960, and 1970) were invited to participate. The OPPHED Health Study participants provided standard blood samples and measurements, and answered the mutual CONOR questionaire that covered the same main topics as for the Oslo Health Study.

In addition to the original invitation, nonresponders received two reminders. Of the 22,000 invited, 12,400 individuals (56%) participated in the survey and provided a blood sample. Two 6 ml full blood samples are stored at −80°C. A 2 ml aliquot is reserved for CONOR.

A cohort including all 15 and 16-year olds in Oppland and Hedmark will be asked to complete two questionnaires at school. They will not be invited to the clinical examination, and no blood samples will be collected.

Abstract (Original Language) I år 2000 og 2001 gjennomførte vi en helseundersøkelse i Hedmark og Oppland (OPPHED). Over 25 000 menn og kvinner fikk invitasjon til å delta. Vi samarbeidet med alle kommunene i de to fylkene om denne store befolkningsundersøkelsen.

Opplysningene fra helseundersøkelsen blir brukt til å lage en oversikt over hedmarkingene og opplendingenes helse. Dataene blir også brukt til medisinsk forskning for å få ny kunnskap om helse og sykdom. Dataene fra OPPHED inngår også i CONOR som er et nettverk av norske helseundersøkelser. Ungdomsundersøkelser i Hedmark og Oppland er kun spørreundersøkelser. Undersøkelsen omfattet seks aldersgrupper, det vil si personer født i 1985, 1970, 1960, 1955, 1940 og 1925. 15-åringene var også med men de svarte kun på spørreskjema på skolen.

Fremmøtet i Hedmark ble noenlunde likt, 57 prosent i Hedmark og 55 i Oppland. I Hedmark hadde Folldal kommune det høyeste fremmøtet med 73 prosent mens Hamar lå lavest med sine 51 prosent. Beste kommunen i Oppland ble Lom med hele 72 prosent, lengst ned på lista havnet Søndre Land og Gjøvik med sine 47 og 49 prosent. Disse fremmøtetallene omfatter alle årsklassene unntatt den yngste (15-åringene).

Deltakerne har fylt ut flere spørreskjema. Alle unntatt den eldste aldersgruppa har fylt ut det vi kaller hovedskjema. De eldste, det vil si personer født i 1925 har fylt ut eldreskjema. I undersøkelsen brukte vi også et såkalt tilleggsskjema.

Det inngår også flere tilleggsundersøkelser i Helseundersøkelsen i Oppland og Hedmark. Noen av undersøkelsene omfatter alle deltakerne i helseundersøkelsen, mens andre tilleggsundersøkelser gjelder bare for spesielle utvalg. Det er prosjektansvarlig for den enkelte tilleggsundersøkelse som offentliggjør disse resultatene etter hvert som de blir klare.

Age Groups

Study population was divided into different groups by their birth year (born in 1985, 1970, 1960, 1955, 1940, or 1925).

The Oslo Health Study

HUBRO

Project Leader

Project Leader	Anne Johanne Sögaard
Address	Norwegian Institute of Public Health
	PO Box 4404 Nydalen
	N-0403 OSLO
	NORWAY
Executing Institution	Norwegian Institute of Public Health
Funding Agency	

Project Information

Start of Project	01/05/2000
End of Project	01/09/2001
Start of Data Collection	01/05/2000
End of Data Collection	01/09/2001
URL	http://www.fhi.no/eway/default0.asp?
	pid=225&oid=0&e=0&trg=Content
	Area_4828&MainArea_4807=4828:0:15,
	2818:1:0:0:4807;4809;::0:0:0&Content
	Area_4828=4812:54464::1:4843:5:4807;4828;::10:0:0
Scope	National

Keywords

Abstract (English) The Oslo Health Study lasted from May 2000 to September 2001. More than 18,000 individuals from various age groups participated in the study. They filled in questionnaires and received a clinical examination. The results will be used to gain a comprehensive overview of the health status of Oslo residents.

As a general overview of health status and conditions of Oslo is lacking, the data generated from this health study will be used to build a health profile (in Norwegian), in other words gain a comprehensive overview of the health status of Oslo residents. This profile was handed over to the municipality of Oslo in August 2002.

The information thus provided will also be a good basis for future health planning and service delivery in the Capital City. In addition, these data will be able to clarify, describe, and explain the variations and differences in health.

Researchers will be able to gain new knowledge about health, disease, and new trends through the data collected in the Oslo Health study. Furthermore, the participants in the health survey have an unique opportunity to discover either the existence of certain diseases or whether they are at risk of developing them in the future.

While the National Health Screening Service now Norwegian Institute of Public Health takes the lead in the implementation of all aspects of the study, a Steering Group with two representatives from each of the three collaborating partners make all the important decisions. The partners are Oslo kommune (Municipality of Oslo), Universitetet i Oslo (University of Oslo), and Nasjonalt folkehelseinstitutt (Norwegian Institute of Public Health).

All men and women residing in Oslo December 1999, from nine different age groups got an invitation. This included persons born in 1924, 1925, 1940, 1941, 1955, 1960, 1970, 1984, and 1985. It was noted that among those born in 1955 and 1970, a lower proportion were willing to participate, compared with the other age groups. Therefore, invitations were also sent to persons born in 1954 and 1969 (additional age groups) to compensate for the low attendance rate from the 1955 and 1970 age groups. A total of 67,000 individuals including the youth cohorts and the two additional age groups received an invitation.

Persons born in the above-mentioned years got a personal invitation in the post in other words, individuals could not apply to participate themselves.

For the youngest participants, i.e., persons born in 1984 and 1985, the two appropriate questionnaires were filled out during school hours in the classroom.

The remaining age groups were invited to participate in the study through a postal invitation including a standard main questionnaire. It was expected that they filled this out before attending the clinical examination. This examination was conducted at a central screening station in the city and included height, weight, and waistline (girth) measurements in addition to blood pressure and pulse recordings. Blood samples were also collected and analysed for lipids, blood sugar, hormones, liver, and kidney functions. Some of the participants had their bone density measured.

The main investigative tool for the study are the different categories of questionnaires. There are three kinds of main questionnaires one for those in the age group 15–16, another one for those in the 30, 40, 45, and 59–60 age group, and one for those aged 75–76 years. There are also supplementary questionnaires for each of the three categories and a second supplementary questionnaire for the adult categories. In other words, the age group 15–16 receive two sets of questionnaires and those between 30 and 76 years receive three sets. The 15 to 16-year olds receive the two sets at school, the adults receive one set with the invitation letter and the rest when they came for the clinical examination.

The first and second supplementary questionnaires included a variety of questions covering everything from use of the health services and diet, to the social network, allergy, and use of medicines.

The additional and extra questionnaires include questions such as muscle and body ailments, insomnia (sleeping problems), housing conditions, pet dogs, and general well-being.

Currently, about 80 supplementary projects are included in the Oslo Health Study. Some projects cover all the participants in the health survey, while others cover only selected groups.

Four weeks after attending the clinical examination, participants received a letter with their test results, informing them of their cholesterol, blood pressure, blood sugar in comparison to the recommended levels. Those at high risk of developing heart disease, cardiac disease, or diabetes were referred to Centre for Preventive Medicine, Ullevl University Hospital for further examinations and follow up.

When the Oslo Health Study was completed, we compiled a report with aggregated results for the entire city and its various districts. The public, district councils, and politicians were then informed about the health situation in Oslo. Those responsible for the supplementary projects will present their findings subsequently.

Abstract (Original Language)

Age Groups

30, 40, 45, and 59–60 age group and 75–76 age group

The Oslo Health Study (HUBRO) – The Youth Part

UNGHUBRO

Project Leader

Project Leader	Anne Johanne Sögaard
Address	Norwegian Institute of Public Health
	PO Box 4404 Nydalen
	N-0403 Oslo
	Norway
Executing Institution	Norwegian Institute of Public Health
Funding Agency	

Project Information

Start of Project	22/03/2000
End of Project	19/02/2001
Start of Data Collection	22/03/2000
End of Data Collection	19/02/2001
URL	
Scope	National

Keywords

Abstract (English) To obtain identifiable data on individual level the Oslo Health Study (HUBRO) was conducted in 2000–2001 (2). To gain more knowledge about the health of children and adolescents, 15 to 16-year olds were also invited. This study was named the youth part of HUBRO (UNGHUBRO).

In 1996, the Norwegian Institute for Research on Adolescence, Welfare, and Aging (NOVA) had carried out a survey of 11,425 youth aged 14–17 years in Oslo (3). Their data was, however, anonymous and the focus was more on well-being than on health and illness. Thus the health authorities wanted more information that could contribute to improved health services for youth in Oslo.

The other aims of UNGHUBRO were to investigate whether or not there were large geographic, ethnic, and social differences in health and illness also among youth, in addition to differences in factors that can influence health and illness later in life.

Abstract (Original Language)

Age Groups

15	16

The Oslo Study I and II

Project Leader

Project Leader	Ingar Holme
Address	Department of Epidemiology and Health Surveillance.
	Centre of Preventive Medicine
	Division of Medicine,
	Ullevål University Hospital
	0407 Oslo
	Norway
Executing Institution	Department of Epidemiology and Health Surveillance
Funding Agency	

Project Information

Start of Project	01/03/2000
End of Project	01/06/2000
Start of Data Collection	01/03/2000
End of Data Collection	01/06/2000
URL	http://www.fhi.no/artikler/?id=54685
Scope	National

Keywords

Abstract (English) The Oslo Study I was conducted in 1972–1973 and the second round in 2000 (Oslo Study II). The study included epidemiological aspects of cardiovascular diseases (CVD) among men aged 20–49 years and how CVD could be prevented. The Oslo Study and the succeeding intervention trial are well known through nearly 100 publications.

FIRST ROUND OF THE OSLO-STUDY: OSLO I

About 30,000 men were invited to attend a health screening for tuberculosis during the period of May 1972 until December 1973. In addition, the screening was aimed at getting more information about risk factors for cardiovascular disease (1). The participants answered a 1-page questionnaire on symptoms, diseases, and risk factors. Height, weight, and blood pressure were measured. A blood sample taken in the nonfasting state was used for measurements of total serum cholesterol, triglycerides, and glucose.

Almost 18,000 men attended the screening. Some of the attendees were, after additional health examination at the Ullevål University Hospital, invited to participate in a cardiovascular disease risk reduction trial. These persons experienced less cardiovascular disease and a lower mortality rate (2). Others were asked to take part in a study on medication for high blood pressure (3). There have been several follow-up studies of the participants regarding CVD disease and death. (4–7).

As one of the first large screenings in the world we got answers to many questions. We got to know that:

- Forty to 49-years-old men with high risk could live longer and get fewer diseases if they consumed more low-fat food and stopped smoking (2).
- Forty to 49-years-old men, who were treated for high blood pressure, had reduced number of strokes (3)
- The risk of myocardial infarction was associated with socio-economical status (4)
- Smoking, high blood pressure, and little physical activity increase the risk of stroke (5)
- Even small changes in ECG led to an increasing risk of dying from cardiovascular disease. Such findings would improve the chance of identifying persons at risk of heart disease (6)
- The screening improved the possibility to find persons that may get cardiovascular diseases (7)

The Oslo-study was the model study for later population-based health studies on cardiovascular risk in Norway. These studies have all contributed much information on risk of myocardial infarction, stroke and diabetes, together with other sufferings and diseases.

SECOND ROUND OF THE OSLO STUDY: OSLO II

The second round of the Oslo-study was conducted in 2000, and was a follow-up screening of The Oslo Study in 1972/1973

Participants in 2000: The data collection was conducted during the spring of 2000 in co-ordination with and prior to the Oslo Health Study (HUBRO). All men previously invited to the Oslo Study in 1972/1973 and who were residents in Oslo and Akershus were invited to the screening in 2000. Men who would be invited to the later HUBRO and MoRo studies in 2000 were not invited, but their data were later added to the Oslo Study-datafile. (MoRo was a survey in parts of Oslo (Romsås and Furuset) and acted as baseline for a community-based intervention project aimed at promoting physical activity and preventing obesity, diabetes, and CHD. The intervention was evaluated with a new survey in 2003).

Neither were persons who already participated in three CHD-prevention projects at Ullevål University Hospital invited, but they were later sent the questionnaires by mail. Data on blood pressure, weight, and height from these three studies as well as results from the lipid analyses from these men, were later linked to the Oslo Study data file. Of men who met to the Oslo Study in 1972/1973, 7,157 participated in the second round of the Oslo-study in 2000.

Questionnaires, data collection, and feedback: The letter of invitation including two questionnaires, a 4-page main questionnaire and a 2-page supplementary questionnaire, was mailed two weeks prior to the appointment. The letter included information on how and where the clinical examination should take place. Both questionnaires were made in two versions, depending on the age of the participants. The main questionnaire was the same as the main questionnaire used in HUBRO and the version for those less than 68 years is translated into English.

The place of appointment was in the central east part of Oslo, as for the HUBRO-study.

The questionnaires were handed in there. All participants signed a letter of consent. Blood samples were stored for research purposes.

About two weeks after the examination, the participants got a feedback-letter by post. The letter informed about the attendants height, weight, body mass index, blood pressure, total serum cholesterol, HDL-cholesterol, triglycerides, and glucose. The letter also contained information about the importance of different risk factors. Persons with a high risk of cardiovascular disease and diabetes were recommended to further control with their local doctor.

Results: The results show considerable changes in risk factors for CHD during the 28 years between the two studies. The variation may be due to changes in lifestyle, use of medication, and/or natural ageing. A substantial decline in the percentage daily smokers was registered. The study showed an increase in weight and body mass index in all age groups examined. The changes were more pronounced in the younger compared with the older age groups.

Abstract (Original Language)

Age Groups

20	29
30	39
40	49

The TROFINN Health Study

TROFINN

Project Leader

Project Leader	Randi Selmer
Address	Norwegian Institute of Public Health
	P.O Box 4404
	Nydalen N-0403 Oslo
Executing Institution	Norwegian Institute of Public Health
Funding Agency	

Project Information

Start of Project	01/01/2001
End of Project	31/12/2003
Start of Data Collection	01/01/2001
End of Data Collection	31/12/2003
URL	http://www.fhi.no/artikler/?id=28259
Scope	National

Keywords

Abstract (English) The population-based TROFINN Health Study (Troms and Finnmark County – except Tromsø) started in 2001 and finished in 2003. The objectives are in principle the same as for the Oslo Health Study.

The TROFINN Study is divided into three parts: the county of Troms except those participating in the 5th Tromsø Study, the county of Finnmark (except the Samii communities), and the Samii Health Study. All men and women in Troms and Finnmark in five different age groups were invited to participate. In Tromsø, this applies to those born in 1926, 1941, 1956, 1961, and 1971, in the rest of Troms, and in Finnmark it applies to those born in 1927, 1942, 1957, 1962, 1972. In addition, all who were invited to the previous Finnmark Studies (I–III) will be invited (born 1925–1969).

This part of TROFINN constitutes about 20,000 invited individuals. Additionally, people aged 35–77 years living in areas with special ethnic settling in Troms and Finnmark (23 000) will be invited (the Samii Health Study). The participation in the TROFINN-part of Tromsø was 56%. In addition to the adult cohorts, all 15- and 16-year olds in Troms and Finnmark will complete two questionnaires at school. They will not be invited to the clinical examination, and no blood samples will be collected.

The blood samples containing 6 ml full blood are stored at –80°C. A 2 ml aliquot is reserved for CONOR. The TROFINN Health Sudy participants provided standard blood samples and measurements, and answered the CONOR-questionnaire that covered the same main topics as mentioned for the Oslo Health Study.

Abstract (Original Language)

Age Groups

Age groups in 30, 40–45, 60, and 75 year

The Tromsø Health Studies

Project Leader

Project Leader	
Address	Norwegian Institute of Public Health
	PO Box 4404 Nydalen
	N-0403 Oslo
	Norway
Executing Institution	Norwegian Institute of Public Health
Funding Agency	

Project Information

Start of Project	01/01/2000
End of Project	01/12/2000
Start of Data Collection	01/01/2001
End of Data Collection	01/12/2001
URL	http://uit.no/tromsoundersokelsen/
Scope	National

Keywords

Abstract (English) The fourth survey was completed in October 1995 and combined for the first time in Norway mass screening with advanced ultrasound technology. A total of 27,163 subjects aged 25+ years participated in the basic examination that was similar to the previous surveys. All persons 55- to 74-years old and 5–10% of participants in the other age groups were asked to return for a more comprehensive examination 4–12 weeks later. A total of 6,889 subjects attended the second visit, which included a number of blood and urine tests, ECG, ultrasonographic examination of the right carotid artery, ultrasonography of abdominal aorta, echocardiography of the heart, and forearm bone mineral densitometry (BMD). In addition to the Phase II participants, all women aged 50–54 years were invited. Thus, the total sample for BMD included 7,948 subjects.

In 2001, 10,429 subjects were invited to the last survey that was completed in December 2001. All subjects who participated in the comprehensive examination in 1994–1995 and were still living in Tromsø (7,071 subjects) were invited and 85% participated.

Abstract (Original Language)

Age Groups

30	34
35	39
40	44
45	49
50	54
55	59
60	64
65	69
70	74
75	79
80	84
85	89
90	and older

The Youth 2004 Study

Youth 2004

Project Leader

Project Leader	
Address	Norwegian Institute of Public Health
	PO Box 4404 Nydalen
	N-0403 Oslo
	Norway
Executing Institution	Norwegian Institute of Public Health
Funding Agency	

Project Information

Start of Project	01/04/2004
End of Project	01/04/2004
Start of Data Collection	01/04/2004
End of Data Collection	01/04/2004
URL	http://www.fhi.no/eway/default0.asp?
	pid=225&oid=0&e=0&trg=Content
	Area_4828&MainArea_4807=4828:0:
	15,2818:1:0:0:4807;4809;::0:0:0&Content
	Area_4828=4812:59810::1:4843:1:4807;4828;::10:0:0
Scope	National

Keywords

Abstract (English) The health survey Youth 2004 was conducted in Oslo and Hedmark counties during spring 2004. The objectives were, among others, to explore how physical activity is related to adolescents' mental health, to study the impact of genes and environment on literacy difficulties (dyslexia), and to investigate mechanisms for social inequalities in health. The survey also focuses on health habits and problems, stressful life-events, use of healthcare services, social networks, education plans, and more. The results will hopefully contribute with important knowledge to improve future health care services for adolescents, and give information about possible health preventive factors. Many of the participants in Youth 2004 also took part in equivalent health surveys three years earlier (UNGHUBRO and UNGOPPHED), allowing for longitudinal analysis.

In Oslo county, Youth 2004 was conducted partly as a school-based survey and partly through mail. All the final year students in every 32 secondary high schools in Oslo were invited to fill out a questionnaire during one school class. The participants in UNGHUBRO (2000–2001) who were not enrolled in the final year of secondary high school in Oslo (2003–2004) were invited by mail to participate in Youth 2004 to follow a cohort of 15- to 16-years old for three years. In Hedmark county, all who participated in UNGOPPHED 2001–2002 were invited to Youth 2004 by mail.

In total, more than 4,700 participated in the survey in Oslo and Hedmark. In Oslo, 3,308 participated (90%) in the school part and 461 participated (43%) by mail. In Hedmark 952 participated (55%).

Of all participants in 2004, 3,316 had also participated in the surveys in 2000–2001 and consented to a linkage between the two datasets.

Abstract (Original Language)

Age Groups

18	19

Portugal

National Health Survey in Portugal

NHSP

Project Leader

Project Leader	Carlos Matias Dias
Address	Av. Padre Cruz
	1649-016
	Lisbon
Executing Institution	Epidemiology and Biostatistic
	Centre of the National Health Institute
	Dr. Ricardo Jorge
Funding Agency	

Project Information

Start of Project	14/09/1987
End of Project	14/09/2006
Start of Data Collection	14/09/2006
End of Data Collection	14/09/2006
URL	http://www.insarj.pt/
Scope	National

Keywords National Health survey; Portugal

Abstract (English) It is a health measurement instrument that gathers information on the health condition of the Portuguese population and studies them throughout the time. Till now 7 surveys have been realized from 1987 until 1999.

Abstract (Original Language)

Age Groups

5	14
15	24
25	44
45	64
65	74
75	84
85	999

Physical Activity of Portuguese population

PA in Portugal

Project Leader

Project Leader	Maria Joäo Branco
Address	National Health Institute Dr. Ricardo Jorge
	Av. Padre Cruz, 1649-016
	Lisboa
	Portugal
Executing Institution	Health National Observatoire
Funding Agency	

Project Information

Start of Project	01/03/2002
End of Project	31/12/2006
Start of Data Collection	10/01/2002
End of Data Collection	01/02/2004
URL	http://www.insarj.pt/
	site/insa_home_00.asp
Scope	National

Keywords Scales of validation; Physical activity; Health determinants

Abstract (English) The aim of the study is to contribute to the characterization of physical global activity of the Portuguese. An observational instrument created by the National Health Observatory was used.

Abstract (Original Language) Foi objectivo deste studo contribuir para caracterizaçao da actividade fisica global dos portugueses. Utilizou-se um instrumento de observação criado pelo Observatório Nacional de Saúde.

Age Groups

18	24
25	29
30	34
35	39
40	44
45	49
50	54
55	59
60	64
65	69
70	74

Romania

Countrywide Integrated Noncommunicable Diseases Intervention – Romania

CINDI – Romania

Project Leader

Project Leader	Dr. Aurelia Marcu
Address	1–3 Dr Leonte Str.; 050463; Bucharest; sector 5
Executing Institution	Public Health Institute, Bucharest
Funding Agency	

Project Information

Start of Project	01/01/2001
End of Project	31/12/2005
Start of Data Collection	31/01/2001
End of Data Collection	31/01/2001
URL	http://euro.who.int/CINDI
Scope	National

Keywords Chronic disease; Prevention and control; Strategic planning; Public health; National health programmes; Programme development; Europe

Abstract (English) CINDI (Countrywide Integrated No Communicable Diseases Intervention) is a programme coordinated by the WHO – Regional Office for Europe in which 29 participating countries are collaborating on the implementation of an integrated approach to chronic disease prevention.

The activities are directed to prevent and control risk factors (such as smoking, high blood pressure, high blood cholesterol, obesity, and excessive alcohol consumption) and to address their social and environmental determinants. It puts existing knowledge to use – first in demonstration programmes in small areas and then countrywide.

Age Groups

20	24
25	29
30	34
35	39
40	44
45	49
50	54
55	59
60	64

Diet and Nutritional Status Survey in Adults and Pregnant Women

NUTRITION

Project Leader

Project Leader	Dr. Elena Popa, MD, hygiene
Address	Str Dr Victor Babes, nr 14, 700465, Iasi Romania
Executing Institution	Institute of Public Health, Iasi, Romania
Funding Agency	

Project Information

Start of Project	15/01/2000
End of Project	31/12/2004
Start of Data Collection	
End of Data Collection	
URL	
Scope	National

Keywords Diet; Nutrition status; Obesity; Pregnancy; Newborn; Breast milk quality

Abstract (English) 1. *Objective*: caloric and nutritive evaluation of adult diet in the actual socio-economic conditions. The methodology was applied according to the methodology of the diet survey – Bucharest, 1980 and validated questionnaires. The results were structured by sex and age. Women registered a lower consumption of milk, fish, fruits, aspect in close relation with dietary customs and family income.

2. The aim of study was to investigate the nutrition of pregnant women in the context of many determinant factors of their health. 263 pregnant women aged between 18 and 39 years were investigated in the first half of pregnancy, in the second half of pregnancy, and about 2 months after delivery. The next aspects were followed: socioeconomic situation, height and weight, nutrition (24-h food recall and food requency questionnaire), mineral supplementation, behavioral factors (smoke, physical exercises, alcohol and coffee consumption), delivery data, lactation data, newborns data, infant at 1 and 6 months data. Laboratory exams identified hematological, nutrition status, oxidative stress, smoking parameters, and nutritive components of mother milk.

Results: Socioeconomic status of pregnant women associated with their nutrition, newborn health, and infant health. Weight gain correlated with lipids and proteins consumption. Majority of pregnant women did not do physical exercises. Mean energy intake was under the recommended values, with a mean carbohydrates intake under normal limit and a mean fats intake over the normal limit. There was an imbalance of food categories, with insufficient fish consumption and a high coffee consumption. Some food consumption of pregnant women associated with newborn parameters and infant health status till 6 months. Majority of pregnant women were supplemented with iron, calcium, and zinc later in pregnancy but this supplementation did not meet the requirements of pregnant or parturient women. Hematological and biochemical parameters showed many associations with food consumption. Newborn and infant health associated with the values of hematological parameters situated in normal domain. Oxidative stress parameters associated with newborn and infant health. Mean serum values of total calcium, magnesium, iron, zinc, and copper were in normal domain during the study; ionic calcium was deficient in all stages, and erythrocyte magnesium and zinc were deficient in late pregnancy. Zinc, calcium, magnesium, and copper were associated with newborn parameters and with newborn and infant health. Twelve percent of women smoked during pregnancy (most of them maximum five cigarettes per day). Smoking associated with coffee consumption, but not with alcohol consumption. Smoking negatively influenced pregnant women nutrition, antioxidant defense, and zinc and copper status and newborn and infant health. At 2 months postpartum, only 62% of mother had sufficient milk to nurse their babies. The mother's nutrition influenced very lightly milk composition. At 1 month of age, the girls were more harmoniously developed comparing with boys but were less healthy.

Conclusion: The nutrition of pregnant women associated with many aspects of their health, and of their newborn and infant health.

Abstract (Original Language) *1. Obiectiv*: evaluarea calorica si nutritiva a dietei adultilor în noile conditii socio-economice. Metodologia utilizata conform cu metodologia de studiu a starii de nutritie - Bucuresti, 1980 si chestionar validat. Rezultatele sunt diferentiate pe sex si vârsta, femeile având un consum mai slab de lapte, peste, fructe, fiind în relatie cu obiceiurile alimentare si starea materiala.

2. Scopul studiului a fost investigarea nutritiei femeilor gravide în contextul determinarii multifactoriale a sanatatii lor. 263 femei gravide în vârsta de 18–39 ani au fost investigate în prima jumatate a sarcinii, în a doua jumatate a sarcinii si la aproximativ 2 luni postpartum. S-au urmarit urmatoarele aspecte: situatia socio-economica, înaltimea si greutatea, nutritia (înregistrarea alimentelor din ultimele 24 ore si frecventa de consum a alimentelor), suplimentarea cu minerale, factori comportamentali (fumat, exercitii fizice, consum de alcool si cafea), date despre nastere, lactatie, nou-nascut si sugar la 1 luna si 6 luni. Examenul de laborator a identificat parametrii hematologici, statusul nutritional, stresul oxidativ, indicatori ai fumatului si componente nutritive ale laptelui matern.

Rezultate: Statusul socio-economic al femeilor gravide s-a asociat cu nutritia lor, cu sanatatea nou-nascutului si a sugarului. Câstigul de greutate s-a corelat cu consumul de lipide si proteine. Majoritatea femeilor gravide n-au facut exercitii fizice. Ingestia medie energetica a fost sub doza recomandata, cu o ingestie medie de carbohidrati sub limita normala si cu o ingestie medie de grasimi peste limita normala. S-a constatat un dezechilibru alimentar, cu un consum insuficient de peste si un consum ridicat de cafea. Consumul unor alimente de catre femeia gravida s-a asociat cu parametrii nou-nascutului si cu starea de sanatate a sugarului pâna la 6 luni. Majoritatea femeilor gravide a primit suplimente de fer, calciu si zinc în a doua jumatate a sarcinii dar acestea n-au fost în concordanta cu necesarul femeilor gravide sau parturiente. Indicatorii hematologici si biochimici au aratat multe asocieri cu consumul de alimente. Sanatatea nou-nascutului si a sugarului s-a asociast cu valorile parametrilor hematologici situati in domeniul normal. Parametrii stresului oxidativ s-au asociat cu sanatatea nou-nascutului sau a sugarului. Valorile serice medii ale calciului total, magneziului, ferului, zincului si cuprului au fost în domeniul normal în timpul studiului; calciul ionic a fost deficient în toate etapele, magneziul si zincul eritrocitar au fost deficiente în a doua jumatate a sarcinii. Zincul, calciul, magneziul si cuprul s-au asociat cu parametrii nou-nascutului si ai sugarului. 12% dintre femei au fumat în timpul sarcinii (cele mai multe dintre ele maxim 5 tigari pe zi). Fumatul s-a asociat cu consumul de cafea dar nu si cu consumul de alcool. Fumatul a influentat negativ nutritia femeii gravide, apararea antioxidanta, statusul zincului si a cuprului si sanatatea nou-nascutului si sugarului. La 2 luni postpartum, numai 62% dintre mame au avut suficient lapte pentru a-si alapta copiii. Nutritia mamei a influentat foarte slab compozitia laptelui. La vârsta de 1 luna fetele erau mai armonios dezvoltate decât baietii dar erau mai putin sanatoase.

Concluzii: Nutritia femeilor gravide s-a asociat cu multe aspecte ale sanatatii lor, ale sanatatii nou-nascutilor si a sugarilor.

Age Groups

20	44
45	60

Gender differences in psychosocial risk factors for cardiovascular disease

Project Leader

Project Leader	Prof. Dr. Adriana Baban
Address	Republicii 37
	Cluj-Napoca 400015
	Romania
Executing Institution	Babes-Bolyai University, Cluj, Romania
Funding Agency	

Project Information

Start of Project	05/01/2001
End of Project	31/10/2001
Start of Data Collection	01/02/2001
End of Data Collection	05/05/2001
URL	
Scope	National

Keywords
Abstract (English)

Abstract (Original Language)

Age Groups

20	57

Monitoring of cardiovascular risk factors in Iasi

MONCARD

Project Leader

Project Leader	Elena Lungu
Address	Victor Babes str, 14, 700465, Iasi
	Romania
Executing Institution	Institute of Public Health, Iasi, Romania
Funding Agency	Ministry of Public Health In the framework of National Program 1.4

Project Information

Start of Project	01/01/2003
End of Project	31/12/2005
Start of Data Collection	10/07/2003
End of Data Collection	25/09/2005
URL	
Scope	National

Keywords Cardiovascular risk factors; Obesity; Waist circumference; HDL-Chol; LDL-Chol; lifestyle

Abstract (English) *Background:* Abdominal obesity became along time an entity both from physiological and clinical point of view. The influence of stress and stimulation of hypothalamo-hypophyso-suprarenal axis followed by a sexual dismorphism is well known, which makes treatment more difficult and less efficiently. The multiendocrin function of the adipose cell, the mechanism of regulation of the energetic balance, and the endocrine hypothesis contribute upon the pharmacological perspectives. The existence of the complex atherogenic picture indicates the need for a simple method, which could be used by family physicians to screen in a rapid and useful manner the associated risks. The complex of the relation between fat tissue and metabolic disorders is measured by anthropometric methods. Waist circumference relates closely to the intraabdominal fat mass and changes in waist circumference reflect changes in cardiovascular risk factors.

Methods: A prevalence study on a sample consisted of 340 patients 20- to 60-years old, in a family medicine unit in the city of Iasi. The studied variables were waist circumference, waist/hip ratio, body mass index (BMI), hypertension values (HTA), total cholesterol, HDL-c, LDL-C, and lifestyle.

Results: Waist circumference higher than 94 cm in men and 80 cm in women has indicated the subjects with a BMI > 25 kg/m2 and a waist/hip ratio > 0.95 in women and >0.80 in men. The values of waist circumference (>94 cm and >80 cm) in men and women who have at least one risk factor (HTA > 160/95, HDL-c <0.9 mmol/l) presented a sensibility of 56% and 68% and a specificity of 74% and 65%, respectively, compared with those subjects with lower waist circumference values (OR 2.4 95% IC 1.9–2.6 in men and OR 1.9 95% CI 1.6–2.3 in women).

Conclusion: Waist circumference is a feasible measurement, which can identify the subjects with high values of blood pressure and low values of HDL-c.

Abstract (Original Language) *Introducere.* Obezitatea abdominala a devenit, de-a lungul timpului, o entitate atit din punct de vedere fiziologic, cit si clinic. Sint bine cunoscute influenta stresului si stimularea axei hipotalamo-hipofizo-suprarenale, urmate de dismorfismul sexual, determinind ineficienta tratamentului medicamentos. Functia multiendocrina a celulei adipoase, mecanismul de reglare a balantei energetice, cit si ipoteza endocrina, contribuie asupra perspectivelor farmacologice. Existenta tabloului aterogenic complex indica necesitatea folosirii unei metode simple utilizata de catre medicul de familie in vederea evaluarii riscurilor asociate intr-o maniera simpla si eficienta. Relatia complexa intre tesutul adipos si tulburarile metabolicese masoara prin metode antropometrice. Circumferinta taliei este legata direct de adipozitatea intra-abdominala, iar modificarile circumferintei abdominale reflecta modificari ale factorilor de risc cardiovascular.

Metoda: Studiu de prevalenta efectuat pe un esantion cuprinzand 340 pacienti cu varste intre 20–60 ani, inscrisi pe lista unui medic de familie din municipiul Iasi. Variabilele luate in consideratie au fost circumferinta abdominala, raportul talie sold, Indicele de masa corporala (IMC), valorile tensiunii arteriale (TA), colesterolul total, LDH-C si LDL-C, varsta si stilul de viata.

Rezultate: Circumferinta abdominala mai mare de 94 cm la barbati si 80 cm la femei a identificat subiectii cu un IMC > 25 kg/m2 si un raport talie sold > 0,95 la femei si > 0,80 la barbati.

Valorile circumferintei abdominale (>94 cm si >80 cm) la barbatii si femeile care au cel putin un factor de risc (TA>160/95 mmHg) au prezentat o sensibilitate de 56% si respectiv 68% si o specificitate de 74%, respectiv 65%., comparativ cu cei la care valorile circumferintei abdominale s-au situat sub limitele mentionate (OR 2,4 95%CI 1,9-2,6 la barbati si OR 1,9 95%CI 1,6-2,3 la femei).

Concluzii. Valorile crescute ale circumferintei abdominale identifica acei pacienti care sunt la risc crescut cardiovascular.

Cuvinte cheie: Factori de risc cardiovascular, obezitate, circumferinta abdominala, LDH-Col, LDL-Col, stil de viata

Age Groups

| 20 | 60 |

Study of Physical Development of Children and Adolescents from Romania (0–18 years)

SDFC

Project Leader

Project Leader	Cordeanu Aurelia, Scientific researcher, University Professor
Address	Institute of Public Health, Dr. Leonte street, nr. 1–3, sect. 5 Bucharest
Executing Institution	Institute of Public Health, Bucharest
Funding Agency	Ministry of Public Health

Project Information

Start of Project	01/01/2006
End of Project	31/12/2008
Start of Data Collection	01/05/2006
End of Data Collection	30/06/2006
URL	
Scope	National

Keywords Physical development; Children

Abstract (English) This study's objective is the evaluation of physical development level of children and adolescents (0–18 years) from Romania, to elaborate national standards necessary for the assessment of the normal physical development. This study is part of a longitudinal study performed from 1950, at 7 years interval. The regular repeated examinations on sections permit the knowledge of changes in physical development level of young people from our country, correlated with external (environmental) factors, for statement and applying the specific measures for children and youths health promotion.

The measurable and ratable objectives are:

- The substantiation of physical development standards for population (0–18 years) through settling of the medium level value and the five zones of variability for a number of four somatic parameters (height, weight, waist circumference, cranial circumference) by age, sex, urban, and rural areas
- The dynamics of physical development in context of existence of acceleration or deceleration phenomena
- Variability of somatically development indices in relation with some social and regional aspects on children and adolescents
- The level of development for secondary sexual characteristics and dentition as indicators of biological maturation
- The level of main physiological parameters (muscular strength, vital capacity, blood pressure, pulse rate, blood group)

The work's objectives allow the elaboration of physical development informative tables, which will be used as reference marks for the diagnosis of individual development of Romanian children. The use of anthropometric data provides for the elaboration of measures to improve and raise the efficiency of medical assistance in children and adolescents. The methods of investigation as somatoscopy, somatometry, physiometry permit the assessment of somatic development, pubertal growth, the development of primary and permanent dentition; social research methods collect data, which will be analyzed through statistical methods. It has been formulated the hypothesis that the present level of physical development for children and adolescents and its characteristics, the variability of parameters, dynamics and trends of evolution reflect the life conditions and important socioeconomic transformation.

The study "Physical development of children and adolescents between 0 and 18 years from Romania" started in 1950 and repeated in 1957, 1964, 1971, 1978, 1985, and 1992 has revealed with extremely convincing data that the physical development level of our children and youth from our country suffer changes at all ages, showing a process of acceleration in the interval 1950–1985. It can be stated that the raising of average values of essential somatic parameters is obvious especially in rural areas. It maintains the differences of development among the research regions remains and significant differences between the average levels of these values for towns and big cities on the one hand and middle and small cities on the other hand have been found. The investigation accomplished in 1985 has revealed that the acceleration phenomenon become null or even negative (deceleration) at certain groups of age, with higher biological fragility. The pubertal growth leap appears now with 1 year and 7 months earlier than in 1950.

The comparative analysis of average height and weight curves "crossing" for boys and girls in prepubertal period indicates a shorting of interval between the two moments. The results of research allowed the elaboration of tables, which include the development data of children and adolescents from our country between 1992 and 1999. The following evaluation will take place in 2006.

Abstract (Original Language) Lucrarea are ca obiectiv evaluarea nivelului de dezvoltare fizica a copiilor si adolescentilor (0–18 ani) din România în vederea elaborarii standardelor nationale pentru aprecierea normalitatii dezvoltarii fizice si se va desfasura în cadrul unui studiu longitudinal efectuat din 1950 la interval de 7 ani.

Repetarea la intervale regulate a examinarilor pe sectiuni permite cunoasterea modificarilor nivelului dezvoltarii fizice a populatiei tinere din tara noastra în relatie cu factorii mezologici în vederea stabilirii si aplicarii masurilor specifice de promovare a starii de sanatate a copiilor si tinerilor.

- Obiectivele masurabile si evaluabile sunt reprezentate de:
- fundamentarea standardelor de dezvoltare fizica a populatiei (0–18 ani) prin stabilirea valorii nivelului mediu si a celor 5 zone de variabilitate, a patru parametri somatici (înaltime, greutate, perimetru toracic, circumferinta craniana) în raport cu vârsta, sexul, mediul urban, mediul rural;

- dinamica dezvoltarii fizice în contextul existentei fenomenului de acceleratie sau deceleratie;
- variabilitatea parametrilor de dezvoltare somatica în relatie cu unele aspecte sociale si regionale la copii si adolescenti
- nivelul dezvoltarii caracterelor sexuale secundare si a dentitiei ca indicatori ai maturizarii biologice.
- nivelul principalilor parametri fiziometrici (forta musculara, capacitatea vitala, tensiunea arteriala, puls, grupa sanguina)
- Obiectivele lucrarii permit elaborarea unor tabele orientative de dezvoltare fizica, ce vor fi folosite ca repere pentru stabilirea diagnosticului de dezvoltare individuala a copiilor din România.

Prin valorificarea datelor antropofiziometrice se pot elabora masuri de ameliorare si crestere a eficientei asistentei medicale în colectivitatile de copii si adolescenti.

- Metodele de investigare somatoscopie, somatometrie, fiziometrie, permit aprecierea dezvoltarii somatice, dezvoltarii puberale, dezvoltarii dentitiei temporare si a celei permanente; metodele de investigatie sociologica, culeg date consemnate în fise care vor fi prelucrate prin metode statistico-matematice.
- S-a formulat ipoteza ca nivelul actual al dezvoltarii fizice a copiilor si adolescentilor, particularitatile lui, variabilitatea parametrilor, dinamica si tendintele de evolutie reflecta conditiile de viata - transformarile profunde socio-economice.
- Cercetarea "Dezvoltarea fizica a copiilor si adolescentilor între 0–18 ani din România" începuta în 1950 si repetata în 1957, 1964, 1971, 1978, 1985 si 1992 a aratat cu date extrem de convingatoare ca nivelul dezvoltarii fizice a copiilor si tinerilor din tara noastra se modifica la toate vârstele, realizând un proces de acceleratie observat în perioada 1950–1985.
- Se poate afirma ca fenomenul de crestere a valorilor medii a parametrilor somatici de baza este evident îndeosebi în mediul rural.
- Se mentine decalajul de dezvoltare dintre regiunile de cercetare si s-au constatat diferente semnificative între nivelele medii ale acestor valori pentru municipii si orase mari fata de orasele mici si mijlocii.
- Investigarea efectuata în 1985 a aratat ca fenomenul de acceleratie devine nul sau chiar negativ (decelerare) la anumite grupe de vârsta, cu fragilitate biologica mai mare.
- Saltul de crestere puberal are loc în prezent cu 1 an si 7 luni mai devreme decât în 1950.

Analiza comparativa a "încrucisarii" curbelor înaltimii si greutatii medii a baietilor si fetelor în perioada prepubertara indica o scurtare a intervalului dintre cele doua momente.

Rezultatele cercetarii au permis elaborarea tabelelor cuprizând datele de dezvoltare a copiilor si adolescentilor din tara noastra în anul 1992 si 1999. Urmatoarea etapa se va desfasura în 2006.

Age Groups

Study on NUTRITIONAL STATUS of Children under 5 Years of Age

Project Leader

Project Leader	Ecaterina Stativa and Michaela Nanu; Project Director Alin Stanescu
Address	Lacul Tei Boulevard no. 120, 2 district
	Bucharest
Executing Institution	A study conducted by "Alfred Rusescu" Institute for Mother
	and Child Care in cooperation and with the support of the UNICEF
	Representative Office in Romania
Funding Agency	

Project Information

Start of Project	01/10/2003
End of Project	31/10/2005
Start of Data Collection	01/02/2004
End of Data Collection	31/07/2004
URL	
Scope	National

Keywords

Abstract (English) Children below 5-years of age are considered to be among the high risk groups. The goal of this survey was to assess the nutritional status of children in general, and particularly the status of iron and iodine micronutrients. The survey starts from the assumption that the child development status, right from the moment of birth, is a very useful indicator for assessing the nutrition status and some specific deficiencies. Health care services targeting these population groups have a major role to play in the early detection of and fight against nutritional disorders; such services should concentrate on monitoring the child's physical and mental development. The overall objectives of the survey were to assess the nutritional status of children under 5-years old, to assess some nutritional practices in the surveyed population, and to evaluate the contribution of health care services in preventing nutritional deficiencies.

Findings from the study:

Iron status:

- High prevalence of anemia in children below 5-years of age
- Higher prevalence in the rural area

Hemoglobin status: Among 12-months-old children, it was identified a higher prevalence of anemia with 59.3%, 14.2% of which with moderate anemia and 0.9% with severe anemia. For 2-years-old children the prevalence of anemia was 56.8% and for 59-months-old children 22.7%.

Growth status:

- High prevalence of infants with low birth weight
- Higher prevalence of low weight for height than in all the other previous surveys, because of some nutritional deficiencies affecting particularly the population aged 2- to 5-years old
- The higher prevalence of high weight for height feeding practices
- 92.2% from children were breast fed but 7.7% did not received human milk

Average time of exclusive breast feeding was 3.9 months and median time 3.2 months. Bottle feeding starts around the average age of 4.2 months.

Average age of weaning is 6.6 months. Average age of complementary food is 4 months.

On the basis of these findings, some recommendations regarding the prevention of iodine deficiency, anemia prevention, the improvement of anthropometric indicators, the development of social and health care integrated services and legislative aspects were made.

Abstract (Original Language) Copiii sub 5 ani sunt considerati printre grupele cu cel mai inalt grad de risc. Scopul acestei anchete a fost de a evalua statusul nutritional al copiilor in general, si in special statusul nutritional in ceea ce priveste aportul de fier si iod. Studiul a pornit de la premiza ca statusul de dezvoltare a copilului, chiar din momentul nasterii este cel mai util indicator pentru evaluarea statusului de nutritie si a unor deficiente specifice. Serviciile de sanatate care se adreseaza acestei grupe de varsta au un rol major in detectarea precoce si combaterea tulburarilor de nutritie; aceste servicii ar trebui sa se concentreze pe monitorizarea dezvoltarii fizice si psihice a copilului. Obiectivele generale ale studiului au fost: sa evalueze statusul nutritional al copiilor sub 5 ani; sa evalueze unele practici alimentare in randul populatiei studiate; sa evalueze contributia serviciilor de sanatate in prevenirea deficientelor nutritionale.

Rezultate:

statusul nutritional in ceea ce priveste fierul :

- prevalenta ridicata a anemiei la copilul sub 5 ani
- prevalenta mai mare in zonele rurale

statusul hemoglobinei : la copii de 12 luni s-a identificat o prevalenta mare a anemiei de 59.3% dintre care 14.2% cu anemie moderata iar 0.9% cu anemie severa. Pentru copiii de 2 ani, prevalenta anemiei a fost de 56.8% si pentru cei de 59 de luni, 22.7%.

statusul dezvoltarii fizice:

- prevalenta ridicata a copiilor cu greutate mica la nastere

- prevalenta mai crescuta fata de studiile anterioare a greutatii scazute fata de inaltime, datorata unor deficiente nutritionale ce afecteaza mai ales populatia de 2–5 ani
- prevalenta ridicata a greutatii crescute fata de inaltime de asemenea datorata unei diete dezechilibrate
- practici alimentare
- 92.2% dintre copii au fost hraniti la san, dar 7.7% un au primit lapte uman
- Durata medie a alaptatului exclusiv la san a fost de 3.9 luni iar durata mediana de 3.2 luni.
- Hranirea cu biberonul incepe la varsta medie de 4.2 luni.
- Varsta medie de intarcare este 6.6 luni.

Pe baza acestor rezultate s-au formulat o serie de recomandari referitor la prevenirea deficitului de iod, prevenirea anemiei, imbunatatirea indicilor antropometrici, dezvoltarea serviciilor sociale si de sanatate integrate si aspecte legislative.

Age Groups

Under 5-years old children:

- 3 months, 3 months plus 7 days
- 6 months, 6 months plus 7 days
- 12 months, 12 months plus 7 days
- 24 months, 24 months plus 7 days
- 36 months, 36 months plus 7 days
- 48 months, 48 months plus 7 days
- 59 months, 59 months plus 7 days

The impact of alcohol consumption on psychosomatic health status of adolescent pupils

Project Leader

Project Leader	Dr. Dumitrache Carmen
Address	Str. Dr. Leonte, nr.1–3, sector 5
	Bucuresti
Executing Institution	Institute of Public Health, Bucharest
Funding Agency	

Project Information

Start of Project	01/01/2001
End of Project	31/12/2005
Start of Data Collection	01/10/2001
End of Data Collection	15/10/2004
URL	
Scope	National

Keywords

Abstract (English) *Introduction:* The aim of this study is to evaluate the real proportion of the phenomena of the alcohol consumption of the teenagers. The process of physical growths are slow down between 14 and 19-years old but, regarding the neuro-psychological evolution, this time is the most intense period. Adolescence periods can become critical regarding social and educational conditions. Our sample consists of 952 pupils from high schools and technical schools.

For these reasons, questionnaires were applied to identify social and cultural data regarding the self-estimate of their health status, another data about the presence or the absence of risk factors, physiological, and pathological data. A general clinical evaluation was carried out, and physiological methods were used.

Results and commentaries:

- A sample comprised 952 pupils from 9th to 12th grade of the high schools and the first and the second grade of the technical schools
- The sample has the following structure: 819 pupils from high schools (86%) and 133 pupils from technical school (14%)
- The following distribution by sexes: 425 male (44.6%) and 527 female (55.4%)
- The alcohol consumption: 94.4% of them (occasional consumption 77.6%, daily consumption 2.1%, weekly consumption 9.1%, and monthly consumption 5.6%)
- Most of them has a starting point of the alcohol consumption around 13.6 years.
- Regarding their preferences we can notice that the teenagers accept almost all of the alcohol categories, and specially, 18.8% of them prefer spirits.
- We found the alcohol consumption without meal in 9.5% of them.

- 99% of the teenagers declare group consumption (with friends) or with their family (48.2%) but it must be noticed that there are also 7.3% of them who declare a solitary consumption
- 95.1% of them prefer to drink alcohol on Saturday and also on Sunday (50.1%)
- The average of alcohol quantity that they declare are around 100 ml and a maximum of 10 l
- 57.8% of those who declare the alcohol consumption recognized a "drunk" situation

Conclusions: The daily or the occasionally alcohol consumption due in the aim to establish a strong social relationship can be the beginning of a serious integration trouble for the teenagers. The phenomena can be found in both samples but mostly in those from high schools. The "pleasure" of the consumption among the friends or the family can produce a false sensation of wellness. This is why, sometimes, the familial model or the group model can be the risk factors for the mentioned behavior.

The society has to be involved in the "fight" for preventing and controlling of hazardous behaviors, by using all its influencing factors and action channels.

Abstract (Original Language) *Introducere:* Lucrarea de fata s-a nascut din necesitatea de a cunoaste la adevarata proportie fenomenul consumului de alcool în rândul adolescentilor. In grupa de vârsta 14–19 ani, procesele de dezvoltare somatica nu mai sunt atât de intense, însa în ceea ce priveste dezvoltarea neuro-psihica – aceasta este perioada cea mai intensa, care culmineaza cu momentul recunoasterii statutului de adult si integrarea în viata sociala. Adolescenta, poate fi transformata într-o perioada de criza numai în anumite conditii sociale si educationale negative. Lotul de adolescenti studiat este de 952 elevi cuprinsi în licee si scoli profesionale, cu vârste între 14 si 19 ani. Pentru a evalua consecintele negative imediate si îndepartate ale consumului de alcool asupra organismului adolescentilor s-au aplicat 4 fise ce urmaresc a identifica date de ordin social, material si cultural, date privind autoaprecierea starii de sanatate, date referitoare la prezenta sau absenta unor factori de risc, date personale fiziologice si patologice. S-a mai efectuat examen clinic general si s-au aplicat doua metode psihologice.

Rezultate si discutii

- Lotul de elevi totalizeaza un numar de 952 subiecti, elevi în clasele a IX-a, a X-a, a XI-a si a XII-a de liceu si anul I, respectiv II de scoala profesionala.
- Lotul este structurat în functie de institutia de învatamânt în care sunt cuprinsi respondentii astfel: din cei 952 de elevi, 819 sunt cuprinsi în institutii liceale – 86,0 %, iar 133 în scolii de arta si meserii – 14,0 %.
- Structura în functie de sexul respondentilor este urmatoarea: din cei 952 de elevi, 425 sunt de sex masculin – 44,6 %, restul 527 sunt de sex feminin – 55,4 %.

- Consuma alcool – 94,4 % dintre adolescenti; acestia se impart pe consumatori ocazionali 77,6 %; consumatori zilnici 2,1 %; consumatori de fiecare saptamâna 9,1 %; consumatori de fiecare luna 5,6 %.
- Vârsta de incepere a consumului de alcool - vârsta medie se situeaza la 13,6 ani.
- Preferintele exprimate au atins intreaga plaja de bauturi alcoolice – 18,8 % consuma distilate.
- Consumul pe stomacul gol (inainte de masa) este prezent la 9,5 % dintre consumatorii de alcool.
- Adolescentii consuma alcool cu prietenii 99,0 %, sau cu familia 48,2 %, cu altii-oricine 13,3 %, dar si singuri 7,3 %.
- Ziua cea mai solicitata pentru "o bauta" ramâne sâmbata folosita de 95,1 % dintre adolescenti pentru a se relaxa in prezenta "unui" pahar cu alcool; nici duminica nu se situeaza foarte departe – 50,1 %.
- Cantitatea de alcool consumata odata variaza intre 100 ml si un maxim de 10 litri.
- La intrebarea "te-ai imbatat" din cei care au declarat ca sunt consumatori de alcool, 57,8 % afirma ca au cunoscut starea de betie, macar odata.

Concluzii: Acest comportament adoptat ocazional sau zilnic pentru a obtine o mai buna integrare sociala ii arunca cu brutalitate pe adolescenti in complexe tulburari de adaptare. Fenomenul este prezent la ambele loturi, dar in proportii mai crescute la elevii de liceu."Placerea" consumului este cu atât mai ingrijoratoare cu cât ea ofera o falsa stare de bine alaturi de prieteni si familie; modelul familial ca si modelul grupului sunt factori de risc care induc comportamentul imitativ. Trebuie antrenata societatea prin toate componentele si canalele sale de actiune in lupta pentru preventia si combaterea comportamentelor cu risc.

Age Groups

14	14
15	15
16	16
17	17
18	18
19	19

Slovenia

CINDI Health Monitor for Slovenia 2001

CHMS SI 2001

Project Leader

Project Leader	Lijana Zaletel-Kragelj
Address	Medical Faculty, Department of Public Health
	Zaloska 4
	SI-1000 Ljubljana
	Slovenia
Executing Institution	University of Ljubljana, Medical Faculty, Department of Public Health
Funding Agency	Ministry of Health of the Republic of Slovenia, Ministry
	of Education,Science and Sports of the Republic
	of Slovenia, CINDI Slovenia

Project Information

Start of Project	15/05/2001
End of Project	30/06/2004
Start of Data Collection	15/05/2001
End of Data Collection	15/05/2001
URL	http://www.javnozdravje.net
Scope	National

Keywords CINDI; Survey; Lifestyle; Risk factors; Cardiovascular diseases

Abstract (English) This survey is conceptually a part of a wider international project in the frame of the WHO CINDI programme. A stratified random sample was drawn from the central population registry of Slovenia. The sampling was performed by the Statistical Office of Slovenia. A self-administered postal questionnaire was used, on the basis of the CHM Core Questionnaire. The response rate was increased by reminding nonrespondents twice (the first reminder contained a new questionnaire form whereas the second was only a new invitation letter) and by a lottery with prizes associated with healthy behavior (visits to health resorts, bicycles, etc.). An extensive media campaign was also mounted at national and regional levels. The total sample sizes were about 15,350, and the age range was 25–64 years. The response rate was 64% (about 9,600 participants).

The questions on behavioral risk factors included several questions on nutrition and physical activity.

Abstract (Original Language) Slovenija se je z raziskavami "Dejavniki tveganja za nenalezljive bolezni pri odraslih prebivalcih Slovenije" v letu 2001 vključila v krog držav, ki spremljajo vedenjski slog odraslih prebivalcev pod okriljem

CINDI pri SZO na nacionalni ravni. Metodologija je bila zastavljena enako kot del širšega mednarodnega projekta CINDI Health Monitor, zato jo imenujemo tudi CINDI Health Monitor za Slovenijo (CHMS SI). Povzeta je po projektu Finbalt Health Monitor. Kljucni nosilec aktivnosti je Katedra za javno zdravje Medicinske fakultete Univerze v Ljubljani, natancneje njen Oddelek za socialno medicino, skupaj s CINDI Slovenije in vsemi devetimi obmocnimi Zavodi za zdravstveno varstvo (ZZV). Slovenija se drži mednarodnih priporocil kolikor se da, kljub temu pa je v družini držav, ki izvajajo tovrstne raziskave, nekaj posebnega. Ker se že dolga leta govori, da zdravje prebivalcev Slovenije ni enako na celotnem obmocju, smo želeli s prvo raziskavo tipa CHM cim bolj natancno ovrednotiti, ali to drži za BSŽ in njihove dejavnike tveganja. Ker smo stremeli k reprezentativnim vzorcem tudi na obmocni ravni, smo imeli skupno število vabljenih v raziskavo vec kot 15.300. Samo zbiranje podatkov je bilo relativno zelo uspešno, saj je bila odzivnost v povprecju 64 %, v najuspešnejši regiji pa celo vec kot 75 %. Za analizo je bilo po vseh preverjanjih uporabnih nekaj vec kot 9.000 vprašalnikov, kar je 3-krat vec, kot so mednarodne zahteve. Vzorec udeležencev se je rahlo razlikoval od populacije po spolu, ni pa se razlikoval v starostni strukturi in strukturi velikosti naselij, iz katerih so prišli udeleženci.

Age Groups

25	29
30	39
40	49
50	59
60	64

CINDI Risk Factor /Process Evaluation Surveys

CINDI RF/PE SI

Project Leader

Project Leader	Jožica Maucec Zakotnik
Address	CINDI Slovenia
	Ulica stare pravde 2
	SI-1000 Ljubljana
	Slovenia
Executing Institution	CINDI Slovenia
Funding Agency	CINDI Slovenia

Project Information

Start of Project	01/01/1990
End of Project	31/03/2003
Start of Data Collection	01/01/1990
End of Data Collection	01/01/1990
URL	http://www.cindi-slovenija.net/raziskave/
Scope	National

Keywords CINDI; Noncommunicable diseases; Risk factors

Abstract (English) Three consecutive cross-sectional surveys, all performed from late autumn to early spring 1990/1991, 1996/1997, and 2002/2003 were carried out in the Ljubljana demonstrational area. All local communities covered by the Community Health Center Ljubljana participated (Brezovica, Dobrova-Polhov Gradec, Dol pri Ljubljani, Grosuplje, Horjul, Ig, Ljubljana, Medvode, Škofljica, Velike Lašce, and Vodice). The simple random samples were drawn from the Central Population Registry, slightly corrected in gender and age (men and younger age groups were slightly overrepresented), to assure that the gender/age distribution of respondents would be similar to the general population distribution as much as possible. The age range was 25–64 years. The sample sizes were 2.436, 2.180, and 2.643, respectively. The sampling was performed by the Statistical Office of the Republic of Slovenia. People were invited to participate in the survey by an invitation letter explaining its rationale and describing its course. The response rates were in 1990/1991: 69.5% (1,692 participants), in 1996/1997: 61.6% (1,342 participants), and in 2002/2003: 52.0% (1,375 participants).

The questions on behavioural risk factors included several questions on nutrition and physical activity.

Abstract (Original Language) Med osnovne dejavnosti mednarodnega programa CINDI sodijo tudi raziskave dejavnikov tveganja in ucinkovitosti ukrepov programa CINDI (CINDI Risk Factors and Process Evaluation Survey)

(CINDI-RF/PES) [8]. Te raziskave imajo, kot že ime samo pove, vec namenov. Na eni strani naj bi se z njimi sledilo gibanju vedenjskih in bioloških dejavnikov tveganja prebivalcev za nenalezljive bolezni, predvsem BSŽ v casu, po drugi strani pa bi se z njimi vrednotila ucinkovitost aktivnosti programa CINDI. Raziskave na splošno potekajo tako, da udeleženci ob pomoci posebej izšolanega izpraševalca najprej izpolnijo vprašalnik o svojih navadah glede kajenja, prehranjevanja, uživanja alkoholnih pijac in gibanja. Dodatno vprašalnik zajema še vprašanja o tem, kje udeleženci dobilo informacije o zdravem nacinu življenja ter še nekatera druga vprašanja. Med njimi so tudi vprašanja o prebolelih boleznih, katerih odgovori pa so podvrženi pristranosti spominjanja. Sledi klinicni pregled, ki je sestavljen iz klinicnega opazovanja, ki ga izvajajo zdravniki in klinicnih meritev, ki jih izvajajo medicinske sestre (npr. meritve krvnega tlaka in telesne teže ipd.). Na koncu sledijo še laboratorijske preiskave krvnega seruma (npr. celokupnega, HDL- in LDL-holesterola, krvnega sladkorja ipd.) [8]. S temi raziskavami naj bi vsaka država, ki pristopi k programu CINDI, najprej naredila posnetek stanja BSŽ, nato pa sledila spremembam v prebivalstvu na približno vsakih pet let. V raziskavo takšne vrste naj bi bilo zajetih vsaj 1.600 udeležencev.

Nosilec raziskav CINDI-RF/PES v Sloveniji je CINDI Slovenije, od sredine devetdesetih let samostojna enota Zdravstvenega doma Ljubljana.

Age Groups

25	29
30	34
35	39
40	44
45	49
50	54
55	59
60	64

Spain

Continued Household Budget Survey

CHBS

Project Leader

Project Leader	
Address	Paseo de la Castellana, 183
	28071-Madrid
	Spain
Executing Institution	National Statistics Institute
Funding Agency	

Project Information

Start of Project	14/09/1958
End of Project	14/09/2006
Start of Data Collection	14/09/2006
End of Data Collection	14/09/2006
URL	http://www.ine.es/
Scope	National

Keywords Private homes; Consumption; Expenses; Household Budget Survey; Spain

Abstract (English) It offers information about consumer expenditures of private homes, estimations of the level and the structure of the annual consumption of homes, and estimations of the quarterly expense of homes.

Abstract (Original Language)

Age Groups

The study involves families.

Dislipemy, Obesity, and Heart Risk study

DORICA

Project Leader

Project Leader	Javier Aranceta
Address	Community Nutrition Unit
	Department of Public Health
	Bilbao
	Spain
Executing Institution	
Funding Agency	

Project Information

Start of Project	13/09/1990
End of Project	13/09/2000
Start of Data Collection	13/09/1990
End of Data Collection	13/09/1990
URL	
Scope	National

Keywords

Abstract (English)

The principal aims of the study are to know the prevalence of global cardiovascular risk factors in the Spanish population and to analyze the impact of the obesity on the above-mentioned factors.

Abstract (Original Language)

Age Groups

25	34
35	44
45	54
55	64

Epidemiología de la obesidad en la edad infantil y juvenil

EnKid

Project Leader

Project Leader	Javier Aranceta Bartrina
Address	Luis Briñas 18, 4th floor
	48013-Bilbao
	Spain
Executing Institution	
Funding Agency	

Project Information

Start of Project	07/09/2006
End of Project	07/09/2006
Start of Data Collection	01/05/1998
End of Data Collection	01/05/1998
URL	
Scope	National

Keywords Children; Youth; Obesity; Food habits; Physical activity; Spain

Abstract (English) The enKid Study was designed to evaluate the food habits and nutritional status of Spanish children and young people and their relationship to sociodemographic and lifestyle factors.

Abstract (Original Language)

Age Groups

2	5
6	9
10	14
15	19
20	24

National Health Survey Spain

NHSS

Project Leader

Project Leader	
Address	Paseo de la Castellana, 183
	28071-Madrid
	Spain
Executing Institution	National Statistics Institute
Funding Agency	Ministry of Health and Consumption

Project Information

Start of Project	14/09/1987
End of Project	14/09/2006
Start of Data Collection	14/09/2006
End of Data Collection	14/09/2006
URL	http://www.ine.es/
Scope	National

Keywords Health Survey; Spain; Autoevaluation

Abstract (English) It is a survey of national area realized by the Ministry of Health and Consumption in the Spanish population. The first one is carried out in 1987 and the last one in 2003. It is a health measurement instrument that gathers information on the health condition of the Spanish population and studies them throughout the time.

Abstract (Original Language)

Age Groups

The age groups are described in two groups. One, younger than 15 years and the other 15 years and older.

Patrón de consumo alimentario actual en España

eVe

Project Leader

Project Leader	Javier Aranceta
Address	Community Nutrition Unit
	Department of Public Health
	Bilbao
	Spain
Executing Institution	
Funding Agency	

Project Information

Start of Project	13/09/1990
End of Project	13/09/1999
Start of Data Collection	13/09/1990
End of Data Collection	13/09/1990
URL	
Scope	National

Keywords Vitamin intake; Food pattern; Spain

Abstract (English) It is a pooled analysis of cross-sectional population nutritional regional studies and metaanalysis of smaller studies in population subgroups performed in Spain between 1990 and 1999. The aim is to describe vitamin intakes in Spanish food patterns, identify groups at risk for inadequacy, and determine conditioning factors that may influence this situation.

Abstract (Original Language)

Age Groups

25	60

Spanish Society for the study of Obesity

SEEDO Study

Project Leader

Project Leader	Javier Aranceta
Address	Community Nutrition Unit, Department of Public Health, Municipality of Bilbao,
	Luis Briñas 18, 4th floor
	48013-Bilbao
	Spain
Executing Institution	
Funding Agency	

Project Information

Start of Project	22/09/1990
End of Project	22/09/2000
Start of Data Collection	22/09/2006
End of Data Collection	22/09/2006
URL	http://www.seedo.es/
Scope	National

Keywords

Abstract (English) The main objetive of the study is to analyse the influence of social and cultural factors in the prevalence of obesity in the Spanish adult population aged 25–60.

Abstract (Original Language)

Age Groups

25	60

Study of Food Consumption

Food Consumption

Project Leader

Project Leader	
Address	Subdirección General de Industrias, Comercialización y Distribución Agroalimentaria
	Infanta Isabel 1-2nd floor
	Madrid
	Spain
Executing Institution	Department of Agriculture, Fishing and Nourishment
Funding Agency	

Project Information

Start of Project	14/09/1987
End of Project	14/09/2006
Start of Data Collection	14/09/2006
End of Data Collection	14/09/2006
URL	http://www.mapa.es/
Scope	National

Keywords Food consumption; Private homes; Commercial and social restoration; Spain

Abstract (English) From 1987, the Department of Agriculture, Fishing, and Nourishment, across the current "Dirección General de Industria Agroalimentaria y Alimentación," takes as one of its aims the study of food consumption in homes (monthly), and in establishments of commercial and social restoration (quarterly) in Spain on the basis of surveys carried out among the consumers and persons in charge of buys of the above-mentioned establishments.The information is offered from 1987 until 2006 month a month and accumulated.

Abstract (Original Language)

Age Groups

The study involves private homes and restoration establishments.

White Book of Elderly People's Nutrition

White book

Project Leader

Project Leader	Mercedes Muñoz Hornillos
Address	Human Nutrition and Dietetic
	Fisiology and Nutrition Department
	University of Navarre
Executing Institution	University of Navarre
Funding Agency	

Project Information

Start of Project	14/09/2003
End of Project	14/09/2003
Start of Data Collection	14/06/2003
End of Data Collection	14/06/2003
URL	
Scope	National

Keywords Nutrition; Food Habits; Health; Elderly; Spain

Abstract (English) This book has two aims: to check the variables that come together in the nourishment and health of the elderly and to evaluate the food habits of the elderly Spanish population across an epidemiological nutritional study realized to 60-year-old major persons.

Abstract (Original Language)

Age Groups

60	69
70	79
80	999

Sweden

Community-Based Study of Physical Activity, Life Style, and Self-Esteem in Swedish School Children

COMPASS

Project Leader

Project Leader	Carin Bokedal
Address	Statens folkhälsoinstitut
	Swedish National Institute of Public Health
	Olof Palmes gata 17
	SE-103 52 Stockholm
	Sweden
Executing Institution	Swedish National Institute of Public Health
Funding Agency	Stockholms läns landsting in corporation with Samhällsmedicin and Statens folkhälsoinstitut

Project Information

Start of Project	01/9/2000
End of Project	01/06/2002
Start of Data Collection	01/09/2000
End of Data Collection	01/06/2002
URL	http://www.fhi.se/templates/Page____1237.aspx
Scope	National

Keywords

Abstract (English) The foundations for people's physical and mental health are laid in childhood. Secure and favorable conditions during childhood and adolescence, good eating habits, and increased physical activity are three of the 11 public health objectives set by the Swedish Parliament in 2003 as part of a new public health policy. It was determined that special attention should be paid to the mental health of children and young people, and to their health behaviors.

The investigation called the "Community-based study of physical activity, life-style, and self-esteem in Swedish school children" (COMPASS) was embarked upon in 2000. Its aim was to survey and analyze the relations among young people's level of physical activity, their self-esteem, eating habits, body size, ethnicity, and socioeconomic circumstances. Further investigated were how body size, level of physical activity and eating habits related to circumstances in the family, the school, participation in organized and unorganized sports, geographic area and infrastructure, and also to policy and decisions made at the municipality level. The target group for COMPASS comprised all boys and girls in School Year 8, starting autumn 2000, and in School Year 9, starting autumn 2001, in municipal schools in south-west Greater Stockholm. Data collection proceeded from the autumn of 2000 through to the spring of 2002.The study covered the municipalities of Botkyrka, Huddinge, Nykvarn, Salem and Södertälje, and the submunicipal administrations of Hägersten, Liljeholmen, Skärholmen and Älvsjö, all within Stockholm County.

Data for this school-based study were gathered from registers, questionnaires administered to pupils, a questionnaire to school personnel, and a questionnaire to officers with responsibility for policy and planning of services within municipalities and submunicipal administrations.The adolescents also participated in a health examination, from which information on body measurements and quantity of body fat was obtained. The target group consisted of 4,188 pupils from all 44 municipal schools in the study area. For 3,142 (75%) of these individuals, there was full information concerning physical activity and body mass index (BMI).The study group comprised 3,142 adolescents, and for 2,604 of whom there was complete information on an overall scale measuring self-esteem.The mean age was 15.2 years. Educational level of the mother was used as a measure of socioeconomic position. The participation rate was somewhat greater among adolescents with a higher educated mother than among the offspring of a mother with lower education.

11.2% of the girls and 14.5% of the boys were found to be overweight, and 3.3% of girls and 3.7% of boys were obese. Obesity was more than three times as common among girls with a lower educated mother than among those with a higher educated mother; for boys, it was almost twice as common for those with a lower educated mother. Adolescents of Swedish background were overweight or obese to a lesser extent than those with a foreign or immigrant background. 14.6% of young people with an immigrant background and 14.6% of those with a foreign background were overweight, which can be compared with a proportion of 11.7% among adolescents of Swedish origin. Obesity was also found to be more common among adolescents of foreign background (4.6%), and of immigrant background (4.4%), than among those of Swedish origin (2.8%).

Girls and boys were sedentary for, on average, 4.6 and 4.9 h, respectively, during weekdays after school. Both boys and girls watched TV or video for an average of 2.1 h per day on weekdays. Young people with a lower educated mother, those in cramped accommodation, and those with immigrant background devoted the most time to sedentary activities. There were substantial intergroup differences in terms of TV/video watching, which may be a significant cause of low personal energy expenditure. For boys with a lower educated mother or with an immigrant background, higher body weight was not explained by less physical activity. On average, boys from these groups showed higher energy expenditure, measured in terms of undertaking moderate and vigorous physical activity, than boys with a higher educated mother or boys with a Swedish background.

Similar socioeconomic and ethnic differences with regard to physical activity were not observed among girls. 64% of girls and 78% of boys achieved the recommended 60 minutes of at least moderate physical activity per day. However, these figures are somewhat uncertain, since – as demonstrated in the validation study – it is difficult accurately to measure the time spent in moderate physical activity. Being involved in organized sports and being physically active in unorganized forms was a good indicator of reaching the recommended activity level.

16.6% of the young people reported that they never walked or cycled to school, and 16.3% reported that they never walked or cycled during leisure time. 4.7% stated that they never walked or cycled either to and from school or during leisure time. Transport to and from school may act as an important supplement to everyday physical activity. Accordingly, the municipality units responsible should formulate objectives to encourage all children and adolescents who are able to walk or cycle to school to actually do so, and to make efforts to identify and remove any obstacles.

On average, boys were considerably more active during physical education classes than girls. The schools should therefore focus more on girls' needs and wishes in physical education, and also make greater efforts in relation to pupils showing a low level of activity.

Summary: During school days most young people had lunch in the school canteen (87.2%), but the proportion was higher among children with a higher rather than a lower educated mother. Young people of Swedish origin more often ate in the school canteen than those with a foreign or immigrant background. A weak positive association was found between the proportion of pupils that liked and ate school meals and the application of the National Food Administration's guidelines for school lunches. Accordingly, the schools should apply these guidelines. In the study, girls were found to have more irregular eating habits than boys. Only two-thirds of girls had breakfast 4 or 5 days a school week, compared with three-quarters of boys. Young people from homes with a lower educated mother, low incomes, and smaller dwellings showed more irregular eating habits than those from homes with better socioeconomic conditions. Adolescents of Swedish origin had more regular eating habits than those with a foreign or immigrant background. Young people who had breakfast on a regular basis took fewer unhealthy snacks between main meals than those who did not, and also watched TV/video to a lesser extent. Also, those who achieved the recommended level of 60 min physical activity of at least a moderate intensity level per day had more regular breakfast habits than others. Overweight and obese youth showed more irregular breakfast habits, and also more irregular eating habits, in general, than the others. The schools should consider offering breakfast to children and adolescents in need of it.

Girls, especially those with a higher educated mother, made a healthier food selection than boys, and more often ate fruit and vegetables. 37.3% of girls and 27.8% of boys ate fruit or vegetables every day. Of the girls, only 11.4% ate both fruit and vegetables every day, and for boys the proportion was as low as 7.9%. This means that only 10% of the young people covered by the study could have reached the recommended level of eating 500 g of fruit and vegetables per day, which is an alarmingly low proportion. Offering fruit at school might increase young people's intake substantially. The dietary patterns of adolescents were analyzed, and three components were identified: "unhealthy food," "healthy food," and "traditional food." Adolescents with a lower educated mother ate "unhealthy food," consisting largely of food items low in nutrients with a high energy density, twice as often as those with a higher educated mother. Girls with a higher educated mother ate "healthy food" more often than the others. When intake of "unhealthy food" was examined among young people of various ethnicities, it was found that a high intake of food of this kind was more common among those with a foreign or an immigrant background.

There are reasons for municipalities and schools to consider how the availability of unhealthy food can be restricted within publicly run services for children and adolescents.

It is known from previous studies that self-esteem is related to mental health. It was found in this study that girls had lower self-esteem than boys, and that the lowest score was on the "psychological well-being" subscale. Adolescents with low self-esteem were found to be more sedentary and less physically active than those with high self-esteem. Those with high selfesteem more often ate "healthy food," whereas those with low self-esteem had more irregular eating habits than the others. Further, boys with low self-esteem had a higher mean BMI and a greater waist circumference than those with high self-esteem.Young people who were overweight or obese showed lower self-esteem than the others, and those who were content with their body size showed higher self-esteem than those who were discontent.

Although this cross-sectional study cannot give definite answers about casuality, there are grounds for believing that poor and irregular eating habits in combination with a sedentary life style (in front of the TV or video) seem to be important factors contributing to the social and ethnic differences in obesity. A low level of physical activity contributes to such differences to only a small extent, or even not at all, but is a problem for all socioeconomic groups. It is likely that low self-esteem gives rise to poor health behaviors.

The COMPASS study has identified a number of factors related to eating habits and physical activity among adolescents. Although the design of the study does not permit far-reaching conclusions to be drawn about causality, it is known from other studies that there are health determinants at all levels of society – ranging from the individual, through the family and school, to the local community's environment and policies. Accordingly, prevention of overweight and obesity should follow an integrated approach across several different levels.The recommendations in this report are relevant at all these levels, and may provide a good foundation for the planning of future efforts designed to promote healthy eating habits and physical activity among the young.

Abstract (Original Language) Människors fysiska och psykiska hälsa grundläggs i barndomen.Trygga och goda uppväxtvillkor, goda matvanor och ökad fysisk aktivitet, är tre av de elva folkhälsomål som riksdagen antog under 2003 i den nya folkhälsopolitiken. Den psykiska ohälsan bland barn och ungdomar ska uppmärksammas, liksom utvecklingen av barns och ungdomars levnadsvanor.

År 2000 initierades studien COMPASS ("Community-based study of physical activity, life style and self-esteem in Swedish school children"). Studien syftade till att kartlägga och analysera relationerna mellan ungdomars fysiska aktivitet och deras självkänsla, matvanor, kroppsstorlek, etnicitet och socioekonomiska förhållanden.Vidare undersöktes hur fysisk aktivitet och matvanor relaterade till familjeförhållanden, skolan, föreningslivet, geografiskt område och infrastruktur samt kommunalpolitiska beslut i relation till detta.

Målgruppen för COMPASS-studien var alla pojkar och flickor som gick i årskurs 8 hösten 2000 eller årskurs 9 hösten 2001 i kommunala skolor i sydvästra Storstockholm. Datainsamlingen pågick från hösten 2000 till våren 2002. Följande kommuner och stadsdelar inom Stockholms stad ingår i studien: Botkyrka, Huddinge, Nykvarn, Salem och Södertälje samt Hägersten, Liljeholmen, Skärholmen och Älvsjö.

Informationen till denna skolbaserade studie hämtades från register, elevenkäter, en enkät till skolpersonal och en enkät till tjänstemän med planeringsansvar inom kommuner och stadsdelar. Ungdomarna medverkade också i en hälsoundersökning där uppgifter om kroppsmått och mängden kroppsfett samlades in. I målgruppen ingick 4 188 ungdomar från samtliga 44 kommunala skolor i studieområdet. För 3 142 (75 %) av ungdomarna finns kompletta uppgifter om fysisk aktivitet och kroppsmasseindex (BMI) och dessa utgör studiepopulationen. För 2 604 av dessa finns kompletta uppgifter om totalskalan för självkänsla. Genomsnittsåldern var 15,2 år. Som ett mått på socioekonomisk ställning valdes moderns utbildningsnivå. Deltagandet i studien var något högre bland ungdomar med högutbildade mödrar än bland dem med lågutbildade mödrar.

11,2 % av flickorna och 14,5 % av pojkarna var överviktiga. Fetma förekom hos 3,3 % av flickorna och 3,7 % av pojkarna. Fetma var mer än tre gånger så vanligt bland flickor med lågutbildade mödrar som bland flickor med högutbildade mödrar, medan det för pojkar var nästan dubbelt så vanligt bland dem med lågutbildade mödrar. Ungdomar med svensk bakgrund var i mindre utsträckning överviktiga och feta, jämfört med ungdomar med Fysisk aktivitet, matvanor, övervikt och självkänsla bland ungdomar 8 utländsk respektive invandrarbakgrund. 14,6 % av ungdomarna med invandrarbakgrund och 14,6 % av dem med utländsk bakgrund var överviktiga, jämfört med 11,7 % av ungdomarna med svensk bakgrund. Fetma var också vanligare hos ungdomar med utländsk bakgrund (4,6 %) och med invandrarbakgrund (4,4 %) än bland ungdomar med svensk bakgrund (2,8 %).

Flickor och pojkar var stillasittande i genomsnitt 4,6 timmar respektive 4,9 timmar per dag på vardagarna efter skoltid. Både flickor och pojkar tittade i genomsnitt på tv/video 2,1 timmar per dag på vardagar. Ungdomar med lågutbildade mödrar och från trångbodda hem samt ungdomar med invandrarbakgrund ägnade mest tid åt stillasittande aktiviteter. Skillnaderna var markanta för tv-/videotittande som kan vara en betydelsefull orsak till låg energiförbrukning. För pojkar med lågutbildade mödrar respektive med invandrarbakgrund förklaras den högre kroppsvikten inte av mindre fysisk aktivitet. Pojkar från dessa grupper hade i genomsnitt högre energiförbrukning på måttlig och hård fysisk aktivitet än pojkar med högutbildade mödrar respektive pojkar med svensk bakgrund. Motsvarande socioekonomiska och etniska skillnader i fysisk aktivitet sågs inte för flickorna. 64 % av flickorna och 78 % av pojkarna klarade rekommendationen om 60 minuter fysisk aktivitet på minst måttlig nivå per dag. Dessa siffror är dock något osäkra, eftersom det är svårt att mäta tiden för måttlig fysisk aktivitet med stor precision, vilket visades i valideringsstudien. Att vara aktiv i någon idrottsförening och fysiskt aktiv på egen hand var en bra markör på om man klarade rekommendationen för fysisk aktivitet.

16,6 % av ungdomarna angav att de aldrig går eller cyklar till skolan och 16,3 % att de aldrig cyklar eller går på fritiden. 4,7 % av ungdomarna angav att de aldrig går eller cyklar vare sig till skolan eller på fritiden.Transport till och från skolan kan ge ett viktigt tillskott till vardaglig fysisk aktivitet. Därför borde kommunerna formulera mål om att alla barn och ungdomar som kan gå eller cykla till skolan verkligen gör det. Pojkar var i genomsnitt betydligt mer fysiskt aktiva på idrottslektionerna än flickor. Skolorna bör därför fokusera mer på flickornas behov och önskemål i idrottsundervisningen och satsa mer på de lågaktiva eleverna.

På skoldagar åt de flesta av ungdomarna i studien lunch i skolmatsalen (87,2 %), men fler av dem med högutbildade mödrar åt lunch i skolmatsalen än av dem med lågutbildade mödrar. Ungdomar med svensk bakgrund åt oftare i skolmatsalen än dem med utländsk eller invandrarbakgrund. Det fanns ett visst positivt samband mellan andelen ungdomar som gillade och åt skolmaten och användandet av Livsmedelsverkets riktlinjer för skollunchen. Skolorna bör följa riktlinjerna. Flickorna i studien hade mer oregelbundna måltidsvanor än pojkarna. Endast två tredjedelar av flickorna åt frukost 4–5 dagar under en skolvecka, jämfört med tre fjärdedelar av pojkarna. Ungdomar från hem med lågut- Smmanfattning 9 bildade mödrar, lägre inkomster och mindre bostäder hade mer oregelbundna måltidsvanor än ungdomar från hem med bättre socioekonomiska förhållanden. Ungdomar med svensk bakgrund hade mer regelbundna måltidsvanor än ungdomar med utländsk eller invandrarbakgrund. Ungdomar med regelbundna frukostvanor åt färre onyttiga mellanmål än dem med oregelbundna frukostvanor och tittade också mindre på tv/video. Ungdomar som klarade rekommendationen om 60 minuter fysisk aktivitet på minst måttlig nivå per dag hade också mer regelbundna frukostvanor än övriga. Överviktiga och feta ungdomar hade mer oregelbundna frukostvanor och överhuvudtaget mer oregelbundna måltidsvanor än de övriga. Skolorna bör överväga att erbjuda frukost till barn och ungdomar i behov av detta. Flickorna, speciellt de med högutbildade mödrar, hade nyttigare livsmedelsval än pojkarna och åt oftare frukt och grönsaker. 37,3 % av flickorna och 27,8 % av pojkarna åt frukt eller grönsaker varje dag. Av flickorna åt bara 11,4 % både frukt och grönsaker varje dag, och endast 7,9 % av pojkarna gjorde det. Detta innebär att högst 10 % av ungdomarna i studien hade möjlighet att nå rekommendationen att äta 500 gram frukt och grönsaker per dag, vilket är alarmerande lågt. Genom att erbjuda frukt i skolorna skulle ungdomarnas intag kunna öka betydligt. Ungdomarnas kostmönster analyserades, och tre komponenter identifierades:

- "onyttig mat", "nyttig mat" och "traditionell mat". Ungdomar med
- lågutbildade mödrar åt dubbelt så ofta "onyttig mat", som i huvudsak
- bestod av näringsfattiga och energitäta livsmedel, jämfört med dem med
- högutbildade mödrar. Flickor med högutbildade mödrar åt oftare "nyttig
- mat" än övriga. När intag av "onyttig mat" undersöktes bland ungdomar
- med olika etnisk bakgrund fann man att ett högt intag var vanligare bland
- dem med utländsk respektive invandrarbakgrund. Det finns anledning för

- kommuner och skolor att överväga hur tillgängligheten av onyttiga livsmedel
- kan begränsas i offentlig verksamhet för barn och ungdomar.
- Från tidigare studier vet man att självkänsla är relaterad till psykisk hälsa.
- I denna studie hade flickorna lägre självkänsla än pojkarna. Lägst värde hade
- ungdomarna på delskalan "psykiskt välmående". Ungdomar med låg självkänsla
- var mer stillasittande och mindre fysiskt aktiva än dem med hög självkänsla.

Ungdomar med hög självkänsla åt oftare "nyttig mat" och ungdomar med låg självkänsla hade mer oregelbundna måltidsvanor än övriga. Pojkar med låg självkänsla hade dessutom högre BMI och större midjeomfångän dem med hög självkänsla. Ungdomar med övervikt och fetma hade lägre självkänsla än övriga, och ungdomar som var nöjda med sin kroppsstorlek hade högre självkänsla än ungdomar som var missnöjda.

Även om denna tvärsnittsstudie inte kan ge definitiva svar om orsakssamband finns fog för bedömningen att dåliga och oregelbundna matvanor i kombination med stillasittande framför tv:n eller videon är viktiga faktorer bakom de sociala och etniska skillnaderna i fetma. Låg fysisk aktivitet Fysisk aktivitet, matvanor, övervikt och självkänsla bland ungdomar 10 bidrar mindre eller inte alls till dessa skillnader utan är ett problem i alla samhällsgrupper. Det är troligt att låg självkänsla orsakar dåliga levnadsvanor.

I COMPASS-studien har ett antal faktorer identifierats som har samband med matvanor och fysisk aktivitet bland ungdomar.Även om studiens uppläggning inte tillåter långtgående slutsatser om orsakssamband, vet man från andra studier att påverkande faktorer finns på alla nivåer – från den individuella, till familjen och skolan och till lokalsamhällets fysiska miljö och policy. Åtgärder för att minska övervikt bland ungdomar bör därför bestå av integrerade insatser på flera olika nivåer. Rekommendationerna i denna rapport rör alla dessa nivåer och kan vara en bra grund för planeringen av framtida insatser för goda matvanor och fysisk aktivitet bland ungdomar.

Age Groups

Different Conditions – Different Health. A Study of Immigrants from Chile, Poland, Iran, and Turkey

SoS

Project Leader

Project Leader	Kerstin Wigzell
Address	Socialstyrelsen
	106 30 Stockholm
	Sweden
Executing Institution	The National Board of Health and Welfare
Funding Agency	The National Board of Health and Welfare and The National Public
	Health Institute, the Swedish Migration Board

Project Information

Start of Project	01/01/1996
End of Project	31/12/1996
Start of Data Collection	01/01/1996
End of Data Collection	31/12/1996
URL	
Scope	National

Keywords

Abstract (English) This report aims to increase the knowledge of the health of four immigrant groups in Sweden. The report forms part of a series of public health reports, and addresses the issue from a public health perspective. Above all, the report highlights the correlation between health and social factors, including certain factors specific to immigrants. However, it is important to identify ill health, which can be attributed to living conditions in Sweden and which it may be possible to remedy.

The report describes the health of four groups, those born in Chile, Iran, Poland, and Turkey who came to Sweden during the 1980s and were aged 20–44 on arrival. Comparing health between these groups and with native Swedes allows the question to be raised of whether health differences are caused by conditions in Sweden or whether they can be explained by differences in background factors from the respective home countries. The analysis is based on the fact that well-established determinants of health are also applicable to the immigrant groups in question.

The study reports statistical correlations and, as this was a cross-sectional study, it is impossible to say that the factors which are clearly linked to the health outcome are also its cause. The correlation may also work in the opposite direction, i.e. the state of health may have an impact on the determinants in question. It is also well known from other studies that these factors are determinants of health and that they are mutually dependent. Comments have only been made on statistically significant correlations and abnormal risks.

Analysing self-reported health and its causes is associated with a number of methodological problems. These questions are always complex, and even more so when respondents come from different cultures. More in-depth analysis is vital but that task has been passed on to researchers in the field.

Interviews on health with people who speak different languages and have different cultural backgrounds also involve a risk of misinterpreting the results. It can be difficult to know for sure whether apparent differences are real or whether it is linguistic and cultural differences which are being measured. On the basis of current knowledge of health and its relationship to social factors and living conditions, this study shows an expected pattern. This suggests that the measurements used and the results do reflect a likely reality.

Summary of results: Health outcome: The study is based on self-reported health and sickness. Measured in this way, there are major health differences between native Swedes and the four groups of immigrants studied, as well as between the immigrant groups. The Swedes are generally in better health than the immigrants. Immigrants from Poland differ least from native Swedes, reporting worse health than the Swedes, but in most respects better health than the other three groups. However, there are cases where the opposite is true. Circulatory diseases are more common among native Swedes than among the immigrant groups, with the exception of Polish men and Iranian women. Native Swedes report allergies to a greater extent than is the case for immigrants from Iran, Poland, and Turkey.

The health differences between men and women are considerable. Across all nationalities the risk of women suffering ill health appears to be one and a half to five times greater than the risk for men. The women from Chile, Iran, and Turkey state significantly more often than the men that they suffer ill health and significantly more often than Swedish women of the same age. This manifests itself most clearly with regard to general health, with over half of Iranian and Turkish women reporting ill health. Long-term illnesses are also common, particularly complaints that are often work-related such as reduced ability to work, reduced mobility, and pain in the back, neck, shoulders, and joints. The gender pattern is basically the same for mental illness. Women report suffering from tiredness, insomnia, anxiety, worry, and nervousness to a greater extent than men. However, insomnia is common among men from Chile, Iran, and Turkey, and there is a significant incidence of anxiety, worry, and nervousness as well as reduced mental well-being particularly among Iranian men.

Significance of determinants: In most cases the same factors/determinants correlate with the health outcome among native Swedes and among the immigrants in the study, although the correlation varies in strength, as does the health outcome. This is also true of background factors such as age, sex, marital status, and education and social factors such as financial problems, employment status, feelings of security, and social support. Factors specific to immigrants such as experiences of discrimination and poor knowledge of Swedish also have an impact on the health outcome in the four immigrant groups. Entered into a regression analysis, these background factors, social factors, and factors specific to immigrants explain many of the differences in health between native Swedes and the immigrants in question, but not all. Unsurprisingly, this suggests that ethnic and cultural differences also have a part to play. However, the differences in health, which can be observed between the four immigrant groups, appear to be wholly explained by the above factors.

Common to all the factors is the fact that a greater proportion of those living in unfavorable conditions have significant ill health than those with good living conditions. This is not unexpected as several of the factors are also mutually dependent. As mentioned earlier, common to all the factors is the fact that it is impossible to establish the direction of the link, i.e., what causes what regarding a proven abnormal risk.

Background factors: Age and health are clearly linked, with worsening health coming with increasing age. In this study, mental ill health is an exception where age does not appear to be of any significance. The age factor has the greatest significance in the Turkish group. In other nationality groups, the age factor is most significant to the risk of suffering functional impairment. Men generally report better health than women, a fact reflected in the immigrant groups. In particular, women are at greater risk than men of suffering functional impairment.

According to the study, being married or cohabiting constitutes some protection against ill health, particularly in the Chilean group. This is also a significant variable for Swedes and Poles.

A low level of education collates strongly with poor health for native Swedes and immigrants from Poland, but is also significant for immigrants from Chile. This applies to all types of ill health except mental ill health.

Social factors: Those in a poor financial situation also report more ill health. This applies to all nationalities regarding many of the types of ill health in question, in particular mental ill health. For example, immigrants from Iran, Chile, or Poland in a poor financial situation run more than double the risk of mental ill health. Being unemployed correlates strongly with ill health among native Swedes and immigrants from Chile and Iran, but to a lesser extent for those from Poland and Turkey. The risk of ill health is greatest among native Swedes. One explanation for this may be that Swedes who are out of work often also have health problems, while immigrants' lack of employment is often unrelated to their health. Insecurity correlates strongly with ill health. Those who are insecure run between a two and three times greater risk of also suffering the types of ill health measured, compared with those who feel secure. This applies to all groups, including the Swedes. For example, immigrants from Iran run a three times greater risk of suffering mental ill health or a serious long-term illness if they feel insecure. Not having a close friend increases the risk of native Swedes and immigrants from Chile suffering general poor health and mental illness.

Factors specific to immigrants: Poor knowledge of Swedish among immigrants from Iran doubles the risk of all types of ill health. The same is true for immigrants from Poland, with the exception of mental health. Feeling discriminated against doubles the risk of suffering mental ill health in all four immigrant groups, compared with not feeling discriminated against.

Sense of coherence: This study shows that a poor sense of coherence correlates with mental ill health in all groups, including native Swedes. In the case of immigrants from Iran, those with a poor sense of coherence ran a 12 times greater risk than those with a strong sense of coherence.

Lifestyle habits: Men and to a certain extent also women in the four immigrant groups are daily smokers to a much greater extent than native Swedes. Daily smoking is most common among men from Turkey at over 50%. Daily smoking is least common among women born in Iran, with one tenth being smokers. Younger people are daily smokers to a greater extent than older people in all four immigrant groups, which is not the case among native Swedes. In the group of native Swedes, the proportion of daily smokers is greatest among those with a low level of education and reduces as the level of education increases. In the other groups, this pattern only applies to men born in Turkey.

Men report being overweight to a greater extent than women in all groups. This is most common among men from Poland, with almost half being overweight. Among the women, more than one third of those from Chile and Turkey are overweight. The proportion of overweight women from Poland is lower than that of native Swedish women. Obesity is most common among men and women from Turkey and is significantly more common among older people than younger people. In almost every group, the proportion of obese people falls as the level of education rises. It is more common for respondents in the four immigrant groups not to take exercise as part of their leisure time than for the Swedes. Approximately, one in ten native Swedes and just under two in ten Poles report this inactivity. Among the other immigrant groups, between 25% and 50% state that they do not get any exercise in their leisure time. Among the Swedes and Poles, it is more common for men not to exercise than for women. Among those born in Chile, Turkey, and Iran, it is more common for women not to exercise at all. In all groups it is more common for those with a low level of education not to exercise in their leisure time than for those with a higher level of education. When it comes to alcohol consumption, the immigrants from Chile, Iran, and Turkey report less alcohol consumption than native Swedes and immigrants from Poland.

Accumulation of unhealthy habits and problems of support: Those who only state one unhealthy habit do not report more health problems. This is probably due to the fact that the respondents are relatively young and that health problems deriving from unhealthy habits have not yet developed to any great extent. The risk is greater in those cases where two or more unfavorable habits, such as daily smoking, lack of exercise, or being overweight, occur at the same time. However, the pattern is not unequivocal.

Immigrants from Turkey show the largest proportion, just over one quarter, of people with two or more unhealthy habits at the same time. However, these Turks show no greater risk of ill health or reduced mental well-being. Nor is there any abnormal risk of ill health, reduced mental well-being, or severe pain among equivalent immigrants from Iran. Otherwise, the risk is almost double and sometimes three or four times as great for all types of ill health both among native Swedes and the other immigrants in question. Those with a poor support system, i.e., those who simultaneously have at least two of the characteristics poor position in the labor market, poor financial situation or poor family relations, report worse health. Immigrants from Chile and Iran who have a poor support system run twice the risk of ill health run by those whose support system is not poor. The same applies to native Swedes. The risk of reduced mental well-being is between two and two and a half times greater for native Swedes and immigrants from Chile and from Poland if they have a poor support system than if they do not.

Health care and dental care: It is more common for immigrants from the four groups, with the exception of men from Poland, to have visited or been visited by the doctor or had contact with a physiotherapist or district nurse in the last three months. It is most common for immigrants from Chile and Turkey to have made various types of health care visit. These differences can mainly be explained by the fact that health care needs to vary. Trust in Swedish health care was greatest among immigrants from Turkey and least among those from Chile. Women appeared to have greater trust in Swedish health care than men. Great or moderate trust varied from half in the Chilean group to around three quarters in the Turkish group. Consumption of prescribed sleeping drugs and antianxiety drugs was greater in all the immigrant groups than among native Swedes, and may partly be explained by the fact that mental problems and insomnia are more common among immigrants. This may be interpreted as the doctors being more inclined to prescribe this type of medicine to immigrants, possibly due to communication problems or to adapting to the expectations of the immigrants. It is more common for immigrants to have chewing problems and dentures or false teeth than for native Swedes. Women from Chile and Turkey have the worst dental health. It is also more common for immigrant groups not to have visited the dentist in the past two years than for native Swedes. The differences in dental health between native Swedes and immigrants may partly be explained by the fact that since the 1950s Swedes have had access to public dental care and the preventive work this has established, which has led to the habit of regular visits to the dentist. People in Poland have also had access to comprehensive preventive initiatives and free dental care.

Conclusions: Avoid generalisations: The report focuses on four groups, those born in Chile, Iran, Poland, and Turkey who came to Sweden during the 1980s and were aged 20–44 on arrival. The interviews were carried out in 1996. The results should not be generalised to cover other immigrant groups. The conclusions must be looked at against the background of the period in question, as well as immigrant policy and the situation in the labor market and housing market in Sweden during this period. Immigrants in this study have worse self-reported health than Swedes. The Swedes generally enjoy better health than the immigrants in the four immigrant groups. The immigrants from Poland differ least from native Swedes with regard to health. There are major differences between men and women in each group. The women run twice the risk of suffering various health problems, particularly musculoskeletal complaints. Mental ill health is common among men and women alike. Generally the same factors as among Swedes, but cultural differences are also significant. The focus is often placed on differences between immigrants and the native population, but there may be cause to point out that there are also major similarities. Factors that constitute unfavorable conditions for health are unfavorable for any one who suffers them. From the point of view of public health, this can highlight the fact that the same health policy is basically valid for the whole population, immigrants, as well as native Swedes. This study shows that, to a large extent, the same factors are linked to the health of native Swedes as to the four immigrant groups included in the study. These factors are age, sex, marital status, education, work, financial situation, security, and social support. Factors linked to being an immigrant, such as feelings of discrimination and the ability to speak and understand Swedish, are also shown to be linked to the health outcome. However, not all the differences in ill health between the four immigrant groups and native Swedes can be explained in relation to the above factors, which suggests that ethnic and cultural differences also play a part. It is also well known from other studies that such factors have their own impact on health among immigrants.

Different conditions are crucial: Generally speaking immigrants and native Swedes are exposed to different conditions in a number of respects. This is also the case between immigrants from different countries and applies to both cultural and socio-economic background. It is also the case that immigrants from the same country differ considerably depending on who immigrates at a certain time, the date, or the reason for coming to Sweden. There are differences, for example, in distribution across age, sex, educational background, and traumatic experiences, depending on the situation in the home country, which prompted emigration. It is important to remember that these differences in origin and living conditions also affect the conditions for health and integration in Sweden of different groups of immigrants. There is a major challenge in finding ways to improve these conditions. The major differences in ill health between the four immigrant groups and between these groups and native Swedes can be seen in the light of the fact that the conditions for health are not the same. As shown in the report, the differences in education, work, finances, and feelings of security are considerable. With regard to education, it should be noted that immigrants from Iran and Poland are more often well educated compared with native Swedes.

Negative attitudes and discrimination prevent participation: Immigrants experience a lack of knowledge of Swedish and feelings of discrimination on grounds of origin. These experiences appear to have an impact on their health. Feelings such as loss of identity in the new country and discrimination, factors that are linked to being an immigrant, have an impact on feelings of security and support. They affect health in general and mental health in particular. Hopefully such problems can be reduced by increasing knowledge and understanding among the population of the difficulties and problems that immigrants encounter in Sweden. Work and the opportunity to provide for oneself is one of the most important factors in feeling part of society. It must be pointed out that well-educated immigrants often find it difficult to find work, which is partly explained by the labor market situation in recent years, but also suggests that Swedish attitudes to immigrants are often negative. Measures to support immigrants' language development and to counter hostile attitudes to immigrants among the Swedish population are important. It must be made easier to find employment. Mental ill health among immigrants must be taken seriously

We know from a number of other studies that mental ill health is widespread among immigrants in Sweden. This survey primarily shows a link between feelings of insecurity and mental ill health. These feelings may partly be due to experiences that have to do with the migration itself, such as traumatic experiences of war or violence and loss and separation from relatives and friends. This should be particularly highlighted as the effects can be treated with the help of health care and other specialist initiatives.

There may be reason to consider how knowledge of such experiences can better be collected, for example, in conjunction with reception in Sweden and the health examination offered to refugees. Mental health problems, for example, can better be dealt with if professional help is offered at an early stage. This places major demands on staff in terms of linguistic and cultural expertise. It is important to improve the reception and living conditions of new immigrants. This would considerably improve the immigrants' chances of enjoying good health and adapting, regardless of whether they stay in Sweden or return to their original country.

Lifestyle and health habits can be influenced: Daily smoking is considerably more common in the four immigrant groups than among native Swedes, a fact that may be worth addressing through preventive initiatives. This mainly applies to men. It should also be noted that in the immigrant groups, it is more common for young people to smoke on a daily basis, whereas among native Swedes, the proportion of daily smokers is larger among older people. The pattern of young people smoking to a greater extent than older people was the case in Sweden around 30–40 years ago. Nowadays in Sweden fewer young people are taking up smoking with each new generation. Daily smoking is comparatively uncommon among Iranian women, but the fact that smoking is twice as common among younger Iranian women compared with the older women gives cause to wonder whether the Western pattern has a crossover effect. It may be worth considering how a successful preventive initiative against tobacco smoking could be targeted at different immigrant groups. When it comes to dental health care and dental health, it is shown that the four immigrant groups, despite significantly worse dental health, are more rarely treated by a dentist. Among the children of the immigrants in question the incidence of caries is also significantly higher than in the children of native Swedes. It is quite likely that significant measures of various kinds are required to remove this inequality. All refugees in Sweden are offered a health examination at the cost of the Swedish state a short time after arrival in Sweden. A similar examination within the dental health care service with free follow-up treatment would probably help to establish regular contact with a dentist for many refugees in Sweden. It is also important that newly-arrived refugee families are offered a preventive dental health programme particularly adapted to their needs. This study appears to show that health care works in a similar way. A greater need for care in the immigrant groups in question could go a long way to explaining why they have used different aspects of the health service more often than native Swedes.

Knowledge is the basis – research is needed: Most studies of immigrants in Europe are characterised by small population samples, mixed groups of foreign-born respondents, limited geographical areas, few social factors, and a lack of good indicators of cultural adaptation. This report, on the basis of a comparatively large sample of immigrants from four different countries who came to Sweden during the

1980s, may help to increase knowledge particularly about the relationship between social factors, living conditions, and to some extent cultural adaptation and health in these groups. Further data and research are needed to increase knowledge of the social conditions and health status of immigrants. Longitudinal studies are needed to study the causal links. Repeated cross-sectional studies also provide a certain amount of guidance. In addition, knowledge of the health situation in the home country and the health of the immigrants in question on their arrival in Sweden is lacking. This could be improved through the systematic collection of certain basic data on arrival. Bearing in mind the major differences between different immigrant groups, each immigrant group should be studied individually as far as possible. However, in Sweden there are no fewer than a hundred ethnic groups and almost as many languages, and it is therefore impossible to study each group separately. Instead groups of immigrants should be found with a common characteristic such as common linguistic area, geography, religion, or cultural distance from Sweden. Linguistic and cultural differences create special difficulties in surveys of immigrants. The need for validation studies of interview questions for different cultures is vital. Such studies can be combined with health examinations and the collection of biological markers. This type of validation study is also needed in the Swedish population. It is vital to increase knowledge of the health situation of immigrants and the fact that there are methodological problems does not mean that we should refrain from trying to measure health and compare different groups.

Abstract (Original Language) Denna rapport syftar till att fördjupa kunskapen om hälsoförhållandena i fyra invandrargrupper i Sverige. Rapporten är ett led i en återkommande folkhälsorapportering och utgår från ett folkhälsoperspektiv. Framför allt belyses hälsans samband med sociala faktorer och med vissa invandrarspecifika faktorer. Det är då viktigt att lyfta fram ohälsa som kan hänföras till levnadsbetingelser i Sverige som kan vara möjliga att åtgärda. Rapporten beskriver hälsan i fyra grupper, nämligen de som är födda i Chile, Iran, Polen och Turkiet och som kom till Sverige under 1980-talet och som var 20–44 år vid ankomsten. Genom att hälsan jämförs dels mellan grupperna, dels med infödda svenskar kan frågan väckas om förhållanden i Sverige orsakat hälsoskillnaderna eller om skillnader i bakgrundsfaktorer från hemlandet är förklaringen. Analysen utgår från att väl kända bestämningsfaktorer för hälsa är giltiga även i de aktuella invandrargrupperna. Det som redovisas är statistiska samband och eftersom det är fråga om en tvärsnittsundersökning, går det inte att säga att de faktorer som har ett tydligt sam band med hälsoutfallet också är dess orsaker. Sambandet kan också ha motsatt riktning, dvs. hälsotillståndet kan ha betydelse för den aktuella bestämningsfaktorn. Det är också väl känt från andra studier att de här aktuella faktorerna är bestämningsfaktorer för hälsa och att det finns ett ömsesidigt beroende mellan bestämningsfaktorerna. Endast statistiskt signifikanta samband och överrisker kommenteras. Många metodologiska problem är förknippade med analyser av självrapporterad hälsa och dess orsaker. Dessa frågeställningar är alltid komplexa och blir det än mer då det rör människor från olika kulturer. Djupare analyser är angelägna men överlämnas till forskarvärlden. Intervjuer om hälsa med människor som har olika språk och ursprung i olika kulturer innebär också risk för feltolkningar av resultaten. Det kann vara svårt att säkert veta om skillnader som påvisas är verkliga skillnader eller om det istället är språk- och kulturskillnader som mäts. Utifrån den kunskap som finns om hälsa och dess relation med sociala faktorer och levnadsförhållanden framträder i denna studie ett förväntat mönster. Detta tyder på att såväl använda mått som resultat ändå speglar en sannolik verklighet.

Sammanfattning av resultaten: Hälsoutfall: Studien bygger på självrapporterad hälsa och sjuklighet. Skillnaderna i ohälsa mätt med dessa mått är stora mellan infödda svenskar och de fyra studerade grupperna av invandrare, men också mellan invandrargrupperna. Svenskarna har i allmänhet bättre hälsa än invandrarna. Invandrare från Polen avviker i hälsohänseende minst från infödda svenskar. De rapporterar sämre hälsa än svenskarna men i de flesta avseenden bättre hälsa än de övriga tre grupperna. Det finns dock exempel på motsatsen. Sjukdomar i cirkulationsorganen är vanligare bland infödda svenskar än i invandrargrupperna, undantaget män från Polen och kvinnor från Iran. Infödda svenskar anger allergier i större omfattning än invandrarna från Iran, Polen och Turkiet. Hälsoskillnaderna är påfallande mellan män och kvinnor. Kvinnor tycks ha mellan en och en halv och tre gånger större risk än män att drabbas av ohälsa. Det gäller samtliga nationaliteter. Kvinnorna från Chile, Iran och Turkiet uppger sig ha något slags ohälsa betydligt oftare än männen och betydligt oftare än svenska kvinnor i motsvarande ålder. Tydligast är det avseende allmänt hälsotillstånd där över hälften av kvinnorna från Iran och Turkiet uppger dålig hälsa. Även långvarig sjukdom är vanligt förekommande, och i synnerhet sådana besvär som ofta är arbetsrelaterade som nedsatt arbetsförmåga, nedsatt rörelseförmåga och smärtor och värk i rygg, nacke, axlar och leder. När det gäller psykisk ohälsa är könsmönstret i stort detsamma. Kvinnorna uppger sig i större omfattning än männen lida av trötthet, sömnbesvär och ängslan, oro eller ångest. Sömnbesvär är dock vanliga bland män från Chile, Iran och Turkiet och ängslan, oro eller ångest samt nedsatt psykiskt välbefinnande är betydande framför allt bland män från Iran.

Bestämningsfaktorernas betydelse: I stort samma faktorer/determinanter har samband med hälsoutfallet såväl bland infödda svenskar som bland här aktuella invandrare, även om sambandet är olika starkt och nivån på hälsoutfallet olika. Det gäller såväl bakgrundsfaktorerna ålder, kön, civilstånd och utbildning som sociala faktorer som ekonomiska problem, sysselsättningsstatus, upplevelse av trygghet och socialt stöd. Invandrarspecifika faktorer som upplevelse av diskriminering och dåliga kunskaper i svenska språket har också betydelse för hälsoutfallet i de fyra invandrargrupperna. Dessa bakgrundsfaktorer, sociala faktorer och invandrarspecifika faktorer förklarar, då de samtidigt ingår i en regressionsanalys, mycket av skillnaderna i ohälsa mellan infödda svenskar och de aktuella invandrarna, dockinte allt. Detta tyder inte oväntat på att även etniska skillnader och kulturskillnader har betydelse. De skillnader i ohälsa som kan observeras mellan de fyra invandrarländerna ser dock ut att helt förklaras av dessa faktorer. Genomgående för samtliga faktorer är att en större andel bland dem med ogynnsamma förutsättningar har signifikant dålig hälsa än bland dem med goda förutsättningar. Detta är inte oväntat eftersom det också finns ett ömsesidigt beroende mellan flera av faktorerna. Genomgående för samtliga faktorer är också, som nämnts ovan, att det inte går att fastställa sambandets riktning, dvs. vad som orsakar vad av en påvisad överrisk.

Bakgrundsfaktorerna: Ålder och hälsa har ett tydligt samband som visar försämrad hälsa med ökande ålder. Psykisk ohälsa utgör i denna studie ett undantag där åldern inte förefaller ha betydelse alls. Åldersfaktorn har störst betydelse i den turkiska gruppen. För övriga nationalitetsgrupper är åldern mest utslagsgivande för risken att drabbas av nedsatt funktionsförmåga.

- Generellt sett uppger män bättre hälsa än kvinnor och så även i de aktuella invandrargrupperna. I synnerhet har kvinnor större risk än män att drabbas av funktionsnedsättning.
- Att vara gift eller sammanboende utgör en skyddsfaktor mot ohälsa i denna studie främst i den chilenska gruppen. Även för svenskar och polacker är detta en betydelsefull variabel.
- Låg utbildningsnivå samvarierar starkt med dålig hälsa för infödda svenskar och invandrare från Polen men är betydande även för de invandrare som kommer från Chile. Detta gäller samtliga typer av ohälsa utom psykisk ohälsa.

De sociala faktorerna

- De som har svag ekonomi rapporterar också mer ohälsa. Det gäller för samtliga nationaliteter avseende flera av här aktuella typer av ohälsa, i synnerhet psykisk ohälsa. Att ha svag ekonomi innebär till exempel mer än fördubblad risk för psykisk ohälsa bland de invandrare som kommer från Iran, Chile eller Polen.
- Att sakna arbete samvarierar starkt med ohälsa bland infödda svenskar, invandrare från Chile och Iran men i mindre utsträckning för dem från Polen och Turkiet. Risken för ohälsa förefaller störst bland infödda svenskar. En förklaring till detta kan tänkas vara att svenskar som saknar arbete ofta också har hälsoproblem men att invandrare ofta saknar arbete oavsett hälsotillstånd.
- Otrygghet samvarierar starkt med ohälsa. Den som är otrygg har mellan dubbelt så stor och drygt tre gånger så stor risk att också ha de typer av ohälsa som mäts jämfört med den som är trygg. Det gäller för alla grupper inklusive den svenska. För invandrare från Iran är exempelvis risken att ha psykisk ohälsa eller lång-varig sjukdom med svåra besvär tre gånger så stor om de är otrygga.
- Att inte ha en nära vän ger för infödda svenskar och invandrare från Chile större risk för allmänt dålig hälsa och psykisk ohälsa. De invandrarspecifika faktorerna • Dåliga kunskaper i svenska innebär för invandrare från Iran mer än dubbelt så stor risk för alla typer av ohälsa och likaså för invandrare från Polen, dock bortsett från psykisk ohälsa.
- Att uppleva sig diskriminerad innebär dubbelt så stor risk att ha psykisk ohälsa i samtliga fyra invandrargrupper jämfört med om de inte upplever sig diskriminerade. Känsla av sammanhang
- Svag känsla av sammanhang har i denna studie samband med psykisk ohälsa i alla grupper, även bland infödda svenskar. Bland invandrarna från Iran var risken 12 gånger större bland dem med svag känsla av sammanhang än bland dem med stark.

Levnadsvanor: Män och i viss mån även kvinnor i de fyra invandrargrupperna är dagligrökare i större omfattning än svenskfödda. Vanligast är dagligrökning bland män från Turkiet med över hälften. Minst vanligt är det bland kvinnor födda i Iran med en tiondel dagligrökare. De yngre är dagligrökare i större omfattning än de äldre i samtliga fyra invandrargrupper, vilket inte är fallet bland infödda svenskar. Bland svenskfödda är andelen dagligrökare störst bland de lågutbildade och minskar med stigande utbildningsnivå. Detta mönster finns i övrigt bara bland män födda i Turkiet. Män uppger övervikt i större utsträckning än kvinnor i alla grupper. Vanligast är det bland män från Polen där nästan hälften är överviktiga. Bland kvinnorna är mer än en tredjedel av dem från Chile och Turkiet överviktiga. Andelen överviktiga bland kvinnor från Polen är mindre än bland svenskfödda kvinnor. Fetma är vanligast bland män och kvinnor från Turkiet. Det är betydligt vanligare bland de äldre än bland de yngre. Andelen med fetma minskar med ökande utbildningsnivå i nästan alla grupper.

Det är vanligare att inte motionera på sin fritid i de fyra grupperna än bland svenskar. I runda tal en tiondel av svenskfödda och inte fullt två tiondelar av dem som kommer från Polen uppger detta. I de övriga invandrargrupperna är det mellan en fjärdedel och hälften som uppger att de inte får någon motion på sin fritid. Det är något vanligare att män inte motionerar än kvinnor bland svenskar och polacker. Bland personer födda i Chile, Turkiet och Iran är det vanligare att kvinnor inte motionerar alls. I samtliga grupper är det vanligare att lågutbildade inte motionerar på sin fritid än att högutbildade inte gör det. Vad avser alkoholkonsumtion rapporterar invandrare från Chile, Iran och Turkiet att de dricker mindre alkohol än infödda svenskar och invandrare från Polen. Ansamling av ohälsosamma levnadsvanor och problem med förankring De personer som enbart uppger en ohälsosam levnadsvana uppger inte fler hälsoproblem. Det beror sannolikt på att intervjupersonerna är relativt unga och att hälsoproblem till följd av ohälsosamma levnadsvanor inte hunnit utvecklas särskilt mycket. Däremot är risken större i de fall då två eller flera ogynnsamma levnadsvanor, såsom dagligrökning, bristande motion eller övervikt, förekommer samtidigt. Mönstret är dock inte entydigt. Störst andel, drygt en fjärdedel, med två eller flera ohälsosamma levnadsvanor samtidigt återfinns bland invandrare från Turkiet. Risken att ej ha god hälsa eller att ha nedsatt psykiskt välbefinnande är dock inte större bland de invandrare från Turkiet som har mer än två ohälsosamma levnadsvanor samtidigt. Inte heller finns någon överrisk att ej ha god hälsa, nedsatt psykiskt välbefinnande eller svår värk bland motsvarande invandrare från Iran. I övrigt är risken nästan dubbelt så stor och ibland tre till fyra gånger så stor för alla typer av ohälsa både bland infödda svenskar och de aktuella invandrarna. De som har svag förankring, med vilket avses att samtidigt ha minst två av egenskaperna svag ställning på arbetsmarknaden, svag ekonomi eller svaga relationer till familjen, uppger sämre hälsa. Invandrare från Chile och Iran har mer än dubbelt så stor risk att ej ha god hälsa om de har svag förankring som om de inte har det. Detsamma gäller för infödda svenskar. Risken att ha nedsatt psykiskt välbefinnande är mellan två och två och en halv gånger så stor för infödda svenskar och invandrare från Chile och från Polen om de har svag förankring än om de inte har det.

Sjukvård och tandvård: Det är vanligare att invandrare från de fyra aktuella invandrargrupperna, med undantag av män från Polen, under den senaste tremånadersperioden har besökt eller haft hembesök av läkare, haft kontakt med sjukgymnast eller distriktssköterska. Vanligast är att invandrare från Chile och Turkiet gjort olika typer av vårdbesök. Dessa skillnader kan i stort förklaras av att vårdbehoven är olika. Förtroendet för svensk sjukvård visade sig vara störst bland invandrare från Turkiet och minst bland dem från Chile. Kvinnorna visade sig ha större förtroende för svensk sjukvård än männen. Stort eller ganska stort förtroende varierade från hälften i den chilenska gruppen till cirka tre fjärdedelar i den turkiska. Konsumtionen av receptbelagda sömnmedel och ångestdämpande medel var större i de fyra invandrargrupperna än bland svenskfödda och förklaras bara delvis av att psykiska besvär och sömnbesvär är vanligare bland invandrarna. Detta kan tolkas som att läkare är mer benägna att skriva ut denna typ av mediciner till invandrare. Det kan tänkas bero på kommunikationsproblem men också på anpassning till invandrares förväntningar. Det är vanligare att invandrare har tuggproblem och att de bär tandprotes helt eller delvis än bland infödda svenskar. Sämst tandstatus har kvinnor från Chile och Turkiet. Det är också vanligare att invandrargrupperna inte besökt tandläkare de senaste två åren än bland svenskarna. Det förefaller troligt att skillnaderna i tandhälsa mellan infödda svenskar och invandrare delvis kan förklaras av att svenskar sedan 50-talet haft tillgång till folktandvård och det förebyggande arbete som denna etablerat vilket lett till inlärt beteende med regelbundna besök i tandvården. Även polacker i Polen har haft tillgång till omfattande förebyggande insatser och gratis tandvård.

Age Groups

Riksmaten 1997–98

Riksmaten

Project Leader

Project Leader	Wulf Becker and Monika Pearson
Address	Livsmedelsverket
	Avdelningen för information och nutrion
	Box 622
	751 26 Uppsala
Executing Institution	Avdelningen för information och nutrion, Livsmedelsverket
Funding Agency	

Project Information

Start of Project	01/01/1997
End of Project	31/12/1998
Start of Data Collection	01/01/1997
End of Data Collection	31/12/1998
URL	http://www.slv.se/templates/SLV_Page____6045.aspx
Scope	National

Keywords

Abstract (English) In 1997–1998, the Statistics Sweden in cooperation with the National Food Adminstration (NFA) carried out the second nation-wide Swedish dietary survey. The survey base consisted of a representative sample of 2,000 households. In each household, one person 18- to 74-years old filled in a precoded 7-d record book. The participants also filled in a questionnaire with information on weight, height, education, occupation, exercise, smoking, and other lifestyle factors.

The precoded record book gives preprinted alternatives (with quantity indications in household measures) for foods, meal components, and facilities for indication of where and when the meals were consumed. Using a portion-guide with photographs, sizes of cooked food portions, and salads eaten at main meals could be estimated. The use of fat spreads on sandwiches was estimated with the help of photographs in a similar way. For snacks and other in-between meal eating was recorded in household measures, pieces, etc., using precoded alternatives. Additional eating was recorded in free text.

Data input and dietary analysis was performed using a commercial software package (MATs) that included food composition data from the NFA (PC-kost 1/98). The preprinted alternatives were directly converted into amounts and NFA food codes. The free text additions were the only data input requiring coding by dieticians.

About 1,200 persons completed the study with a participation rate of about 60%. Participation was lower in larger cities and surrounding areas than in rural areas and lower among young as well as older house-holds.

The results indicate that certain changes in dietary habits have occurred since the first survey carried out in 1989 (Hulk-survey). In Riksmaten, a more frequent consumption of juice and nectar, pizza, rice, pasta, nuts, and snacks and sweets were seen for both men and women. Women also more often consumed vegetables, milk, meat and poultry, and alcoholic beverages, and men more often consumed jam, icecream, softdrinks, etc. A less frequent consumption was seen for cheese, offal, bread, sweet bakery products, spreads, cream, sugar (as additional foods), and desserts. Men also less frequently consumed eggs, fish, pulses, and porridge.

The observed differences in consumption frequency were mostly reflected in consumed amounts. Exceptions were bread and sweet bakery products. A higher consumption was also seen for vegetables (men), sausages (men and women), meat, and poultry (men). Part of these differences could be explained by changes in the standard portion sizes used in the record book.

The dietary fat content was on average about 34 energy percent (E%), which is lower than in the Hulk-survey, but still higher than the recommended level of 30 E%. The differences among sex and age groups were generally small, but the youngest age group (18–24 year) tended to have a lower fat percentage. The proportion of saturated fatty acids was 14 E%, also lower than in Hulk. Together with trans-fatty acids "hard fat" contribute 15 E%, considerably higher than the recommended level of 10 E%.

Carbohydrates provided on average 47 E% and 46 E% among women and men, respectively. The proportion was higher in the youngest age group. The proportion of sucrose in the diet was higher among women than among men. The average intake of fiber was 17–18 g/d, corresponding to 1.8 g/MJ among men and 2.0 g/MJ among women, which is about two thirds of the recommended level of 3 g/MJ. The intake has not changed compared to the Hulk-survey.

The alcohol intake was higher among men than among women and provided on average 4 E% and 3 E%, respectively. The intake of sodium from food and drink (excl. salt added at the table, etc.) was 2.8 and 3.6 g/d among women and men, respectively.

The average intakes of vitamins and minerals were generally close to or above the recommended daily intakes (RI). The intake of vitamin D was lower than recommended for older persons, while the intake of folate was about 75% of the RI. The intake of iron among women in fertile ages was about two thirds of the RI. The selenium intake was about three fourths of the RI. The intake of retinol was lower in Riksmaten than in Hulk, while the intake of vitamin C was higher. The iron intake was lower than in the Hulk-survey because of the termination of iron fortification of flour in 1995.

Pronounced age differences in dietary habits were seen. Older people eat more of "traditional" foods like potatoes, root vegetables, fish, offal and blood, porridge, and sweet bakery products, while young people eat and drink more of more "modern" foods, e.g., pasta, rice, pizza, sweets, nuts and snacks, and softdrinks. Older people also eat more fruit and vegetables. Women eat more fruit and vegetables than men do. There were generally small differences in the nutrient composition of the diet between men and women.

Low education among men was linked to a lower consumption of e.g., fruit and vegetables and a higher intake of spreads. Men with low education consumed a diet with higher fat content compared with well-educated men (35 E% and 33 E%, respectively). No such difference was observed for women. High education was linked to a higher alcohol intake, in both sexes. High education was linked to a higher intake of beta-carotene (women only), vitamin C, and folate compared with low education. Similar tendencies, although less pronounced, were seen when the participants were classified into socio-economic groups.

Although certain improvements in the dietary pattern have occurred since the late 1980s, the main problem with an imbalance between fat (and fat quality) and complex carbohydrates remains. Factors like smoking and low education are still associated with poorer dietary habits, especially among men, while a certain equalisation seems to have occurred among women in this respect. For the population as a whole the general advice, that part of the dietary fat, mainly hard fat, should be replaced by complex carbohydrates, is still valid. On a food level this means increased consumption of fruit, berries, vegetables, bread and cereal products, to replace high fat meat and dairy products with fat-reduced alternatives, and to limit the consumption of high fat bakery products and sugar containing products like soft-drinks and sweets. Soft or fluid edible fats should replace hard fats to a larger degree. An increased physical activity in the population is equally important. However, it should be stressed that the degree and magnitude of desirable changes in dietary habits varies between different groups and individuals. Methods and advice to promote changes should be adapted according to the context and conditions/prerequisites relevant for the group or individual.

Abstract (Original Language) I samarbete med Livsmedelsverket genomförde Statistiska centralbyrån under 1997–98 kostundersökningen Riksmaten. Undersökningen ingick i SCBs Utgiftsbarometer och omfattade ett riksrepresentativt urval av cirka 2 000 hushåll. I varje hushåll fick en person i åldern 18–74 år registrera matintag under en vecka med hjälp av en s k menybok, en förenklad 7-dagarsregistrering med förtryckta alternativ. Drygt 1 200 personer (cirka 60 procent) deltog i undersökningen. Riksmaten är en uppföljning av undersökningen "Hushållens livsmedelsinköp och kostvanor" (Hulk), som genomfördes 1989.

Resultaten pekar på att vissa förändringar i matvanorna skett sedan Hulk-undersökningen. Kvinnor åt t ex oftare grönsaker, kött och fågel, pizza m m, ris, pasta, nötter och snacks, sötsaker och drack oftare juice och nektar, mjölk och fil samt alkoholhaltiga drycker jämfört med i Hulk. Däremot var konsumtionsfrekvensen för ost, inälvsmat, matbröd, bullar och annat kaffebröd, matfett (på smörgås), grädde (som tillbehör), söta soppor och efterätter samt socker (som tillbehör) lägre. Män åt oftare pizza m m, ris, pasta, glass, nötter och snacks, sötsaker samt drack oftare juice och nektar samt saft och läsk. Konsumtionsfrekvensen var lägre för baljväxter, ost, ägg, fisk och skaldjur, inälvsmat, matbröd, gröt och välling, bullar och annat kaffebröd, matfett (på smörgås), grädde (som tillbehör), söta soppor och efterätter, marmelad och sylt samt socker. De skillnader som ses i konsumtionsfrekvenser återspeglas till viss del i konsumerade mängder. Det gäller grönsaker (kvinnor), juice och nektar, ost, inälvsmat, gröt och välling (män), pizza m m, ris, pasta, matfett, grädde (män), nötter och snacks, söta soppor och efterätter, marmelad och sylt, sötsaker, saft och läsk samt drycker. För livsmedel där en signifikant ändring av konsumtionsfrekvensen inte avspeglas i en motsvarande signifikant ändring i konsumerade mängder kan variationer i angiven portionsstorlek vara en viktig förklaring.

Fetthalten i kosten var i genomsnitt cirka 34 energiprocent (E%), vilket är lägre än i Hulk men fortfarande över rekommenderad nivå på 30 E%. Skillnaderna mellan de olika köns- och åldersgrupperna var små, men de yngsta (17–24 år) tenderade att ha en lägre fettenergiprocent än åldersgruppen 25–44 år. Andelen mättade fettsyror var cirka 14 E%, också lägre än i Hulk. Tillsammans med transfettsyror uppgår intaget av "hårt fett" till 15 E%, vilket är betydligt över rekommenderad nivå på 10 E%. Kolhydrater bidrog i genomsnitt med 47 E% för kvinnor och 46 E% för män. Andelen var högre i den lägsta åldersgruppen, 17–24 år. Kostens sockerinnehåll var högre bland kvinnor än bland män och högst bland de yngsta. Fibreintaget var 17–18 g/d, motsvarande 1,8 g/MJ för män och 2,1 g/MJ för kvinnor, vilket är cirka två tredjedelar av den rekommenderade nivån (3 g/MJ). Intaget har inte förändrats nämnvärt jämfört med Hulk.

Alkoholintaget var högre bland män än bland kvinnor och utgjorde i genomsnitt 4 respektive 3 E%. Nivån är något högre än i Hulk. Intaget av koksalt (exklusive saltning vid bordet m m) var 7 g/d bland kvinnor och 9 g/d bland män vilket är något högre än i Hulk. Det faktiska intaget är högre.

Intaget av vitaminer var som regel tillfredsställande. Intaget av vitamin D var lägre än rekommenderad nivå bland äldre, medan intaget av folat var cirka 75 procent av rekommendationen. Även det genomsnittliga intaget av mineralämnen var som regel i nivå med eller över rekommenderad nivå. Intaget av järn var däremot lågt hos kvinnor i fertil ålder, cirka två tredjedelar av rekommendationen. Selenintaget var cirka tre fjärdedelar av rekommenderad nivå, både för män och kvinnor. Intaget av retinol var lägre i Riksmaten än i Hulk, medan intaget av vitamin C var högre. Järnintaget var lägre än i Hulk beroende på att järnberikningen av siktat mjöl upphörde 1995.

Åldersskillnader i matvanorna var för flera livsmedel betydande. Äldre äter mer av "traditionella" livsmedel såsom potatis och rotfrukter, fisk, inälvs- och blodmat, gröt och kaffebröd än yngre gör, som i sin tur äter och dricker mer "moderna" livsmedel såsom pasta, ris, pizza, godis, nötter och snacks samt läsk och juice. Äldre äter däremot mer frukt och grönsaker än yngre och tycks alltså bättre ha tagit till sig kostbudskapet. Kvinnor har i vissa avseenden bättre matvanor än män, t ex var frukt- och grönsakskonsumtionen högre. Skillnaderna i näringsintag mellan män och kvinnor var relativt små.

Låg utbildning var kopplad till en lägre konsumtion av bl a grönsaker och frukt och hos män till ett högre intag av matfett. Lågutbildade män åt en kost med en högre fetthalt i kosten än högutbildade gjorde (35 respektive 33 E%) medan någon sådan skillnad inte förelåg bland kvinnor. Hög utbildning var kopplad till ett högre alkoholintag. Välutbildade kvinnors kost innehöll mer beta-karoten, vitamin C och folat än de lågutbildades. Välutbildade mäns kost innehöll mer vitamin C och folat än lågutbildade mäns kost. Liknande tendenser, dock mindre uttalade, sågs när personerna grupperades efter hushållets socioekonomiska status.

Rökare, främst män, hade sämre matvanor än icke-rökare med bl a en lägre konsumtion av frukt och grönsaker. Rökande män åt en fetare kost än icke-rökare (36 E% respektive 34 E%). Män som snusade drack mer alkohol jämfört med dem som aldrig snusat.

Vissa regionala skillnader i kostmönster noterades men som regel var skillnaderna inte uttalade. Bland annat var intaget av frukt och grönsaker lägre i Norrland jämfört med Stockholmsområdet, medan intaget av matfett, mjölk och fil var högre. Andelen fett och mättat fett i männens kost var högre i Norrland än i Stockholmsområdet, medan intaget av alkohol var högre i Stockholmsområdet. Intaget av kalcium bland män och kvinnor var högre i Norrland än i Stockholms län och i Sydsverige, medan intaget av askorbinsyra hos män och kvinnor var högre i Stockholm än i mellersta och övre Norrland. I övrigt var de regionala skillnaderna små.

Age Groups

18	24
25	34
35	44
45	54
55	64
65	74

Sweden on the move 2001

Sätt Sverige i rörelse 2001

Project Leader

Project Leader	Johan Tranquist
Address	National Institute of Public Health
	Olof Palmes gata 17
	103 52 Stockholm
	Sweden
Executing Institution	National Institute of Public Health
Funding Agency	National Institute of Public Health

Project Information

Start of Project	01/01/2001
End of Project	31/12/2001
Start of Data Collection	01/01/2001
End of Data Collection	31/12/2001
URL	
Scope	National

Keywords

Abstract (English) *Sweden on the move 2001*: People in modern-day society have become less and less physically active, which has well-documented negative consequences for health and well-being. There is a growing awareness at all levels of society, and many countries show a need for action to follow development. Physical inactivity has become an important public health issue that must be highlighted at the local, regional, and national level.

A long-term strategy of change: Sweden on the move – 2001 was a national programme that focuses on people's need for physical activity to promote health and well-being. The National Institute of Public Health was commissioned by the Government to plan for a physical activity year 2001 in collaboration with a number of government agencies and organisations. This year was the start of a long-term strategy of change with the aim of promoting health and preventing disease by increased physical activity. In 1999 a joint steering group established the objectives and organisation of the work. The aims and objectives were based on the Ottawa charter and the five strategies: Strengthen community action; develop personal skills; reorient health services, create supportive environments; and build healthy public policy, and on the National Public Health Committee's proposals for aims for physical activity.

The government commission: "The National Institute of Public Health shall, in broad consultation with the relevant authorities and organisations, turn 2001 into a year of physical activity."

Aims: To introduce through various social and structural measures a long-term national programme of change with the purpose of increasing the level of physical activity in Sweden. To spread knowledge to decision-makers and professional groups of the health consequences of decisions that affect the external environment, leisure, preschool/school, healthcare, and the workplace. To deepen understanding of the great importance of daily physical exercise for public health. To develop everyday environments so that they support safe forms of physically active behavior. To make the population more physically active, with the emphasis on the most inactive groups in society.

Overall objectives: The knowledge, interest, and the prerequisites for physical activity are to be increased for everyone. Health is to be specially improved for the groups that are exposed to the greatest health risks. All people regardless of social position, gender, age, ethnicity, and disability are to be given the prerequisites for physical activity and movement.

Specific objectives: Children of preschool age are stimulated to daily physical activity and play indoors and outdoors. Children and adolescents are stimulated to a positive attitude to physical activity, and are to be given the opportunity of taking part every day in some activity that appeals to them. School is a supportive environment for physical activity. Adults are encouraged and given the opportunity to daily physical activity. The residential environment is a supporting environment for physical activity. The recreational venues for physical activity are developed from the perspective of accessibility, equality of opportunity, equity, and integration. The work place is a supporting environment for healthy physical activity. Health care staffs have a broad knowledge of the preventive effects of physical activityand apply this knowledge for disease prevention. Guidelines for physical activity are used for different patient categories with regard to prevention and reactivation.

Research on physical activity and its importance for public health is to be stimulated. Regarding setting oriented strategic initiatives, two parallel approaches have been developed to implement this. One involves strategic measures via four settings and the other involves the encouragement and creation of opportunities for local and regional initiatives. The four setting-oriented groups were producing proposals during the spring of year 2000 on strategic and structural initiatives for the settings preschool and school, workplace, health care, and leisure time on the basis of the aims and overall objectives. Efforts will concern increase of knowledge and knowledge dissemination, education, method development, research, and evaluation.

As regards the work of local and regional players within the municipalities and county councils and organisations, the National Institute of Public Health's intention was that the regional and local level would be inspired and encouraged by the work of the arena groups to develop local strategies for increased physical activity in society. The National Institute of Public Health has also collaborated with the Swedish Association of Local Authorities in the run up to 2001 to producing method guidance for local public health work relating to physical activity. Each region/county has recruited a "messenger" via the social-medicine units. The messenger has been responsible during the year for regional communication and to take on the task of creating regional networks to coordinate the measures.

Target group: The measures and activities have been primarily geared toward professional groups that can help to create supportive environments for health-promoting physical activity with the purpose of creating equal conditions for the population to make healthy choices. Measures and activities directly geared toward the general public have primarily come about through players other than the National Institute of Public Health.

Message: The main emphasis of the message have been the health-promotive importance of daily exercise also including exercise, sport, and recreation. The message have been based on the principle that 30 min of daily physical activity can prevent a wide range of illnesses and that inactivity in Sweden is one of the major factors behind premature death and preventable illness.

The role and responsibility of the National Institute of Public Health: The National Institute of Public Health has coordinated the planning of the year, with the responsibility for the coordination of the national measures. The Institute has been responsible for common marketing and communication and also for evaluation and follow-up. We have checked to ensure that equality aspects are being observed and part-financing the measures. The Institute has also coordinated the support and encouragement of local and regional initiatives primarily through the messenger system at regional level, but also through method development and network support. The National Institute of Public Health has although been responsible for material production and for supporting certain research measures.

Evaluation: In the short term, the recommended focus for the evaluation has been the implementation of "Sweden on the move 2001," on the basis of the objectives formulated by each arena group for its activity and the activity initiated locally in the country's municipalities and regions. Primarily, this involves studying whether it has been possible to implement the planned measures and, if so, what factors made that possible.

After a number of years, it is also important to study the distribution effect and how measures that have been initiated are maintained and developed. In the longer term, after about five years, it is also important to study the degree to which the overall objectives and the specific objectives of the programme have been achieved. To gain an understanding of both the process and the outcome in the form of short-term, desirable and any undesired effects, various methods and strategies have been and will be used in the evaluation process with both quantitative and qualitative study methodology.

Result: Some results of the SoM-year. More than 70 different nongovernmental and governmental organisations have been collaborating during the year. Over 80 national conferences have been arranged, and the first national conference of health enhancing physical activity had over 900 participants. As many as 162 municipalities (out of 289) have been participating in 15 regional conferences. All 21 county councils have been actively involved in the work with the SoM-year, at least one "SoM-messenger" from each county council have been selected for this mission. A total of 205 (out of 289) municipalities were familiar with the physical activity year and 65% had planned their own activities. Over 200 companies, with 50, 000 employees all together, are involved in a certification process of becoming a health promotion company. Sweden is now in the Guinness Book of Record for having brought together a total of 64,782 people doing aerobics simultaneously. Nearly 3,000 mass media features on the physical activity year have been spotted during the SoM-year as well as news on how to be physical. Over 20 official publications have been produced and distributed to different target groups. National recommendation for health enhancing physical activity has been set – "At least 30 min of physical activity per day on a moderate intensity." A lot of schools are involved in the process to increase the physical activity to consist of at least 30 min every day. A number of conferences have been held throughout the country. Pamphlets on best practice as well as several activity catalogues for children regarding activities in school have been produced. Physical activity on prescription is emerging, and the results have been good so far. A handbook for GP on how to prescribe physical activity is about to be published. Please visit http://www.fyss.org for more information in Swedish. Health enhancing physical activity is at the top of the agenda. The status of physical activity has increased. Physical activity has become one of the most important public health issues. This year's good results have led to a new commission from the Government – "Keep Sweden Moving." The commission instructs the National Institute of Public Health to continue their work with health enhancing physical activity troughout year 2003 and 2004. The comission also includes a request for a proposed national strategy for increased physical activity in society.

Abstract (Original Language) Det växande problemet i västvärlden med fysisk inaktivitet, som är en bidragande orsak till övervikt och fetma och dess följdsjukdomar, kom alltmer i fokus under senare delen av 90-talet. Regeringen gav därför 1998 Folkhälsoinstitutet i uppdrag att ta fram underlag för hur man skulle kunna vända den negativa hälsoutvecklingen. Resultatet blev rapporten "Fysisk aktivitet för nytta och nöje", som innehåller en genomgång av nationella och internationella studier och onsensusrapporter rörande fysisk aktivitet och hälsa. Dessa visar ett mycket tydligt samband mellan omfattningen av fysisk aktivitet och hälsotillståndet. Folkhälsoinstitutet fick därefter ett nytt regeringsuppdrag, att "i samråd med berörda myndigheter och organisationer göra 2001 till ett fysiskt aktivitetsår". Satsningen fick namnet "Sätt Sverige i rörelse 2001" (SSIR).

Syftet med SSIR var att inleda ett långsiktigt arbete med att förändra inställningen i samhället till fysisk aktivitet och så småningom få en beteendeförändring i befolkningen.

Satsningen har engagerat organisationer och myndigheter samt ledare och personal inom många olika samhällssektorer. Inriktning, syfte, mål och strategier liksom namn och budskap fastslogs av en styrgrupp med bred representation.

Två parallella ansatser för genomförandet utvecklades. Den ena ansatsen avsåg strategiska insatser via fyra arenor; arbetsplatsen, förskolan/skolan, fritiden och hälso- och sjukvården. Den andra avsåg möjliggörande och uppmuntran till lokala och regionala initiativ, med stöd av regionala s.k. "budbärare".

Även i genomförandet har funnits ett brett engagemang från och samverkan mellan myndigheter och organisationer, på såväl nationell som regional och lokal nivå. Mycket av det samarbete som startats kommer att fortleva efter projektets slut.

Omgivningens intresse för SSIR var stort så fort det blivit klart att FHI fått uppdraget. Planeringsarbetet kom därigenom att genomföras under tidspress. Det breda samarbetet innebar också att många myndigheter och organisationer inspirerades till egna insatser. Sådana spridningseffekter är förstås glädjande men innebär också att projektet inte blev så välavgränsat som man ur utvärderingssynpunkt kunnat önska.

SSIR har inte haft någon speciell budget för reklaminsatser men trots det har aktiviteterna inom ramen för projektet rönt jämförelsevis mycket stor uppmärksamhet i media.

Age Groups

The Choice of Lunch: Study

Val av lunchrätt – En orienterande studie

Project Leader

Project Leader	Clara Westman and Marie Skans
Address	The National Food Administration
	Box 622
	751 26 Uppsala
	Sweden
Executing Institution	The National Food Administration
Funding Agency	

Project Information

Start of Project	01/03/2001
End of Project	31/03/2001
Start of Data Collection	01/03/2001
End of Data Collection	31/03/2001
URL	
Scope	National

Keywords

Abstract (Original Language) Ätandet på restauranger ökar och en relativt stor del av den vuxna befolkningen äter lunch på restaurang flera gånger i veckan. På uppdrag av Livsmedelsverket har Sifo Research & Consulting AB genomfört en undersökning vars syfte var att kartlägga yttre och individrelaterade faktorer som bestämmer gästernas val av maträtter och tillbehör i lunchrestauranger. De faktorer som Livsmedelsverket primärt önskade få belysta i denna process var:

- Inställning och förhållningssätt till lunch på restaurang
- Kunskap och medvetenhet om kostens betydelse för hälsan
- Hälsoaspekter vid lunch på restaurang
- Nyckelhålsmärkning av rätter
- Betydelsen av utbud för val av lunchrätt och tillbehör

Undersökningen har genomförts i två delar, en med kvantitativa och en med kvalitativa metoder. Den kvantitativa delen syftar till att visa omfattning av olika aspekter kring lunchätande. Den kvalitativa delen syftar till att skapa förståelse av de olika aspekterna och ge förståelse för varför.

Lunchätandet fyller till stor del en social funktion; att få ett avbrott i arbetsdagen och tid attsamtala med sina kollegor. Att restaurangen ligger nära arbetsplatsen är därför betydelsefullt. Lunchen utgör också för många en stor del av det dagliga kostintaget. Valet av lunchrestaurang påverkas därmed av att flera personer i ett sällskap ska kunna hitta en lunchrätt som de kan tänka sig att äta, att restaurangen serverar prisvärd mat (god kvalitet och smak till rätt pris) och att inomhusmiljön är trevlig. Dagens rätt är ett sådant erbjudande som ofta betraktas prisvärt när sallad, bröd och dryck ingår.

Valet av maträtt styrs av aspekter som att man önskar variera sin kost, bli mätt och njuta, dvs äta något man förväntar sig ska vara gott och som stämmer överens med egna värderingar (vegetariskt, hälsosamt, ekologiskt odlat). När man kommer till den faktiska valsituationen har matens utseende stor betydelse. Man vill äta mat som ser ut att vara tillagad av råvaror med god kvalitet. En hjälp i detta val är att se hur maten ser ut på övriga restauranggästers tallrikar eller i förekommande fall på provtallrikar.

Att kunna välja tillbehör som potatis (kokt/ stekt), ris eller pasta visar sig inte vara centralt för val av maträtt i denna undersökning. Har man möjligheten, väljer man det tillbehör man själv upplever smakmässigt passar bäst till maten eller det man av erfarenhet upplever håller bäst kvalitet i storkökstillagning.

Matens innehåll är man intresserad av och det finns också ett stigande matintresse. I enlighet med detta finns ett behov av att veta mer om matens ursprung och produktion. Nyckelhålsmärkning uppfattas vara en vägvisare till den som vill välja fettsnål mat, men en utvidgad innehållsdeklaration för maträtter efterfrågas och skulle sannolikt underlätta valet för den alltmer medvetne lunchätaren.

Age Groups

20	34
35	64

The National Public Health Report 2005

Folkhälsorapport 2005

Project Leader

Project Leader	Gudrun Persson
Address	Socialstyrelsen
	S-106 30 Stockholm
	Sweden
Executing Institution	Centre for Epidemiology, National Board of Health and Welfare
Funding Agency	

Project Information

Start of Project	01/01/2005
End of Project	31/12/2005
Start of Data Collection	01/01/2005
End of Data Collection	31/12/2005
URL	http://www.socialstyrelsen.se/Om_Sos/organisation/
	Epidemiologiskt_Centrum/Enheter/A/Folkhalsorapportering.htm
Scope	National

Keywords

Abstract (English) Health in Sweden – the National Public Health Report 2005 is number six in a series of public health reports commissioned by the Swedish government. The purpose of these reports is to monitor and analyse the development of health in various groups of the population. By doing this the public health reports form a basis for evaluation and improvements of health policies. Overall social change, living conditions, and behaviors are of major significance for health; and in the report these are related to health development. The prerequisites for epidemiological research as for monitoring public health are particularly good in Sweden thanks to several extensive national health registers of high quality, which also include unique personal identification numbers for each citizen. The national Public Health Report is a fine illustration of the use of registers, and we hope the Report will be of interest to an international audience.

The Report is intended primarily for politicians at national, regional, and local levels whose decisions, in different ways, can create the preconditions for favorable public health development. The Report is also directed toward organizations and authorities responsible for improving the health of the population, toward local public-health workers, toward health-oriented study programmes in uppersecondary schools and universities, and toward interested members of the public. Bearing this in mind some parts of the Report – e.g., some fact boxes of descriptions of methods and measures – might seem rather basic especially to an international scientific public. The overall development of health, of mortality, of the major public health-problems as well as of living habits constitutes the central core of the Report. Topics such as working life and the importance of the work environment, and the significance of the external environment for public health, each has their own chapters. A concluding chapter forecasts how health might develop in the future. The development of social differences in health is also discussed, as well as the role of medical care for future health, particularly among the elderly. The consequences of increased alcohol consumption and of increased obesity for public health are other issues dealt with. Moreover, it is debated whether snuff-taking is contributing to reduced smoking, and also how developments in society and public health are linked.

Abstract (Original Language) Folkhälsorapporten utarbetas på uppdrag av regeringen. Den beskriver hur svenska folkets hälsa utvecklas samt hur levnadsvanor och faktorer i omgivningen hänger samman med hälsoutvecklingen. Vanliga folksjukdomar belyses för hela befolkningen, i olika åldrar och för män och kvinnor. Av särskilt intresse är hälsans samband med sociala faktorer och exponering som individen inte själv kan påverka men som kan vara möjliga att påverka med politiska åtgärder. Att se mönster i ohälsan och följa utvecklingen över tid förbättrar möjligheterna att förstå vad som orsakar ohälsa och att se hur hälsoproblemen kan angripas.

Folkhälsorapport 2005 som publicerades i slutet av mars 2005 är den sjätte i raden av nationella folkhälsorapporter. Tidigare rapporter har utgivits åren, 1987, 1991, 1994, 1997 och 2001.

Folkhälsorapport 2005 ger en bred översikt över hur svenska folkets hälsa utvecklas och hur den påverkas av levnadsvanor och omgivningsfaktorer. Den beskriver folkhälsoläget övergripande samt fördelningen i befolkningen efter kön, ålder, socioekonomisk grupp m.m. Den ger även ett internationellt perspektiv på folkhälsan i Sverige. När det gäller de största folkhälsoproblemen har det i denna folkhälsorapport gjorts en fördjupning med avseende på utvecklingen av diabetes samt övervikt och fetma. Även barns hälsa behandlas mer ingående än tidigare, bland annat genom att kapitlet om den yttre miljön har ett särskilt fokus på barns hälsa.

Dessutom introduceras ett för svenska folkhälsorapporter nytt ämne: reproduktiv hälsa, som i Sverige har en mer begränsad betydelse för folkhälsan i stort men är en mycket väsentlig del av framför allt kvinnors hälsa. Folkhälsan beskrivs vidare i ett livscykelperspektiv; hur ser hälsan ut bland barn och ungdomar respektive bland yngre och äldre pensionärer? I övrigt behandlas befolkningens levnadsvanor, som alkohol- och tobaksvanor, matvanor, fysisk aktivitet etc. Hälsa sätts även i relation till arbetslivet och arbetsmiljön. Rapporten avslutas med ett kapitel som kommenterar hälsoutvecklingen och blickar framåt – vad kan vi vänta oss av av folkhälsoutvecklingen i framtiden?

Age Groups

16	24
25	34
35	44
45	54
55	64
65	74
75	84

The Netherlands

Dutch Food Consumption Survey 1992

VCP-2

Project Leader

Project Leader	Dr. K. Hulshof
Address	P.O. Box 360,
	3700 AJ Zeist
Executing Institution	TNO Quality of Life
Funding Agency	Ministry of Health, Welfare and Sport and Ministry of Agriculture,
	Nature and Food quality

Project Information

Start of Project	01/01/1992
End of Project	31/12/1992
Start of Data Collection	01/01/1992
End of Data Collection	31/12/1992
URL	
Scope	National

Keywords Food Consumption Survey-2; The Netherlands; Dietary intake; DNFCS-2; Food intake; Energy; Macronutrients; Micronutrients

Abstract (English) The Dutch National Food Consumption Survey (DNFCS) is a comprehensive survey of food consumption in a representative sample of the Dutch population. In 1992, the second national survey was conducted (DNFCS-2). Data collection was performed by a marketing research institute experienced in nationwide surveys. The surveys were financially supported and carried out under the authority of the Ministry of Agriculture, Nature Management & Fisheries, the Ministry of Welfare, Health and Culture.

From an existing panel, households were selected. Institutionalised individuals, households with a person with inadequate fluency in the Dutch language and children younger than 1 year were not eligible. In DNFCS-2, 6,218 subjects aged 1–92 years participated (response 72%).

The food consumption data were collected through a two-day dietary record method. The foods consumed indoors were recorded in a household diary for all members of the household by the person usually engaged in preparation of the meals. Outdoor consumption was recorded by every participant on a personal diary (children less than 13 were assisted by a parent or both parents). In each survey, food consumption data were collected during 40 weeks per year and evenly distributed over the season and the days of the week. No field work was conducted during (public) holidays because low response levels were expected on these days and in these periods. Specially trained dietitians were responsible for the field work, including contacting participants, instructions regarding completion of the diaries, checks on completeness of data and estimates of capacity of household utensils (common household measures and foods regularly used were weighed), and coding of the data. For more information see Hulshof et al., 1991.

Hulshof KFAM & Staveren WA van (1991). The Dutch national food consumption survey: design, methods and first results. Food Policy 16, 257–260.

Anonymous: Zo eet Nederland, 1998. Resultaten van de Voedselconsumptiepeiling 1997–1998 (1998): Netherlands Nutrition Centre, The Hague.

Abstract (Original Language) Voedselconsumptiepeilingen in Nederland De voedselconsumptiepeiling (VCP) is een uitgebreid onderzoek naar de voedselconsumptie bij een representatieve steekproef van de Nederlandse bevolking (circa 6000 personen). De eerste landelijke VCP is in 1987–1988 uitgevoerd in opdracht van het ministerie van Volksgezondheid, Welzijn en Sport en het ministerie van Landbouw Natuurbeheer en Visserij. In 1992 volgde de tweede peiling. Ook deze peiling werd uitgevoerd in opdracht van en met financiële steun van voornoemde ministeries.

Gegevens VCP: De deelnemers van de VCP zijn afkomstig van een representatief panel van huishoudens (GfK Scriptpanel) met een huisvrouw of -man jonger dan 75 jaar. Personen die in instellingen verblijven (bijvoorbeeld ziekenhuis of verzorgingshuis), personen zonder vaste woon- of verblijfplaats, personen die de Nederlandse taal onvoldoende beheersen en kinderen jonger dan 1 jaar vallen buiten de steekproef van de VCP.

Verspreid over het gehele jaar (vakantieperiodes uitgezonderd) noteerden de deelnemers aan de VCP ieder twee aaneensluitende dagen alles wat zij aten en dronken. Het veldwerk van het onderzoek, waaronder het leggen van contacten met de deelnemers, het instrueren over het invullen van de dagboekjes, het controleren en coderen van de gegevens werd uitgevoerd door speciaal voor het onderzoek getrainde diëtisten. De binnenshuis gebruikte voedingsmiddelen werden door iedere deelnemer afzonderlijk in een persoonsboekje genoteerd. Naast informatie over de voeding werden specifieke gewoonten (bijvoorbeeld volgen van een dieet, gebruik van voedingssupplementen) en enkele persoonsgegevens (bijvoorbeeld lengte en gewicht) nagevraagd. Overige gegevens van de deelnemers zoals samenstelling van de huishouding, opleiding en woonplaats, waren reeds bij het onderzoeksbureau GfK bekend.

Aan VCP-2 is deelgenomen door 6218 personen.

Age Groups

1	4
4	7
7	10
10	13
13	16
16	19
19	22
22	50
50	65
65	and older

Injuries and Physical Activity in the Netherlands

IPAN

Project Leader

Project Leader	Wil Ooijendijk
Address	TNO Kwaliteit van Leven,
	Bewegen en Gezondheid
	Postbus 2215
	2301 CE Leiden
Executing Institution	TNO Quality of Life
Funding Agency	Ministry of Health, Welfare and Sport

Project Information

Start of Project	01/01/2000
End of Project	
Start of Data Collection	01/01/2000
End of Data Collection	
URL	
Scope	National

Keywords Physical activity; Health; Fitness; Guidelines for physical activity

Abstract (English) PURPOSE: Continuous monitoring of physical activity (PA), body mass index (BMI), and health was initiated in 2000 to study trends in physical activity (PA), obesity, and their determinants in the general Dutch population. This abstract refers to this monitor on the period 2000–2004.

Methods:

- Representative rolling sample of the adult Dutch population ($n = \pm 8.000$ yearly)
- Interviews by telephone (mean response rate: 54 %)
- Questions on
- Demographic characteristics
- Physical activity (PA)
- Height/weight
- Determinants of PA

Results: In 2004, 60% met one or both PA-recommendations; this percentage increased during the last two years. Groups that show much lower rates were:

- Persons with overweight
- Younger persons and students
- Elderly persons
- Lower educated persons
- Unemployed persons

- Workers with sedentary work
- Persons with chronic diseases.

The percentage respondents with overweight (BMI 25) was higher in persons who did not comply with the PA-recommendations.

Abstract (Original Language)

Age Groups
4   and older

Local and National Public Health Monitor

LNM

Project Leader

Project Leader	Carolien den Brink (interim projectleader)
Address	P.O. Box 1
	3720 BA Bilthoven
	the netherlands
Executing Institution	RIVM (The National Institute for Public Health and the Environment)
Funding Agency	Ministry of Health

Project Information

Start of Project	01/01/2002
End of Project	
Start of Data Collection	01/01/2004
End of Data Collection	
URL	http://www.monitorgezondheid.nl
Scope	National

Keywords

Abstract (English) The project "Local and National Public Health Monitor" was launched in 2002 as a joint venture of the regional Community Health Services, the National Institute of Public Health and the Environment, and the Netherlands Association of Community Health Services. Its major aim is to bring about a uniform collection of regional data by the Community Health Services. This will enable both a comparison of regional data and a comparison of regional with national reference data, ultimately to support health policies at a local and national level. The project also entails the development of a support structure and database, to store the information collected and to generate national and regional reference data.

Abstract (Original Language)

Age Groups

4	12
12	19
19	64

Longitudinal Aging Study Amsterdam

LASA

Project Leader

Project Leader	Mw. Prof. Dr. Dorly J.H. Deeg
Address	EMGO instituut, VUmc-LASA
	Van der Boechorststraat 7
	1081 BT Amsterdam
Executing Institution	EMGO Institute, Vrije Universiteit
Funding Agency	Ministry of Health, Welfare and Sport; Vrije Universiteit

Project Information

Start of Project	01/01/1992
End of Project	
Start of Data Collection	01/01/1992
End of Data Collection	
URL	http://ssg.scw.vu.nl/lasa/
Scope	National

Keywords

Abstract (English) *Objectives*: LASA is designed to be an interdisciplinary, longitudinal study. Although basically scientific in nature, the study should provide a basis for developing and evaluating (central and local government) policy in the field of aging. The global objective of current policy in the field of aging can be formulated as enhancing the autonomy and quality of life of older persons. It is expected that by using longitudinal data, policy relevant aspects of aging can be identified and new policy aims can be developed. Moreover, assumptions from which policy measures are developed can be tested, and effects of policy changes can be assessed prospectively. LASA is primarily an observational study; the data-base will allow testing of various specific hypotheses. Full intervention studies will not be included in LASA.

Central questions: LASA's main topics of concern are autonomy and quality of life of older persons. Autonomy is operationally defined as functioning, i.e., observable behavior; quality of life is defined as the evaluation by older persons of their functioning. Four components of functioning are distinguished: physical, cognitive, emotional, and social. The four components will have different contributions to autonomy and quality of life. However, this distinction does not intend to deny any interrelation between these components. The study focuses primarily on predictors of change in these components of functioning, on trajectories of functioning, and on consequences of change in functioning. The following central questions have been formulated:

1. Among older persons, what changes over time take place in the physical, cognitive, emotional, and social components of functioning?
2. What are the predictors of change for each of the four components of functioning?
3. How are changes in the four components of functioning interrelated?
4. What are the consequences of changes in functioning in terms of older persons' contributions to society, their adjustment, and their need for care?

More detailed research questions are formulated, some of which make use of additional data collected in specific subsamples. The most important of these side studies are on the course of depression, and on predictors of falls and fractures.

Sample: The initial sample was weighed according to expected mortality at mid-term within each sex and age group, so that after five years equal numbers of men and women were expected to be alive in the ages 55–59, 60–64, 65–69, 70–74, 75–79, and 80–85 years. This design was expected to provide sufficient opportunity for multivariate research and for obtaining adequate subsamples for special studies. In addition, it should leave sufficient participants to be examined after a period of 10 years.

Municipal registries provided the sampling frame. The sample was constructed so as to reflect the national distribution of urbanization and population density. The sample was based in three culturally distinct geographical areas in the West, North-East, and South of the Netherlands. Each area consists of one middle to large-size city and two or more rural municipalities, which border on the city. The municipalities included in the sample are: Amsterdam, Wormerland, Waterland (three municipalities in the West), Zwolle, Ommen, Genemuiden, Zwartsluis, Hasselt (North-East), and Oss, Uden, Boekel (South). Within follow-up observations, subjects who moved out of the municipality were traced and reinterviewed.

Time schedule: The LASA baseline was carried out separately from September 1992 to September 1993, an average of 11 months following the LSN baseline. In 1995–1996, 1998–1999, and 2001–2002 almost identical follow-up data collections were conducted. The data collection among the new cohort has been completed in 2003. In a limited number of side studies of specific subsamples, topics are studied for which additional data collection is needed with more frequent intervals.

Approach of respondents: Trained interviewers who use laptop computers for data entry visit the respondents at home. Interview and tests take one and a half hour approximately. To obtain additional data, respondents are asked to fill out a written questionnaire separately. After having obtained the consent of the respondent, a separate visit is made by a nurse interviewer to draw blood and to take clinical measurements (the "medical interview").

Age Groups

| 55 | and older |

National Panel of People with Chronic Diseases and Handicaps

NPCG

Project Leader

Project Leader	Dr Mieke Rijken
Address	P.O Box 1568
	3500 BN Utrecht
	The Netherlands
Executing Institution	Netherlands Institute for Health
	Services Research (NIVEL)
Funding Agency	Ministry of Health, Welfare and Sports
	and Ministry of Social Affairs and Employment

Project Information

Start of Project	01/01/2004
End of Project	
Start of Data Collection	01/01/2004
End of Data Collection	
URL	http://www.nivel.nl/npcg
Scope	National

Keywords

Abstract (English) NPCD is a nationwide research programme investigating the consequences of chronic illness and physical handicaps for patients and their families in the Netherlands. Patients were recruited via a representative sample of general practices and via two population surveys. Every year the panel is refreshed because persons dropped out. Data are collected by postal questionnaires. Data on physical activity are measured by frequencies of activities and by type of activity. Data on food are only limited collected: the panel members are asked how they take account of their food

Age Groups

Data are collected from persons 15 years and older

National Survey Musculoskeletal Complaints

Project Leader

Project Leader	Dr. Ir. A.M.J. Chorus
Address	P.O. box 2215
	2301 CE Leiden
Executing Institution	TNO Quality of Life
Funding Agency	Ministry of Health, Welfare and Sport,
	Dutch Arthritis Association

Project Information

Start of Project	01/01/2006
End of Project	31/12/2008
Start of Data Collection	01/05/2006
End of Data Collection	
URL	
Scope	National

Keywords Rheumatic diseases; Musculoskeletal complaints; Quality of life; Prevalence

Abstract (English) Objective of the study is collecting new data on the prevalence and societal impact of musculoskeletal conditions and specifically, rheumatic diseases in the Netherlands. At this moment data are analysed. First results will be presented in October 2006.

Abstract (Original Language) Doel van het project is nieuwe cijfers te verzamelen over het voorkomen en de maatschappelijke gevolgen van klachten van het bewegingsapparaat en specifiek reumatische aandoeningen in Nederland. Op dit moment vinden de analyses plaats. De eerste resultaten zullen oktober 2006 gepresenteerd worden.

Age Groups

15	and older

NL: *Kinderen in Prioriteitswijken: Lichamelijke (in)Activiteit en Overgewicht; ENGLISH: Children in disadvantaged neighbourhoods: Physical (in)Activity and Overweight*

NL: Wijk en Jeugd English: SPACE Study (Spatial Planning And Children's Exercise study)

Project Leader

Project Leader	Dr. Ir. Ingrid Bakker
Address	TNO Kwaliteit van Leven,
	Preventie en zorg,
	Bewegen en Gezondheid,
	Postbus 2215
	2301 CE Leiden
	Nederland
Executing Institution	TNO Kwaliteit van Leven; Bewegen en Gezondheid (TNO Quality of Life)
Funding Agency	Ministry of Health, Welfare and Sport; Ministry of Housing, Spatial Planning and the Environment

Project Information

Start of Project	01/07/2004
End of Project	01/10/2005
Start of Data Collection	01/10/2004
End of Data Collection	01/01/2005
URL	
Scope	National

Keywords Physical activity; Children; Obesity; Built environment; Accelerometer

Abstract (English) *Background*: The rapid increase in the prevalence of overweight and obesity in children has attracted the attention of the public health community and raised the awareness of children's physical activity levels. The lack of evidence for an increased energy consumption by children implies their physical activity level has declined and their physical inactivity level has increased in recent years. Nowadays, children have less space to play outside. Building offices, houses, and car parks often get higher priority in urban planning than realizing playgrounds. To date, the effects of these decisions on children's physical activity levels and the successive increase in the prevalence of overweight and obesity are unknown.

Objectives: The objective of the Spatial Planning and Children's Exercise (SPACE) study was to investigate the association between neighborhood characteristics and children's physical (in)activity level in order to guide urban planners in remodeling "non-activity friendly" into "activity-friendly" neighborhoods

Methods: The SPACE study involved 1,228 6- to 11-year-old children recruited from 20 elementary schools in ten Dutch neighborhoods. Five of these neighborhoods have received priority from the Dutch Ministry of Housing, Spatial Planning and the Environment for spatial restructuring in the near future. The other five were matched on type of buildings, construction period, socioeconomic status, and age distribution. Physical activity was assessed by activity diaries and ActiGraph accelerometers. Neighborhood characteristics were scored using a checklist. Multivariate analyses were used to examine the association between neighborhood characteristics and children's physical (in)activity level.

Results: More than 600 children completed the activity diary ($n = 625$; 6–11 yr; 22% overweight; 9% obese; 51% girls). Three percent of the subjects met the physical activity guideline to accumulate a minimum of 60 min of moderate-intensity activity per day. The number of days on which the children met the guideline significantly increased with the presence of sport grounds, low-rise buildings, residential areas with limited access to traffic, green facilities, water, and car parks. Parking places in the street, intersections, heavy bus and lorry traffic, and the presence of a tram in the neighborhood were negatively associated with the number of days on which children met the physical activity guideline.

Conclusions: This is the first study in the Netherlands in which subjective and objective physical activity data has been gathered and related to neighborhood characteristics in this age group. In this study, the percentage of children meeting the 60 min guideline is considerably lower than what has been found in national surveys. In addition, compared with national surveys, a much higher prevalence of overweight and obesity have been found. Physical (in)activity levels of 6- to 11-year-old children are associated with neighborhoods characteristics of disadvantaged Dutch neighborhood.

Future research: The study should be extended to more "activity-friendly" areas. Furthermore, the measurements of the SPACE study should be repeated in the ten neighborhoods after spatial restructuring of five of them, to investigate its effect on children's physical (in)activity levels and the prevalence of overweight and obesity.

Abstract (Original Language) *Achtergrond*: Steeds meer kinderen in Nederland zijn te dik door een verstoorde energiebalans: het energieverbruik is te laag ten opzichte van de energie-inname. Er is sprake van een toenemende lichamelijk inactieve leefstijl: kinderen kijken meer televisie, zitten veel achter de computer en worden vaker met de auto naar school gebracht. Bovendien bestaat de indruk dat er steeds minder buiten wordt gespeeld, mede doordat de buitenspeelmogelijkheden steeds schaarser worden. DoelTNO Kwaliteit van Leven heeft met financiering van de Ministeries van VWS en VROM onderzocht of er een cross-sectioneel verband bestaat tussen kenmerken van de gebouwde omgeving en de lichamelijke (in)activiteit van kinderen in Nederlandse stadswijken.

Tien stadswijken zijn onderzocht: vijf stadswijken uit het dossier '50-wijkenaanpak' van het Ministerie van VROM en vijf vergelijkbare controlewijken. Ruim 1200 kinderen uit groep 3 t/m 7 van twintig reguliere basisscholen hebben tussen oktober 2004 en januari 2005 deelgenomen aan het onderzoek.

Methoden: Om de prevalentie van overgewicht en obesitas te bepalen, is bij alle kinderen de lichaamslengte en het lichaamsgewicht gemeten. De kinderen hebben samen met hun ouders gedurende een week een beweegdagboekje bijgehouden. Een aantal kinderen heeft daarnaast ook een beweegmeter gedragen. De energie-inname van de kinderen is gemeten met behulp van een voedselfrequentievragenlijst. De kenmerken van de gebouwde omgeving van de tien stadswijken zijn door twee observatoren in kaart gebracht met behulp van een checklist. Tevens is een aantal kringgesprekken met kinderen en ouders gehouden om een indruk te krijgen van hun wensen en behoeften omtrent het 'beweegvriendelijk' (her)inrichten van hun stadswijk.

ResultatenIn: de onderzochte stadswijken voldeed 3% van de kinderen aan de Nederlandse Norm Gezond Bewegen. Daarnaast was het percentage te dikke kinderen in deze stadswijken (31%) hoger dan gemiddeld in Nederland (±15%). De gemiddelde energie-inname uit de voeding was in overeenkomst met de gemiddelde energiebehoefte van Nederlandse leeftijdsgenootjes. Ook het energiepercentage dat uit tussendoortjes gehaald werd, was niet hoger dan landelijke cijfers.Verder bleek dat hoe meer sportvelden, laagbouw, woonerven en woongebieden met autoluwe zones, groen, water en gegroepeerde parkeerplaatsen en hoe minder hondenpoep en druk en zwaar verkeer in de wijk, des te actiever de kinderen.

Het onderzoek: biedt stedenbouwkundigen en beleidsmedewerkers handvatten voor het 'beweegvriendelijk' (her)inrichten van stadswijken voor kinderen. Na herinrichting van de vijf stadsvernieuwingswijken zal een nameting plaatsvinden.

Age Groups

6	6
7	7
8	8
9	9
10	10
11	11

Permanent Onderzoek Leefsituatie, Module Gezondheid (Permanent Survey on Living Conditions)

POLS_Gezo

Project Leader

Project Leader	J. van den Berg (interim)
Address	P.O Box 4481
	6401 CZ Heerlen
Executing Institution	Centraal Bureau voor de Statistiek
	(CBO) (Statistics Netherlands)
Funding Agency	CBS

Project Information

Start of Project	01/01/2001
End of Project	
Start of Data Collection	01/01/2001
End of Data Collection	
URL	http://www.cbs.nl
Scope	National

Keywords Health survey; Health lifestyle; Health care

Abstract (English) *Aim*: To monitor trends in health, lifestyle factors and consumption of health care in the general Dutch population. Methods: A continuous face-to face health survey in the Dutch population (>12 years) containing the self-administered SQUASH questionnaire and questions about alcohol consumption.

Results: Physical activity: In 2005, the Dutch population spend 55 min/week to commuter traffic, 885 min/week to activities at school or work, 649 min/week to household activities, 426 min/week to leisure time activities, and 138 min/week to sports. In 2005, 53% of the Dutch populated lived according the Dutch guideline of physical activity. Alcohol: In 2005, the average number of alcohol consumption each day was 1.1 glass/day while 18.6% of the Dutch population consumed no alcohol, and 10.8 % of the population consumed at least once a week more than 6 glasses of alcohol.

*Conclusion*s: In 2005, more subjects met the Dutch guideline of physical activity compared the average of

Aim: To monitor trends in health, lifestyle factors, and consumption of health care in the general Dutch population. *Methods*: A continuous face-to-face health survey in the Dutch population (>12 years) containing the self-administered SQUASH questionnaire and questions about alcohol consumption.

Results: Physical activity: In 2005, the Dutch population spend 55 min/week to commuter traffic, 885 min/week to activities at school or work, 649 min/week to household activities, 426 min/week to leisure time activities, and 138 min/week to sports. In 2005, 53% of the Dutch populated lived according the Dutch guideline of physical activity. Alcohol: In 2005, the average number of alcohol consumption each day was 1.1 glass/day while 18.6% of the Dutch population consumed no alcohol and 10.8% of the population consumed at least once a week more than 6 glasses of alcohol.

Conclusions: In 2005, more subjects met the Dutch guideline of physical activity compared, the average of 2001–2004. For alcohol consumption, the percentage of heavy drinkers slightly decreases compared with the previous years.

Abstract (Original Language) *Doel*: Het bestuderen van trends in gezondheid, leefstijl en gebruik van gezondheidszorg in de Nederlandse bevolking.

Methoden: Face to face gezondheidssurvey, waarbij de SQASH vragenlijst en vragen over alcohol consumptie zijn opgenomen in een aanvullende schriftelijke vragenlijst. Deze is jaarlijks afgenomen bij een steekproef van de Nederlands bevolking van 12 jaar en ouder (ca 9000 personen)

Resultaten: Lichamelijke activiteit: In 2005 heeft de Nederlandse bevolking gemiddeld 55 minuten per week gespendeerd aan woon/werk of woon/school verkeer, 885 minuten per week aan activiteiten op werk of school, 649 minuten per week aan huishoudelijke werkzaamheden, 426 minuten per week aan vrijetijdsactiviteiten en 138 minuten per week aan sport. Gemiddeld 55 % van de bevolking voldeed aan de Nederlandse Norm van Gezond Bewegen. Alcohol: In 2005 bedroeg het gemiddelde aantal glazen alcohol per dag per persoon 1.1 glas/dag. In 2005 dronk 18.6% van de bevolking dronk geen alcohol en 10.8% van de bevolking dronk minstens 1 keer per week 6 of meer glazen alcohol per dag drinken.

Conclusie: Iets meer personen voldoen aan de Nederlandse Norm voor Gezond Bewegen dan het gemiddelde in de periode 2001–2004. Het overmatige alcoholgebruik was procentueel iets lager dan in de voorgaande jaren.

Age Groups

Data are collected from the age of 12 years up

The Second Dutch National Survey of General Practice

NS-2

Project Leader

Project Leader	Prof. Dr. F Schellevis
Address	Postbus 1568
	3500 BN
	Utrecht
Executing Institution	NIVEL
Funding Agency	Ministry of Health, Welfare and Sport

Project Information

Start of Project	01/01/1998
End of Project	31/12/2003
Start of Data Collection	01/01/2001
End of Data Collection	31/12/2002
URL	http://www.nivel.nl/nationalestudie
Scope	National

Keywords

Abstract (English) The second Dutch National Survey in General Practice was mainly conducted in 2001. In all, 195 general practitioners (GPs) from 104 practices across the Netherlands recorded all contacts with patients during 12 consecutive months. Data included diagnosis made during one year by general practitioners, derived from the electronic medical records, prescriptions for medication and sociodemographic characteristics collected via a postal questionnary (response 76%). Complementary, around 5% of the total patient population was interviewed, which led to a total of 12,699 persons. In interview, questions were asked about lifestyle factors, such as physical activity, smoking behavior, and food consumption. Several groups were identified with a less health food consumption such as scholars, unemployed persons, and persons with a lower social economic status. Groups with a lower level of physical activity were allochtonous persons, persons living in urban areas, and persons incapacitated for work.

Abstract (Original Language)

Age Groups

12	19
20	29
30	39
40	49
50	59
60	69
70	and older

Voedselconsumptiepeiling 2003 bij Jongvolwassenen; Dutch Food Consumption Survey 2003 Among Young Adults

VCP-2003

Project Leader

Project Leader	Dr. ir. Marga C Ocké
Address	P.O. Box 1,
	3720 BA Bilthoven
Executing Institution	RIVM (National Institute for Public Health and the Environment)
Funding Agency	Ministry of Health, Welfare and Sport

Project Information

Start of Project	01/07/2003
End of Project	10/10/2004
Start of Data Collection	20/10/2003
End of Data Collection	13/12/2003
URL	http://www.voedselconsumptiepeiling.nl
Scope	National

Keywords 24-h recalls; Dietary monitoring; Food consumption; Telephone interviews; Young adults

Abstract (English) Among young Dutch adults consumption of vegetables and fruits is grossly inadequate. With regard to dietary fat intake, intake of satured fats is still too high whereas average intake of trans fatty acids is almost at the recommended level. A great gain in public health can be achieved by improving dietary habits to recommendation levels, i.e., by increasing vegetable and fruit consumption and improving the fatty acid profile in the diet. Food consumption was assessed in 750 Dutch adults 19–30 years of age. Given the recommendation of 150–200 g vegetables per day, only 2% of the research population consumed 150 g daily and nobody consumed 200 g daily. Less then 10% of the population consumed the recommended 200 g of fruit per day. Over half of the respondents (53% of the women and 58 of the men) consumed a diet with less than 35 energy% fat. The recommendation to use a diet with less than 10 energy% saturated fatty acids was met by few: 11% of the men and 6% of the women. Almost 60% of the men and 28% of the women used a diet that contained less than one energy% of trans fatty acids. On the basis of these results, we advise that nutrition policy should remain focussed on increasing vegetable and fruit consumption, and decreasing intake of saturated fatty acids.

Abstract (Original Language) Nederlandse jongvolwassenen consumeren veel te weinig groenten en fruit. Met betrekking tot de vetinneming is met name de inneming van verzadigde vetzuren te hoog, terwijl de inneming van transvetzuren de aanbeveling gemiddeld benadert. Er valt veel gezondheidswinst te behalen wanneer de voedingsgewoonten in lijn zouden zijn met de aanbevelingen, met name door de groente- en fruitconsumptie te verhogen en het vetzuurprofiel in de voeding te verbeteren. In dit onderzoek zijn de voedingsgewoonten van 750 19-30 jarige Nederlanders gemeten. Uitgaande van de aanbeveling van 150–200 gram groenten per dag, bleek dat slechts 2% van de deelnemers (5,5% van de mannen en 0,2% van de vrouwen) minstens 150 g per dag consumeerde en niemand gewoonlijk 200 gram groente of meer gebruikte. Op basis van gebruikelijke consumptie voor de groep 'vruchten' bleek dat slechts 7–8% de aanbevolen 200 gram at. Ruim de helft van de deelnemers (53% van de vrouwen en 58% van de mannen) gebruikte een voeding met minder dan 35 energie% vet. De richtlijn om minder dan 10 energie% verzadigde vetzuren te gebruiken werd slechts door weinigen bereikt: namelijk door 11% van de mannen en 6% van de vrouwen. Bijna 60% van de mannen en 28% van de vrouwen gebruikten een voeding die minder dan één energie% transvetzuren bevatte. Op basis van deze resultaten wordt geadviseerd om het voedingsbeleid te blijven richten op het stimuleren van de groente- en fruitconsumptie en het verminderen van de hoeveelheid verzadigde vetzuren in de voeding.

Age Groups

19	31

Voedselfconsumptiepeiling 1997/1998; Food Consumption Survey 1997/1998

VCP-3

Project Leader

Project Leader	Dr. K. Hulshof
Address	P.O. Box 360
	3700 AJ Zeist
Executing Institution	TNO Quality of Life
Funding Agency	Ministry of Health, Welfare and Sport; Ministry
	of Agriculture, Nature Management & Fisheries

Project Information

Start of Project	01/04/1997
End of Project	01/03/1998
Start of Data Collection	01/04/1997
End of Data Collection	01/03/1998
URL	
Scope	National

Keywords Food Consumption Survey-3; The Netherlands; Dietary intake; DNFCS-3; Food intake; Energy; Macronutrients; Micronutrients

Abstract (English) The Dutch National Food Consumption Survey (DNFCS) is a comprehensive survey of food consumption in a representative sample of the Dutch population. In 1997–1998, the third national survey was conducted (DNFCS-3). Data collection was performed by a marketing research institute experienced in nationwide surveys. The surveys were financially supported and carried out under the authority of the Ministry of Agriculture, Nature Management & Fisheries, the Ministry of Welfare, Health and Culture.

From an existing panel households were selected. Institutionalised individuals, households with a person with inadequate fluency in the Dutch language, and children younger than 1 year were not eligible. In DNFCS-3, 6,250 subjects aged 1–97 years participated (response 68.5%).

The food consumption data were collected through a two-day dietary record method. The foods consumed indoors were recorded in a household diary for all members of the household by the person usually engaged in preparation of the meals. Outdoor consumption was recorded by every participant on a personal diary (children less than 13 were assisted by a parent or both parents). In each survey food consumption data were collected during 40 weeks per year and evenly distributed over the season and the days of the week. No field work was conducted during (public) holidays because of low response levels were expected on theses days and in these periods. Specially trained dietitians were responsible for the field work, including contacting participants, instructions regarding completion of the diaries, checks on completeness of data and estimates of capacity of household utensils (common household measures and foods regularly used were weighed), and coding of the data. For more information see Hulshof et al, 1991.; Löwik et al, 1994; Löwik et al, 1998; Anonymous, 1998.

Hulshof KFAM & Staveren WA van (1991). The Dutch national food consumption survey: design, methods and first results. Food Policy 16, 257–260.

Anonymous: Zo eet Nederland, 1998. Resultaten van de Voedselconsumptiepeiling 1997–1998 (1998): Netherlands Nutrition Centre, The Hague.

Abstract (Original Language) Voedselconsumptiepeiling 1992

Voedselconsumptiepeilingen in Nederland: De voedselconsumptiepeiling (VCP) is een uitgebreid onderzoek naar de voedselconsumptie bij een representatieve steekproef van de Nederlandse bevolking (circa 6000 personen). De eerste landelijke VCP is in 1987–1988 uitgevoerd in opdracht van het ministerie van Volksgezondheid, Welzijn en Sport en het ministerie van Landbouw Natuurbeheer en Visserij. In 1992 volgde de tweede peiling en in 1997–1998 de de. Ook deze peiling werd uitgevoerd in opdracht van en met financiële steun van voornoemde ministeries.

Gegevens VCP: De deelnemers van de VCP zijn afkomstig van een representatief panel van huishoudens (GfK Scriptpanel) met een huisvrouw of -man jonger dan 75 jaar. Personen die in instellingen verblijven (bijvoorbeeld ziekenhuis of verzorgingshuis), personen zonder vaste woon- of verblijfplaats, personen die de Nederlandse taal onvoldoende beheersen en kinderen jonger dan 1 jaar vallen buiten de steekproef van de VCP.

Verspreid over het gehele jaar (vakantieperiodes uitgezonderd) noteerden de deelnemers aan de VCP ieder twee aaneensluitende dagen alles wat zij aten en dronken. Het veldwerk van het onderzoek, waaronder het leggen van contacten met de deelnemers, het instrueren over het invullen van de dagboekjes, het controleren en coderen van de gegevens werd uitgevoerd door speciaal voor het onderzoek getrainde diëtisten. De binnenshuis gebruikte voedingsmiddelen werden door iedere deelnemer afzonderlijk in een persoonsboekje genoteerd. Naast informatie over de voeding werden specifieke gewoonten (bijvoorbeeld volgen van een dieet, gebruik van voedingssupplementen) en enkele persoonsgegevens (bijvoorbeeld lengte en gewicht) nagevraagd. Overige gegevens van de deelnemers zoals samenstelling van de huishouding, opleiding en woonplaats, waren reeds bij het onderzoeksbureau GfK bekend.

Aan VCP-3 is deelgenomen door 6250 personen.

Age Groups

1	4
4	7
7	10
10	13
13	16
16	19
19	22
22	50
50	65
65	97

Turkey

2000 Population Census

Project Leader

Project Leader	Turkish Statistical Institute (Turkstat),
Address	Necatibey Cad. No:114 Bakanliklar/ANKARA
Executing Institution	Republic of Turkey Prime Ministry Turkish
	Statistical Institute (Turkstat)
Funding Agency	The Government of Republic of Turkey

Project Information

Start of Project	01/01/1999
End of Project	31/12/2003
Start of Data Collection	22/10/2000
End of Data Collection	22/10/2000
URL	http://www.tuik.gov.tr/VeriBilgi.do (nüfus, konut ve demografi)
	(population, housing and demography)
Scope	National

Keywords Population; Census; Demography; Education

Abstract (English) The first population census in Turkey was carried out in 1927. The next population censuses were carried out between 1935 and 1990 regularly, in years ending with 0 and 5. After 1990, population censuses have been decided to be carried out in years ending with 0 by a law and in this regard, the fourteenth population census was carried out on 22 October 2000.

The purpose of the census is to determine completely and correctly the size and the distribution by the administrative division and the demographic, social, and economic characeristics of the population.

The population of Turkey was found to be 67,803,927 in 2000. The percentage of the populaion who live in urban area was found to be 64.9%. The literacy rate in Turkey shows a continous increase for both sexes. Illiteracy rate increasased to 93.9% or males, 80.6% for females in 2000.

The proportion of at least primary education graduates (at least 8 years of educaion) was 43.6% for males and 26.6% for females. The proportion of the population who have been graduated from university (tertiary) was found to be 10.2% for males and 5.4% for females.

Abstract (Original Language) Türkiye'deki ilk nüfus sayimi 1927 yilinda gerçeklestirilmistir. Daha sonraki nüfus sayimlarinin 1935 ile 1990 yillari arasinda düzenli olarak sonu 0 ve 5 ile biten yillarda uygulanmasi kanunla belirlenmis ve bu kapsamda 22 Ekim 2000 tarihinde Türkiye'de ondördüncü Genel nüfus sayimi gerçeklestirilmistir.

Nüfus sayiminin amaci uygulama tarihinde Türkiye sinirlarinda bulunan nüfusun büyüklügünün, idari bölünüse göre dagilimini ve baslica demografik, sosyal ve ekonomik niteliklerini tam ve dogru olarak tespit etmektir.

Türkiye nüfusu 2000 yilinda 67 803 927 kisi olarak saptanmistir. Kentsel yerlesim yerlerinde yasayan nüfus orani% 64.9'dur.

Türkiye'de okuma yazma bilenlerin orani her 2 cinsiyet için de sürekli artis göstermektedir. Bu oran 2000 yilinda erkeklerde % 93.9, kadinlarda % 80.6 olarak saptanmistir. Ilk ögretim okulu (8 yillik egitim) mezunu olanlar erkeklerde % 43.6, kadinlarda % 26.6'dir. Üniversite mezunu olanlarin orani ise erkeklerde % 10.2, kadinlarda % 5.4'dür.

Age Groups

5	9
10	14
15	19
20	24
25	29
30	34
35	39
40	44
45	49
50	54
55	59
60	64
65	69
70	74
75	79
80	84
85	and older

Current Agricultural Statistics

Project Leader

Project Leader	Yavuz Akova
Address	Necatibey Cad. No:114 Bakanliklar/ANKARA
Executing Institution	Republic of Turkey Prime Ministry Turkish Statistical Institute (Turkstat)
Funding Agency	Turkish Republic Government

Project Information

Start of Project	
End of Project	
Start of Data Collection	01/01/2005
End of Data Collection	31/12/2005
URL	Bulletin of news http://www.tuik.gov.tr/VeriBilgi.do?null (tarim)(agriculture)
Scope	National

Keywords Current Agricultural Statistics; Fruit production; Vegetable production; The number of livestock; The number of milked animal; Milk production; The number of slaughtered animals; Meat production; Chicken meat production

Abstract (English) Agricultural statistics are compiled through Current Agricultural Statistics and General Agricultural Censuses in Turkey. Current Agricultural Statistics compiled annually cover data related to the agricultural structure, and General Agricultural Censuses are conducted to measure the changes in agricultural structure as well as to collect data on the structure of agricultural holdings, which are not obtained through Current Agricultural Statistics. Data related to field crops, vegetables, fruits, number of livestock, animal products and agricultural equipment, and machinery on the basis of 81 provinces and all the districts are compiled. 2004 yilinda total production of field crops was found to be 59,794,857 tons. Total production of potatoes was 4,800,000 tons. Total vegetable production was 23,140,672 tons. Meat production was 190,806 tons for cattle, while they were 174 193, 1,751, 198, 32,685, 37,030, 10,300 tons for calf, buffalo, buffalo calves, sheep, lamb, and goat and kid, respectively.

Abstract (Original Language) Türkiye'de tarim istatistikleri, Cari tarim istatistikleri ve genel tari sayimlari olmak üzere iki sekilde derlenmektedir. Cari Tarim istatistikleri ile her yil Türkiye'nin tarimsal varligina iliskin veriler derlenmekte, Genel Tarim Sayimlariyla ise her on yilda bir tarimsal yapida meydana gelen degisiklikler ölçülmekte ve Cari tarim Istatistikleri ile elde edilemeyen Tarimsal isletmelerin yapilarina iliskin bilgiler elde edilmektedir.

81 il ve tü ilçeler bazinda tarla ürünleri, sebzeler, meyveler, hayvan sayilari, hayvansal ürünler ve tarimsal alet ve makineler hakkinda bilgiler derlenmektedir. 2004 yilinda toplam tarla ürünleri üretimi 59 794 857 ton olarak gerçeklesmistir. Toplam patates üretimi 4 800 000 tondur. Toplam sebze üretimi 23 140 672 tondur. Et üretimi sigir için 190 806 ton olarak saptanmis olup, dana, manda,manda yavrusu, koyun, kuzu ve keçi ve oglagi için sirasiyla 174 193, 1 751, 198, 32 685, 37 030, 10 300 ton olarak saptanmistir.

Age Groups

Age data are not applicable for this study.

Household Budget Survey

Project Leader

Project Leader	Enver Tasti
Address	Necatibey Cad. No:114 Bakanliklar/ANKARA
Executing Institution	Republic of Turkey Prime Ministry Turkish Statistical Institute (Turkstat). (The State Institute of Statistics (SIS) was officially renamed as the Republic of Turkey Prime Ministry Turkish Statistical Institute (Turkstat) in 2006)
Funding Agency	The Government of Republic of Turkey

Project Information

Start of Project	
End of Project	
Start of Data Collection	01/01/2005
End of Data Collection	31/12/2005
URL	http://www.tuik.gov.tr/VeriBilgi.do (gelir dagilimi, tüketim ve yoksulluk) (income distribution, consumption and poverty)
Scope	National

Keywords Income; Expenditure; Consumption; Income distribution; Household budget survey

Abstract (English) In Turkey, the consumption patterns and income levels of the individuals and the households are determined through the "Household Budget Survey" for each socio-economic sector, population stratum, and region. Through these surveys information on the household size, employment conditons of the individuals in the households, the total household income, sources of income, consumption expenditure types, consumption patterns are gathered.

The survey aimed to determine the items to be included in consumer price indices and the base year weights; to monitor the changes of households' consumption patterns with the time; to compile the data that will help in forecasting private final consumption expenditues used in the national income calculation; to obtain equired data for the determination of poverty line and other socioeconomic analysis; to obtain necessary information to enable the minimum wage to be determined according to recent conditions. These data on "relative poverty" (household income as the percentage of households with a total income below 50% of the median income of the country) indicated that 15.5% of the population were poor (11.3% in urban and 22.1% in rural).

Abstract (Original Language) Türkiye'de bireylerin ve bunlarin olusturdugu hanehalkinin tüketimlerini, gelir düzeylerini, sosyoekonomik kesimler ve nüfus tabakalarina ve bölgelere göre ortaya çikaran çalismalar "Hane Halki Bütçe Anketleri'dir. Bu anketlerle, hanehalki büyüklükleri, hanehalki fertlerinin isgücü ve çalisma durumlari, hanehalkinin toplam geliri, gelir kaynaklari, tüketim harcama türleri, tüketim kaliplari hakkinda bilgiler derlenmektedir. Hane Halki Bütçe Anketinden elde edilen tüketim harcamalari bilgileri ile; tüketici fiyat endekslerinde kullanilacak maddelerin seçimi ve temel yil agirliklarinin elde edilmesi; hanelerin tüketim kaliplarinda zaman içinde meydana gelen degisikliklerin izlenmesi; milli gelir hespalmalarinda özel nihai tüketim harcamalari tahminlerine yardimci olacak verilerin derlenmesi; yoksulluk sinirinin belirlenmesi vb. diger sosyoekonomik analizler için gerekli verilerin elde edilmesi; asgari ücret tespit çalismalari için gerekli verilerin elde edilmesi amaçlanmaktadir.

Göreli yoksulluk (esdeger kisi basina tüketim harcamasi medyan degerinin % 50sinin altinda olan kisi yüzdesi) ile ilgili veriler, Türk toplumunun % 15.5'inin yoksul oldugunu göstermekte olup, bu veri kentsel yerlesim yerlerinde % 11.3, kirsal yarlesim yerlerinde % 22.1'dir.

Age Groups

15	999

Household Labor Force Survey

HLFS

Project Leader

Project Leader	Enver Tasti
Address	Necatibey Cad. No:114 Bakanliklar/ANKARA
Executing Institution	Republic of Turkey Prime Ministry Turkish Statistical Institute (Turkstat)
Funding Agency	The Government of Republic of Turkey

Project Information

Start of Project	
End of Project	
Start of Data Collection	01/01/2005
End of Data Collection	31/12/2005
URL	http://www.tuik.gov.tr/VeriBilgi.do &$$$;((istihdam, issizlik ve ücret) (employment, unemployment, salary)
Scope	National

Keywords Unemployed; Unemployed rate; Status in employment; Branch of economic activity

Abstract (English) The main objective of the Household Labor Force Survey (HLFS) is to obtain information on the structure of the labor force in the country. This includes information on economic activity, occupation, status in employment and hours worked for employed persons; and information on the duration of the unemployment and occupation sought by the unemployed.

According to results of Household Labor Force Surveys, unemployed rate is 10.3% in Turkey in 2005 (12.7% in urban areas and 6.8% in rural areas). Unemployed rates were similar between men and women (10.3% vs. 10.3%).

These data on employed persons by status in employment indicated that 50.0% of men and 38.2% of women were regular employee, 7.8% of men and 5.6% of women were casual employee, 6.6% of men and 0.01% of women were casual employer, 28.5% of men and 13.6% of women were self employed, 7.1% of men and 41.7% of women were unpaid family worker. These data on employed persons by branch of economic activity for men indicated that 48.0% of men were employed in services, 26% of men were employed in agriculture and 26% of men were employed in industry. The figures were 29%, 14%, and 57% for women, respectively.

Abstract (Original Language) Hane Halki Isgücü Anketinin (HiA) amaci, ülkedeki isgücünün yapisi konusunda bilgi elde etmektir. Bu bilgiler, iktisadi faaliyet, meslek, isteki durumu ve istihdam edilenlerin çalisma süresi; issizlerin is arama süresi ve issizlerin aradiklari meslek konusundaki bilgileri kapsamaktadir.

Hane Halki Isgücü Anketi sonuçuna göre, 2005 yilinda Türkiye'de issizlik orani % 10.3'tür. Bu ran kadinlarda ve erkelerde ayni olarak bulunmustur.

Istihdam edilenlerin isteki durumuna göre dagilimina bakildiginda, erkeklerin % 50'sinin ve kadinlarin % 38.2'sinin ücretli veya maasli olarak istihdam edildigi, erkelerin % 7.'i ve kadinlarin % 5.6'sinin yevmiyeli (mevsimlik) olarak istihdam edildigi, erkeklerin % 6.6'si ve kadinlarin % 0.01'inin isveren oldugu, erkeklrin % 28.5'inin ve kadinlarin % 13.6'sinin kendi hesabina çalistigi ve erkeklerin % 7.1'i ve kadinlarin % 41.7'sinin ücretsiz aile isçisi olarak çalistigi saptanmistir.

Istihdam edilenlerin ekonomik faaliyete göre dagilimina bakildiginda ise, erkeklerin % 48'inin hizmet sektöründe, % 26'sinin tarim sektöründe ve % 26'sinin sanayi sektöründe çalistigi saptanmistir. Kadinlarin ise % 29'u hizmet sektöründe, % 57'si tarim sektöründe ve % 14'ü sanayi sektöründe çalismaktadir.

Age Groups

15	24
25	44
45	64
65	and older

National Food and Nutrition Strategy (Working Group Report)

National Food and Nutrition Strategy

Project Leader

Project Leader	Taylan Kiymaz
Address	Devlet Planlama Teskilati Müstesarligi
	Necatibey Cad. No:108 06100 YÜCETEPE - ANKARA
	Tel: 00 90 312 294 50 00
Executing Institution	T.R. Prime Ministry State Planning Organization (SPO)
Funding Agency	SPO and UN during report preparation period

Project Information

Start of Project	01/04/2001
End of Project	01/11/2001
Start of Data Collection	
End of Data Collection	
URL	http://ekutup.dpt.gov.tr/gida/ugbs/beslenme.pdf,
	http://ekutup.dpt.gov.tr/gida/strateji.pdf
Scope	National

Keywords Food security; Food safety; Nutrition; National policies; Turkey

Abstract (English) The existing agricultural structure, scale of enterprises, inadequate use of agricultural technology and insufficient input productivity are the most significant problems of agricultural sector in Turkey.

The most significant issue on food accessibility is the income distribution. Poverty studies conducted on minimum food expenses show that 8.4% of the individuals live below poverty threshold.

Government's role in developing food safety programme is very important. The next stage after policy formation is the risk analysis.

On the one hand, we can observe macro and micronutrient deficiencies in some communities because of household food insecurity and low consumption of animal products. On the other hand, FAO statistics indicate that food supply in Turkey is adequate to provide daily requirement of energy intake.

If food energy and nutrition elements in Turkey are examined, it can be seen that the proportion of families having inadequate energy intake is low. Total protein consumption is adequate but most of the protein intake is of vegetable origin.

When formulating policies on ensuring food security and safety, protecting and improving health, preventing diseases, protecting environment, and ensuring socio-economical development, food and health concepts should be considered together.

Abstract (Original Language) Bu çalismada, gida güvencesi, gida güvenligi ve beslenme konularinda Türkiye'de mevcut durum ayrintili olarak incelenerek, ulusal gida ve beslenme politikalarinin uygulanmasi ve yeni politikalarin olusturulmasina yönelik önerilerde bulunulmasi amaçlanmistir.

Ülkemizdeki mevcut tarimsal yapi ve isletme büyüklügü ile tarimda yeterli ölçüde teknoloji kullanilamamasi ve kullanilan girdilerden istenilen verimlilik saglanamamasi, tarim sektöründe üretime yönelik en önemli sorunlar olarak gözükmektedir.

Gidanin ulasilabilirligini etkileyen önemli bir konu gelir dagilimindaki adaletsizliktir. Minimum gida harcamasi yöntemiyle yapilan yoksulluk çalismalarina göre, Türkiye'de fertlerin %8,4'ü yoksulluk sinirinin altinda yasamaktadir.

Toplumun bazi kesimlerinde hane halki gida güvencesizligi ve hayvansal ürünlerin az miktarda tüketimine bagli olarak makro ve mikro besin ögeleri eksikligi görülmektedir. Öte yandan, FAO verilerine göre, Türkiye'de kisi basina günlük enerji alimina yetecek gida arzi bulunmaktadir.

Türkiye'de, enerji ve besin ögeleri yönünden beslenme durumu incelendiginde yetersiz düzeyde enerji alan aile orani düsüktür. Toplam protein tüketimi kisi basina yeterli düzeydedir ancak proteinin çogu bitkisel kaynaklidir.

Gida güvencesi ve güvenliginin saglanmasi, sagligin korunmasi ve gelistirilmesi, hastaliklarin önlenmesi, çevrenin korunmasi ve sosyo-ekonomik gelismenin saglanmasi amaciyla politikalar olusturulurken gida ve saglik kavramlarinin birlikte ele alinmasi gerekmektedir.

Age Groups

Age data are not applicable for this study.

Turkey Demographic and Health Survey 2003

TDHS-2003

Project Leader

Project Leader	Prof.Dr. Sabahat Tezcan
Address	Hacettepe Üniversitesi
	Merkez Kampüsü Sihhiye
	06100 Ankara
	Tel: 00 90 312 305 11 15
	Fax: 00 90 312 311 81 41
	hips@hacettepe.edu.tr
Executing Institution	Hacettepe University Institute of Population Studies
	Ankara, Turkey
Funding Agency	Government of Turkey, European Union

Project Info1rmation

Start of Project	01/01/2002
End of Project	31/12/2004
Start of Data Collection	01/12/2003
End of Data Collection	01/05/2004
URL	http://www.hips.hacettepe.edu.tr/tnsa2003/
	anaraporenglish.htm, http://www.hips.hacettepe.edu.tr/
	tnsa2003/analizrapor.htm
Scope	National

Keywords Fertility; Child mortality; Mother and child health

Abstract (English) Turkey Demographic and Health Surveys are nationally representative sample surveys designed to provide information on levels and trends on fertility, infant and child mortality, family planning, and maternal and child health, which are carried out every 5 years. The last survey is the 2003 Turkey Demographic and Health Survey (TDHS 2003). Survey results are presented at the national level, by urban and rural residence, and for each of the five regions in the country. The TDHS-2003 sample also allows analyses for some of the survey topics for the 12 geographical regions (NUTS1), which were adopted at the second half of 2002 within the context of Turkey's move to join the European Union.

Educational level of household population: The majority of the population in Turkey has attended school. Among the population with schooling, about one-third of both males and females have completed at least second level primary school. The proportion of population with at least high school education is 23% for males and 14% for females. However, the indicators for successive cohorts show a substantial increase over time in the educational attainment of both men and women.

Breastfeeding and supplemental feeding: Breastfeeding is almost universal in Turkey; 97% of all children are breastfed for some period of time. Complementary feeding is common among very young children. In the first two months of life, only

44% are exclusively breastfed. The median duration of breastfeeding for all children is 14 months. Among children who are breastfeeding and younger than six months, 18% received infant formula.

Iodization of Salt: Iodine deficiency contributes to higher rates of childhood morbidity and mortality. According to tests conducted during the survey, the table salt in 30% of the households did include neither iodide nor iodate. Iodized salt is not used in about half of rural households. Less than half of the households in Central and Southeast Anatolia use iodized salt.

Nutritional Status of Children: By age five, 12% of children are stunted (short for their age), compared with an international reference population. Stunting is more prevalent in rural areas, in the East, among children of mothers with little or no education, among children who are of higher birth order, and among those born less than 24 months after a prior birth. Wasting is a less serious problem. Four percent of children are underweight for their age.

Nutritional Status of mothers: Obesity is a problem among mothers. According to BMI calculations, 57% of mothers are overweight, of which 23% are obese. BMI increases rapidly with age, exceeding 25.0 for the majority of women aged 25 and older.

Abstract (Original Language) 2003 Türkiye Nüfus ve Saglik Arastirmasi (TNSA-2003) dogurganlik düzeyi ve degisimi, bebek ve çocuk ölümlülügü, aile planlamasi ve anne ve çocuk sagligi konularinda bilgi saglamak üzere tasarlanmis ulusal düzeyde bir örneklem arastirmasidir. Arastirma sonuçlari ulusal düzeyde, kentsel ve kirsal alanlar ile bes cografi bölge düzeyinde sunulmaktadir. TNSA-2003 örneklemi ayrica arastirma kapsamindaki bazi konular için 2002 yilinin ikinci yarisinda Avrupa Birligi'ne katilim sürecinde olusturulan 12 cografi bölge (NUTS1) düzeyinde de analize izin vermektedir.

Hane Halki bireylerinin egitim düzeyi: Türkiye'de nüfusun çogunlugu okula gitmektedir. Okula gidenler arasinda hem erkeklerin hem de kadinlarin üçte biri en az ilkögretimin ikinci kademesini tamamlamistir. En az lise mezunu olan nüfusun orani erkeklerde yüzde 23, kadinlarda yüzde 14'tür. Daha genç kusaklar için hesaplanan göstergeler, gerek erkeklerde gerekse kadinlarda egitime devam etmenin zaman içinde sürekli arttigini göstermektedir.

ÇOCUKLAR VE KADINLAR IÇIN BESLENME GÖSTERGELERI

Emzirme ve Ek Gida: Emzirme Türkiye'de çok yaygindir; tüm çocuklarin yüzde 97'si bir süre emzirilmistir. Destekleyici besleme çok genç yastaki çocuklar arasinda yaygindir. Yasamlarinin ilk iki ayinda çocuklarin sadece yüzde 44'ü sadece anne sütü ile beslenmistir. Tüm çocuklar için ortanca emzirme süresi 14 aydir. Emzirilen ve 6 ayliktan daha küçük olan çocuklarin yüzde 18'ine hazir mama verilmistir.

Tuzun Iyotlanmasi: Iyot eksikligi çocukluk dönemi hastaliklari ve ölüm hizlarinin artmasina yol açmaktadir. Arastirma sirasinda yapilan testlere göre, hanelerde kullanilan sofra tuzunun yüzde 30'u ne iyodür ne de iyodat içermektedir. Kirsal hanelerin yarisinda iyotlu tuz kullanilmamaktadir. Orta ve Güneydogu Anadolu bölgelerindeki hanelerin yarisindan azi iyotlu tuz kullanmaktadir.

Çocuklarin ve Annelerin Beslenme Durumu: Bes yasina kadar olan çocuklarin, yüzde 12'si, uluslararasi referans nüfusla karsilastirildiginda bodurdur (yasina göre kisa). Bodurluk kirsal alanlarda, Dogu Bölgesinde ve annesi egitimsiz veya çok az egitimli olan çocuklar arasinda, daha yüksek dogum sirasi olan çocuklarda ve bir önceki dogumla arasinda 24 aydan daha kisa süre olan çocuklar arasinda daha yaygindir. Zayiflik daha önemsiz bir sorundur. Çocuklarin yüzde dördü yaslarina göre zayiftir. Obezite anneler arasinda varolan bir problemdir. BMI hesaplamalarina göre, annelerin yüzde 57'si sisman, bunlarin yüzde 23'ü de obezdir. BMI yasla birlikte hizli bir sekilde artmakta, 25 yas ve üzeri kadinlarin çogunda 25.0'i asmaktadir.

Age Groups

The results related "breastfeeding," "malnutrition among children" and "antropometric data of the reproductive aged women" were presented for different age groups.

Age groups for the data on "breastfeeding":

(<2 months), (2–3 months), (4–5 months), (6–7 months), (8–9 months), (10–11 months), (12–15 months), (16–19 months), (24–27 months), (28–31 months) and (32–35 months)

Age groups for the data on "malnutrition among children" :

(<6 months), (6–9 months), (10–11 months), (12–23 months), (24–35 months), (36–47 months) and (48–59 months)

Age groups for the data on "antropometric data of the reproductive aged women":

(15–19 years), (20–24 years), (25–29 years), (30–34 years), (35–39 years), (40–44 years), (45–49 years)

Turkish Adult Risk Factor Study

TEKHARF study

Project Leader

Project Leader	Prof Dr. Altan Onat
Address	Türk Kardiyoloji Dernegi Merkezi
	Darülaceze Cd. Fulya Sk.
	Eksioglu Is Merkezi, No:9/1 Okmeydani 34384, Istanbul
Executing Institution	Turkish Society of Cardiology
Funding Agency	2 (Türk Kardiyoloji Dernegi (Turkish Cardiology Society)
	and Unilever TURKEY

Project Information

Start of Project	01/01/1990
End of Project	01/01/1991
Start of Data Collection	01/07/1990
End of Data Collection	10/09/1990
URL	
Scope	National

Keywords Coronary heart disease; Cardiovasculer risk factors; Total cholesterol; Triglyceride profiles; BMI; WHR; WC

Abstract (English) The first population based study in Turkey, Turkish Adult Risk Factor Study (TEKHARF), was undertaken in the year 1990.

The aim of the study was to determine the prevalence of coronary heart disease and cardiovasculer risk factors in a random sample of Turkish adults. The plasma total cholesterol and triglyceride profiles among Turkish adults were also measured.

On the basis of a probability-related point score, age-adjusted clinical coronary heart disease was estimated to prevail in 5.8% of men and 5% of women ($P > 0.5$). The overall prevalence of obesity in adults was 18.6% in the year 1990. It is found 21.1% among males and 43.0% in females. Among male subjects mean BMI, WHR, WC are found $26.8 \pm 3.9\,kg/m^2$, 0.93 ± 0.07, $91.8 \pm 10.6\,cm$ and in females $29.2 \pm 5.3\,kg/m^2$, 0.86 ± 0.70, $89.4 \pm 12.1\,cm$, respectively. BMI was found as an independent risk factor for CVD in men and the cardiovascular event risk were found to be increasing 9% in every $1\,kg/m^2$ BMI increment.

Hypercholesterolaemia (> or = $6.5\,mmol/l$, $250\,mg/dl$) prevailed in 8.5%, and hypertriglyceridaemia (>$2.25\,mmol/l$, $200\,mg/d$) in 16.6% among men and women aged 40–59 years. Age adjusted total cholesterol values were $4.8\,mmol/l$ ($185\,mg/dl$) in men and $5\,mmol/l$ ($192\,mg/dl$) in women.

Abstract (Original Language) Türk Eriskinlerinde kalp sagligi, risk profili ve kalp hastaligi çalismasi bu konuda yürütülen ulusal düzeydeki ilk çalismadir. Çalisma 1990 yilinda yürütülmüstür. Çalismanin amaci Türk eriskinlerinde koroner kalp hastaligi prevalansini ve kardiyovaskuler risk faktörlerini saptamaktir. Arastirma kapsaminda ayrica plasma kolesterol düzeyi ve trigliserid profili de belirlenmistir. Olasiliga dayali puanlama degerine göre yasa göre düzeltilmis klinik koroner hastalik sikligi erkelerde % 5.8, kadinlarda % 5 olarak saptanmistir (P > 0.5)

Obesite prevalansi % 18.6 olup, bu oran erkeklerde % 21.1, kadinlarda % 43.0 olarak saptanmistir. Erkeklerde Vücut kitle indeksi, bel kalça orani, bel çevresi $26.8\pm3.9\,kg/m^2$, 0.93 ± 0.07, $91.8\pm10.6\,cm$ olup kadinlarda bu oranlar sirasiyla $29.2\pm5.3\,kg/m^2$, 0.86 ± 0.70, $89.4\pm12.1\,cm$ olarak saptanmistir. VKI erkelerde kardiyovaskuler hastaliklar için bir risk faktörü olarak saptanmis olup, VKI'deki her $1\,kg/m^2$ artisin kardiyovaskuler hastalik riskini % 9 arttirdigi saptanmistir.

40- 59 yas arasindaki kisilerde hiperkolesterolemi (> or = $6.5\,mmol/litre$, $250\,mg/dl$) % 8.5, hipertrigliseridemi (> $2.25\,mmol/litre$, $200\,mg/dl$) % 16.6 olarak saptanmistir. Yasa göre düzeltilmis total kolesterol degeri erkeklerde $4.8\,mmol/litre$ ($185\,mg/dl$) olup, bu oran kadinlarda $5\,mmol/litre$ ($192\,mg/dl$)'dir.

Age Groups

20	29
30	39
40	49
50	59
60	69
70	And older

Turkish Diabetes Epidemiology Study

TURDEP

Project Leader

Project Leader	Prof Dr Ilhan Satman
Address	Istanbul Faculty of Medicine, Diabetes Division, P.K. 75, Millet Caddesi, Çapa 34 272, Istanbul Turkey.
Executing Institution	Istanbul Faculty of Medicine, Diabetes
Funding Agency	Istanbul Faculty of Medicine; Turkish Statistical Institute (Turkstat);Ministry of Health, Ankara, Turkey; Bayer Turk Pharma; Pepsi Cola Turk.

Project Information

Start of Project	01/10/1995
End of Project	01/09/2001
Start of Data Collection	01/09/1997
End of Data Collection	01/05/1998
URL	
Scope	National

Keywords Diabetes epidemiology; Obesity; Hypertension; Type 2 diabetes mellitus

Abstract (English) *Objectives*: To investigate for the first time the prevalence of diabetes and impaired glucose tolerance (IGT) nationwide in Turkey; to assess regional variations and relationships between glucose intolerance and lifestyle and physical risk factors.

Research design and methods: The Turkish Diabetes Epidemiology Study (TURDEP) is a cross-sectional, population-based survey that included 24,788 subjects (age $\geq$ 20 years, women 55%, response 85%). Glucose tolerance was classified according to World Health Organization recommendations on the basis of 2-h blood glucose values.

Results: Crude prevalence of diabetes was 7.2% (previously undiagnosed, 2.3%) and of IGT, 6.7% (age-standardized to world and European populations, 7.9 and 7.0%). Both were more frequent in women than men ($P < 0.0001$) and in those living in urban rather than rural communities ($P < 0.001$). Prevalence rates of hypertension and obesity were 29 and 22%, respectively. Both were more common among women than men ($P < 0.0001$). Prevalence of diabetes and IGT increased with rising BMI, waist-to-hip ratio (WHR), and waist girth ($P < 0.0001$). Multiple logistic regression analysis revealed that age, BMI, WHR, familial diabetes, and hypertension were independently associated with diabetes, age, BMI, WHR, familial diabetes, and hypertension with IGT (except for familial diabetes in women with IGT). Education was related to diabetes in men but was protective for diabetes and IGT in women.

Socioeconomic status appeared to decrease the risk of IGT in men while it increased the risk in women. Smoking had a protective effect for IGT in both sexes. *Conclusion*: Diabetes and IGT are moderately common in Turkey by international standards. Associations with obesity and hypertension have been confirmed. Other lifestyle factors had a variable relationship with glucose tolerance.

Abstract (Original Language) AMAÇ: Ulusal düzeyde Türkiye'de ilk olarak diyabet ve bozulmus glukoz toleransi prevalansini saptamak; bölgesel farkliliklari ve bozulmus glukoz toleransi ve yasam sekli ve fiziksel risk faktörleri arasindaki iliskileri incelemek

Gereç ve Yöntem: Türkiye Diyabet Epidemiyolojisi çalismasi (TURDEP) toplum tabanli bir kesitsel çalsmadir. Çalismaya 20 yasin üzerinde 24 788 kisi katilmis olup, yanit orani % 85'dir. Çalismaya katilan kisilerin % 55'i kadindir. Glukoz toleransinin degerlendirilmesinde, Dünya saglik Örgütü'nün önerdigi degerlere göre 2. Saatte ölçülen kan sekeri düzeyi degerlendirilmistir.

Bulgar: Kaba diyabet prevalansi % 7.2 (ilk kez tani alma için % 2.3) ve bozulmus glukoz toleransi % 6.7 (yasa standardize edilmis hizlar sirasiyla % 7.9 ve %7.0) olarak saptamistir. Diyabet ve bozulmus glukoz toleransi kadinlarda (P<0.0001) ve kentsel yerlesim yerlerinde yasayanlarda (P<0.0001) daha sik görülmektedir.

Hipertansiyon ve obesite prevalansi sirasiyla % 29 e % 22 olarak saptanmistir. Hipertanso,iyon ve obesite kadinlarda erkeklere göre daha sik olarak saptanmistir (P<0.0001). Diyabet ve bozulmus glukoz toleransi VKI, bel- kalça orani ve bel çevresi arttikça artmaktadir (P< 0.0001). Çoklu regresyon analizi sonucunda yas, VKI, Bel-kalça orani, ailede diyabet öyküsünün bulunmasi ve hipertansiyon diyabetle iliskili faktörler olarak saptanmistir. Yas, VKI, Bel-kalça orani, ailede diyabet öyküsünün bulunmasi ve hipertansiyon bozulmus glukoz toleransi ile de iliskili faktörler olarak saptanmistir. Egitim erkeklerde diyabetle ilskili bir risk faktörü olarak saptanmistir. Kadinlarda ise egitim diyabet ve bozulmus glukoz toleransi açisindan koruyucudur. Bozulmus glukoz toleransi açisindan sosyoekonomik durum erkeklerde koruyucu etkiye sahip olup, kadinlarda ise bir risk faktörü olarak saptanmistir. Her 2 cinsiyette de sigara içme bozulmus glukoz toleransi açisindan koruyucu etkiye sahiptir.

Sonuçlar: Uluslarasi verilerle karsilastirildiginda Türkiye'de diyabet ve bozulmus glukoz toleransi ort düzeyde görülmektedir. Dyabet ve bozulmus glukoz toleransi ile obesite ve hipertansiyon arasindaki ilski bu çalisma kapsaminda da gösterilmistir. Diger yasam sekli degiskenleri, bozulmus glukoz toleransi ile farkli iliskilere sahiptir.

Age Groups

20	29
30	39
40	49
50	59
60	69
70	999

Turkish Obesity and Hypertension Study

TOHS

Project Leader

Project Leader	Prof Dr Hüsrev Hatemi
Address	Aksaray 34303, Istanbul, Turkey
Executing Institution	Istanbul University Cerrahpasa Medical Faculty
Funding Agency	ABBOT Pharmaceuticals

Project Information

Start of Project	01/01/1999
End of Project	31/12/2001
Start of Data Collection	15/04/1999
End of Data Collection	15/04/2000
URL	
Scope	National

Keywords Body weight; Height; Body mass index; Systolic blood pressure; Diastolic blood pressure

Abstract (English) The objectives of this study were to determine the prevalence of overweight and obesity in Turkey, and to investigate their association with age, gender, and blood pressure. A crosssectional population-based study was performed. A total of 20,119 inhabitants (4,975 women and 15,144 men, age > 20 years) from 11 Anatolian cities in four geographic regions were screened for body weight, height, and systolic and diastolic blood pressure between the years 1999 and 2000. The overall prevalence rate of overweight was 25.0% and of obesity was 19.4%. The prevalence of overweight among women was 24.3% and obesity 24.6%; 25.9% of men were overweight, and 14.4% were obese. Mean body mass index (BMI) of the studied population was $27.59 \pm 4.61 \, \text{kg/m}^2$. Mean systolic and diastolic blood pressure for women were 131.0 ± 41.0 and $80.2 \pm 16.3 \, \text{mmHg}$, and for men 135.0 ± 27.3 and $83.2 \pm 16.0 \, \text{mmHg}$. There was a positive linear correlation between BMI and blood pressure, and between age and blood pressure in men and women. Obesity and overweight are highly prevalant in Turkey, and they constitute independent risk factors for hypertension.

Abstract (Original Language) Toplum tabanli kesitsel çalisma, Türkiye'de "fazla kiloluluk" ve "obesite" prevalansini ve ilgili parametrelerin yas, cinsiyet ve kan basinci ile iliskisini arastirmak üzere yürütülmüstür. 1999 ve 2000 yillarinda 4 farkli cografi bölgedeki 11 ilden yaslari 20'nin üzerinde olan 20119 kisiye ulasilarak (4975 kadin, 15144 erkek) boy, kilo ve kan basinci ölçümleri yapilmistir. Fazla kilolu olanlarin orani % 25.0 olup, obesite prevalansi ise % 19.4 olarak saptanmistir. Bu veriler sirasiyla kadinlarda % 24.3 ve % 24.6; erkeklerde % 25.9 ve % 14.4 olarak saptanmistir. Arastirma grubunda Vücut kitle

indeksi (VKI) ortalamasi 27.59 ± 4.61 kg/&$$$;m2'dir. Ortalama sistolik ve dias-
tolik kan basinci ortalamasi sirasiyla kadinlarda 131.0 ± 41.0 ve 80.2 ± 16.3 mm
Hg, erkeklerde ise 135.0 ± 27.3 ve 83.2 ± 16.0 mm Hg olarak saptanmistir. VKI
ile kan basinci arasinda pozitif yönde dogrusal bir iliski bulunmaktadir. Obesite
ve fazla kiloluluk Türkiye'de oldukça yaygindir. Obesitenin hipertansiyon için bir
risk faktörü oldugu belirlenmistir.

Age Groups

21	30
31	40
41	50
51	60
61	70
71	999

United Kingdom

Health and Wellbeing Survey

Project Leader

Project Leader	Central Survey Unit
Address	Central Survey Unit
	McAulay House
	Castle Street
	Belfast
	Northern ireland
Executing Institution	Northern Ireland Statistics and Research Agency
Funding Agency	

Project Information

Start of Project	01/01/2001
End of Project	31/07/2001
Start of Data Collection	01/01/2001
End of Data Collection	31/07/2001
URL	http://www.csu.nisra.gov.uk/surveys/survey.asp?id=5&details=0
Scope	National

Keywords

Abstract (English) Household survey followed by individual interview of every person in household aged over 16 years. Sample of 5,000 households.

Age Groups

16	24
25	34
35	44
45	54
55	64
65	74

Low Income Diet and Nutrition Survey

LIDNS

Project Leader

Project Leader	Mark Bush
Address	Food Standards Agency
	Aviation House
	125 Kingsway
	London WC2B 6NH
	United Kingdom
Executing Institution	Food Standards Agency
Funding Agency	Food Standards Agency

Project Information

Start of Project	01/09/2003
End of Project	31/03/2007
Start of Data Collection	01/11/2003
End of Data Collection	31/01/2005
URL	
Scope	National

Keywords

Abstract (English) The Food Standards Agency has commissioned a diet and nutrition survey of low-income consumers. The purpose of the survey is to provide for the first time robust, nationally representative, baseline data on food consumption, nutrient intake and nutritionally factors affecting these in low-income/materially-deprived consumers. Data from the survey will feed directly into work by the Agency, other Government departments and non-Government bodies to understand and address barriers to the uptake of healthy balanced diet by low-income groups.

The survey will include over 3,600 people, both adults and children, throughout the UK. It will collect detailed quantitative information on food consumption (by 4× multiple pass 24-h recall) and nutrient intake. Other components are physical measurements (e.g., height, weight, blood pressure), a blood sample for analysis of nutritional status indices, a detailed interview to collect information on socio-economic, demographic and lifestyle characteristics, and assessments of physical activity and oral health by questionnaire.

A feasibility study was undertaken during the summer of 2002. Following further discussions on how to address the predicted low response rates, and to reexamine how the survey data could be interpreted, fieldwork for the mainstage of the survey commenced innovember 2003. Fieldwork will be completed in early 2005, with results expected in 2006.

Age Groups

National Diet and Nutrition Survey

NDNS

Project Leader

Project Leader	
Address	
Executing Institution	Office for National Statistics
Funding Agency	

Project Information

Start of Project	01/07/2000
End of Project	30/06/2001
Start of Data Collection	01/07/2000
End of Data Collection	30/06/2001
URL	http://www.food.gov.uk/multimedia/pdfs/ndns5full.pdf
Scope	National

Keywords

Abstract (English) This survey, of a national sample of adults aged 19–64 years, is one of a programme of national surveys with the aim of gathering information about the dietary habits and nutritional status of the British population. The results of the survey will be used to develop nutrition policy and to contribute to the evidence base for Government advice on healthy eating.

Age Groups

19	24
25	34
35	49
50	64

National Diet and Nutrition Survey: Adults Aged 19–64 Years

NDNS Adults 19–64 Years

Project Leader

Project Leader	
Address	Food Standards Agency
	Aviation House
	125 Kingsway
	London WC2B 6NH
Executing Institution	
Funding Agency	Food Standards Agency and the Department of Health

Project Information

Start of Project	01/10/1998
End of Project	31/12/2004
Start of Data Collection	01/07/2000
End of Data Collection	30/06/2001
URL	http://www.food.gov.uk/science/101717/ndnsdocuments/ printedreportpage
Scope	National

Keywords

Abstract (English) A survey of the diets and nutritional status of adults aged 19–64 living in private households in Great Britain was carried out between July 2000 and June 2001. Information was collected from interviews, 7-day dietary records, physical measurements, and analysis of blood and urine samples. The findings from this survey are presented into a series of five volumes. The results are broken down by age, sex, region, and households in receipt of benefits.

Volume 1: The National Diet & Nutrition Survey: adults aged 19–64 years – Types and quantities of food consumed – presents the findings on food consumption – the proportions eating different foods during the survey week and the quantities consumed. An analysis of the number of portions of fruit and vegetables consumed is also included in this volume.

Volume 2: The National Diet & Nutrition Survey: adults aged 19–64 years – Energy, protein, carbohydrate, fat, and alcohol intake – presents findings on the intakes of energy and macronutrients. Intakes are compared with the current UK Dietary Reference Values and the contribution of food groups to intakes is detailed.

Volume 3: The National Diet & Nutrition Survey: adults aged 19–64 years – Vitamin and mineral intake and urinary analytes – presents findings on the intakes of micronutrients – vitamins and minerals. Intakes are compared with the current UK Dietary Reference Values and the contribution of food groups to intakes is presented.

Volume 4: The National Diet & Nutrition Survey: adults aged 19–64 years – Nutritional status (anthropometry and blood analytes), blood pressure and physical activity – presents findings on nutritional status, assessed by physical measurements (height, weight, waist and hip circumferences) and a range of biochemical indices measured in the blood; and on blood pressure and physical activity. Results are compared with reference values where appropriate.

Volume 5: The National Diet & Nutrition Survey: adults aged 19–64 years – Summary report

This report summarises the key findings from the first four volumes.

Age Groups

National Diet and Nutrition Survey: Children Aged 1½–4½ Years

NDNS Children 1½–4½ Years

Project Leader

Project Leader	
Address	Food Standards Agency
	Aviation House
	125 Kingsway
	London WC2B 6NH
Executing Institution	
Funding Agency	Ministry of Agriculture, Fisheries and Food, Department of Health

Project Information

Start of Project	01/01/1989
End of Project	31/12/1995
Start of Data Collection	01/07/1992
End of Data Collection	30/06/1993
URL	
Scope	National

Keywords

Abstract (English) This report presents the findings of a survey of the diet and nutrition of children aged 1½–4½ years living in private households in Great Britain carried out over 12 months beginning July 1992.

The results from the survey are presented in tabular form, accompanied by graphical illustrations and commentary. These results are taken from interview questionnaires, four-day weighed intake dietary records, body measurements, including height and weight, and from analyses of blood samples.

Information is given on the intakes by the children of food, energy, and more than 40 nutrients and the results of assays for more than 30 blood analytes are presented. Nutrient intakes are compared with reference values where these have been previously determined. For several nutrient levels in blood, this survey provides, for the first time, information against which the status of children in the future can be matched. Results are shown for children classified according to various characteristics such as family type, social class, and region.

An accompanying volume reports on the dental health of the same group of children: National Diet and Nutrition Survey: children aged 1½–4½ years. Volume 2: Report of the dental survey.

Age Groups

National Diet and Nutrition Survey: People Aged 65 Years and Over

NDNS 65 Years and Over

Project Leader

Project Leader	
Address	Food Standards Agency
	Avaition House
	125 Kingsway
	London WC2B 6NH
Executing Institution	
Funding Agency	Ministry of Agriculture, Fisheries and Food,
	and the Department of Health

Project Information

Start of Project	01/01/1993
End of Project	31/10/1998
Start of Data Collection	01/10/1994
End of Data Collection	30/09/1995
URL	
Scope	National

Keywords

Abstract (English) This report presents the findings of a survey of the diet and nutritional status of British adults aged 65 years and above carried out between October 1994 and September 1995. The survey included both people living in private households (free-living group) and people living in residential or nursing homes (institution group).

Information was collected from interviews, 4-day dietary records, physical measurements, and analysis of blood and urine samples. The results are presented in tabular form, accompanied by commentary and graphical illustrations. Results are presented separately for the free-living and the institution groups.

Results are given for food consumption, intakes of energy and over 40 nutrients and for more than 30 biochemical indices of nutritional status. Nutrient intakes are compared with the current UK Dietary Reference Values, and the nutritional status indices are compared with reference values where these are available. Results are also presented for people classified into characteristics such as region, social class, and income.

An accompanying volume reports on the oral health of the same group of adults: National Diet and Nutrition Survey: people aged 65 years and over. Volume 2: Report of the oral health survey.

Age Groups

568

National Diet and Nutrition Survey: Young People Aged 4–18 Years

NDNS 4–18 Years

Project Leader

Project Leader Address	Food Standards Agency Aviation House 125 Kingsway London WC2B 6NH
Executing Institution Funding Agency	Ministry of Agriculture, Fisheries and Food, and the Department of Health

Project Information

Start of Project	01/01/1996
End of Project	31/12/2000
Start of Data Collection	01/01/1997
End of Data Collection	31/12/1997
URL	http://www.food.gov.uk/news/pressreleases/2000/jun/nationaldiet
Scope	National

Keywords

Abstract (English) This report presents the findings of a survey of the diet and nutritional status of young aged 4–18 years living in private households in Great Britain and carried out between January and December 1997.

Information was collected from interviews, 7-day dietary and physical activity records, physical measurements, and analysis of blood and urine samples. The results are presented in tabular form, accompanied by commentary and graphical illustrations. Most results are presented separately for boys and girls in four age groups, 4–6, 7–10, 11–14, and 15–18 years.

Results are given for food consumption, intakes of energy and over 40 nutrients, and for more than 40 biochemical indices of nutritional status indices. Nutrient intakes are compared with the current UK Dietary Reference Values, and the nutritional status indices are compared with reference values where these are available. Results are also presented for young people classified by characteristics such as region, social class of head of household and income.

An accompanying volume reports on the oral health of the same group of young people: National Diet and Nutrition Survey: young people aged 4–18 years. Volume 2: Report of the oral health survey.

Age Groups

Welsh Health Survey

Project Leader

Project Leader	Alice McGee
Address	Welsh Assembly Government Statistical Directorate
Executing Institution	National Centre for Social Research
Funding Agency	Welsh Assembly Government

Project Information

Start of Project	01/10/2003
End of Project	30/09/2005
Start of Data Collection	01/10/2003
End of Data Collection	30/09/2005
URL	http://www.natcen.ac.uk/natcen/pages/publications/ Welsh_Health_Technical_Report.pdf
Scope	National

Keywords

Abstract (English) A household survey on a range of health issues

Age Groups

16	24
25	34
35	44
45	54
55	64
65	74

References

[1] Association of Schools of Public Health in the European Region (ASPHER), http://www.aspher.org (accessed 3 February 2007)

[2] Casperson CJ, Powell KE, Christensen GM: Physical activity, exercise, and physical fitness. Public Health Reports 1985, 100, 125–131(the original reference); and Pate PR, Pratt M, Blair SN, et al. Physical Activity and Public Health: A recommendation from the Centre for Disease Control and Prevention and the American College of Sports Medicine. JAMA 1995, 273, 402–407.

[3] Cavill N, Kahlmeier S, Racioppi F: Physical activity and health in Europe: Evidence for action; World Health Organization, Copenhagen, 2006, available online at http://www.euro.who.int/document/e89490.pdf (accessed 1 February 2007)

[4] Data Food Networking (DAFNE), http://www.nut.uoa.gr/english/dafne/DafneEN.htm (accessed 1 February 2007)

[5] European Academy of Nutritional Sciences (EANS), http://www.eans.net (accessed 3 February 2007)

[6] European Commission (EC), http://ec.europa.eu/health/ph_information/reporting/analysing_reporting_en.htm (accessed 22 January 2007)

[7] European Commission (EC), http://ec.europa.eu/health/ph_programme/programme_en.htm (accessed 22 January 2007)

[8] European Commission (EC), http://ec.europa.eu/health/ph_overview/overview_en.htm (accessed 22 January 2007)

[9] European Commission (EC), http://ec.europa.eu/health/ph_information/information_en.htm (accessed 22 January 2007)

[10] European Food Information Council (EUFIC), http://www.eufic.org (accessed 3 February 2007)

[11] European network for the promotion of health-enhancing physical activity (HEPA), http://www.euro.who.int/hepa/ (accessed 3 February 2007)

[12] European Platform on Mobility Management (EPOMM), http://www.epomm.org (accessed 3 February 2007)

[13] European Public Health Association (EUPHA), http://www.eupha.org (accessed 3 February 2007)

[14] European Society for Social Paediatrics and Child Health (ESSOP), http://www.essop.org (accessed 3 February 2007)

[15] Federation of European Nutrition Societies (FENS), http://www.fensweb.org (accessed 3 February 2007)

[16] Health Behaviour in school-aged children (HBSC), http://www.hbsc.org (accessed 1 February 2007)

[17] International Physical Activity Questionaire (IPAQ), http://www.ipaq.ki.se/ (accessed 1 February 2007)

[18] International Society for Behavioral Nutrition and Physical Activity (ISBNPA), http://www.isbnpa.org (accessed 3 February 2007)

[19] National Public Health Institute, http://www.ktl.fi/portal/english/osiot/research,_people_programs/health_promotion_and_chronic_disease_prevention/projects/finbalt/roskaa/finbalt_health_monitor/ (accessed 1 February 2007)

[20] Oja P, Borms J (eds.): Health Enhancing Physical Activity. In Perspectives. The Multidisciplinary Series of Physical Education and Sport Science, Vol. 6, 2004.

[21] de Onis M, Wijnhoven TMA, Onyango AW: Worldwide practices in child growth monitoring. Journal of Paediatrics, 2004, 144, 461–465.

[22] Rigby M: Principles and challenges of child health and safety indicators; International Journal of Injury Control and Safety Promotion 2005, 12, 2; 71–78.

[23] Sjöström M, Yngve A, Poortvliet E, Warm D, Ekelund U: Diet and physical actitvity – interactions for health; Public Health Nutrition in the European Perspective. Public Health Nutrition 1999, 2, 453–459

[24] Sjöström M, et al.: Making way for a healthier lifestyle in Europe. Monitoring Public Health Nutrition in Europe. List of Indicators. Summary Report – final version. European Commission, 2003

[25] Smolin LA, Grosvenor MB: Nutrition: Science & Applications, Third Edition, 2000.

[26] The Nutrition Society (NS), http://www.nutritionsociety.org (accessed 3 February 2007)

[27] Transport, Health and Environment Pan-European Programme (THE PEP), http://www.thepep.org/en/welcome.htm (accessed 3 February 2007)

[28] World Health Organization (WHO), http://www.who.int/mediacentre/factsheets/fs311/en/ (accessed 1 February 2007)

[29] World Health Organization (WHO), http://www.who.int/chp/steps/GPAQ%20Instrument%20and%20Analysis%20Guide%20v2. pdf (accessed 1 February 2007)

[30] World Health Organization (WHO), http://www.who.int/chp/steps/GPAQ/en/index.html (accessed 1 February 2007)

[31] World Health Organization (WHO), http://www.who.int/ncd_surveillance/infobase/web/InfoBaseCommon/ (accessed 1 February 2007)

[32] World Health Organization (WHO), http://www.who.int/ncd_surveillance/infobase/web/surf2/start.html (accessed 1 February 2007)

[33] World Health Organization (WHO), http://www.who.int/ncd_surveillance/infobase/web/surf2/reg_tables.pdf (accessed 1 February 2007)

[34] World Health Organization (WHO): The European health report 2005. Public health action for healthier children and populations. World Health Organization, 2005

[35] World Health Organization (WHO): Global Strategy on Diet, Physical Activity and Health; World Health Organization, Geneva, 2004 available online at http://www.who.int/dietphysicalactivity/strategy/eb11344/strategy_english_web.pdf (accessed 1 February 2007)

[36] World Health Organization (WHO): The World Health Report 2002. Reducing Risks, Promoting Healthy Life. World Health Organization, 2002

[37] World Health Organization (WHO): Development of Indicators for Monitoring Progress towards Health for All by the Year 2000. World Health Organization, Geneva, 1981

[38] World Health Organization, Regional Office for Europe (WHO Europe), http://www.euro.who.int/obesity (accessed 1 February 2007)

[39] World Health Organization, Regional Office for Europe (WHO Europe), http://www.euro.who.int/Nutrition (accessed 1 February 2007)

[40] World Health Organization, Regional Office for Europe (WHO Europe), http://www.euro.who.int/healthtopics/HT2ndLvlPage?HTCode=physical_activity (accessed 1 February 2007)

[41] World Health Organization, Regional Office for Europe (WHO Europe), http://www.euro.who.int/obesity/conference2006 (accessed 1 February 2007)

[42] World Health Organization, Regional Office for Europe (WHO Europe), http://www.euro.who.int/nutrition/20060612_3 (accessed 1 February 2007)

[43] World Health Organization, Regional Office for Europe (WHO Europe), http://www.euro. who.int/nutrition/Publications/NutPolicyWho (accessed 1 February 2007)

[44] World Health Organization, Regional Office for Europe (WHO Europe), http://www.euro. who.int/CINDI (accessed 1 February 2007)

[45] World Health Organization, Regional Office for Europe (WHO Europe), http://www.euro. who.int/Document/NUT/Instanbul_conf_%20ebd02.pdf (accessed 1 February 2007)

[46] World Health Organization, Regional Office for Europe (WHO Europe), http://www.euro. who.int/Document/E89567.pdf (accessed 1 February 2007)

[47] World Health Organization, Regional Office for Europe (WHO Europe), http://www.euro. who.int/Document/NUT/Instanbul_conf_edoc09.pdf (accessed 1 February 2007)

[48] World Health Organization, Regional Office for Europe (WHO Europe): Food and Health in Europe: a New Basis for Action; World Health Organization, Copenhagen, 2002

Index